National Strategies for Health Care Organization

A World Overview

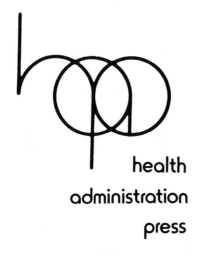

health
administration
press

Health Administration Press was
established in 1972 with the support
of the W.K. Kellogg Foundation and
is a nonprofit endeavor of The
University of Michigan Program
and Bureau of Hospital
Administration.

Milton I. Roemer

National Strategies for Health Care Organization

A World Overview

Health Administration Press
Ann Arbor, Michigan 1985

Library of Congress Cataloging in Publication Data

Roemer, Milton Irwin, 1916–
    National strategies for health care organization.

    Consists mainly of works previously in various sources.
    Includes bibliographies and index.
    1. Medical policy. 2. Medical care. I. Title.
[DNLM: 1. Health Policy—collected works. 2. Health Services—organization & administration—collected works.
W 84.1 R715n]
RA393.R5935 1984   362.1   84–12878
ISBN 0–914904–99–X

Health Administration Press
School of Public Health
The University of Michigan
1021 East Huron
Ann Arbor, Michigan 48109

Contents

Part One
Background and Overview

Part Two
Developing Countries

Part Three
Industrialized Countries

Part Four
Socialist Countries

Part Five
General Health Policy Issues

List of Tables
and Figures

TABLES

FIGURES

Preface

Everywhere in the world, health services are becoming more organized. Most obvious is the increased organization of patterns of health care delivery, but greater organization also characterizes the means of health care financing, the development of resources (personnel, facilities, and so on), the process of planning and regulation, and the entire structure for arranging health programs to meet the diverse needs of national populations. The reasons for this trend are found both in society and in the health sciences.

Each nation's approach to the organization of health services varies with its economic development and its general political ideology, and is further influenced by its history. As a result, every country has its own more or less unique national health care system.

A comprehensive analysis of the health care systems of the world's 160 nations remains to be done. In this volume I offer accounts of significant strategies in a number of those systems. Perhaps it will help countries that are facing problems to see how other countries have tackled the same problems effectively. In many aspects of health service, of course, nations have long learned lessons from one another, with both positive and negative results: foreign ideas must obviously be adapted to varying national settings.

The 25 chapters in this book present the viewpoint of one observer. Insofar as this viewpoint is biased, the bias is toward regarding health care as a human and social right, not just a market commodity. Much of the organizational strategy of countries in their health care systems is designed to reduce the dependence of health services on market dynamics, so that it becomes a social benefit available to all.

Strategies change over time. It is virtually impossible to describe a health care system—or even one program within it—without changes having occurred by the time the words are in print. The chapters in this volume are all based on work done since 1976, and half of them date from 1980 or later.* Thirteen of the 25 chapters, furthermore, are based entirely or mainly on field observations in the countries described. The other 12 chapters are reviews and interpretations of major health care strategies (such as health insurance or organized ambulatory care) from a comparative, cross-national perspective.

The book is organized in five parts. First are three chapters offering historical background and an overview of health care organization. Part two consists of seven chapters on developing countries—five of them on specific countries and two on certain aspects of developing countries as a whole. Part three is devoted to industrialized countries—three chapters on selected nations and three on strategies and their effects on groups of such countries. Part four offers analyses of four Socialist countries—two of which are industrialized and developed and two of which are more agricultural and less economically developed. Part five contains chapters that examine five features of all health care systems as they are implemented under various national strategies.

In a work of this type, which analyzes health care organization both according to country and according to subject, some duplication is inevitable. The health insurance program of Norway, for example, must be part of an account of that country's health care system, as well as part of a worldwide review of health insurance strategies. Perhaps such repetition may contribute to the clarification of complexities.

For providing me the opportunity to observe various national health care systems, I must acknowledge my debt to the World Health Organization and the U.S. government. To the national governments of numerous countries and to countless health workers goes my gratitude for furnishing information and guidance. For the interpretation of topics or issues, of course, I take responsibility. I hope that readers of every nationality may find some strategies of other countries that can help them improve their own health care systems.

MILTON I. ROEMER, M.D.

---

*An earlier volume, *Health Care Systems in World Perspective* (Ann Arbor: Health Administration Press, 1976), presented papers done prior to 1976.

Part One

Background and Overview

1

Major Health Care Trends
Since 1900

Current national strategies for health care organization can be better understood by considering their historical development. All history has influenced the current world, but, in the health services, events since 1900 have been particularly important.

To summarize worldwide developments in the health services in this century, one must resort to oversimplification. Now that four-fifths of the twentieth century has passed, furthermore, one can look back and identify a number of major developments that help to explain significant features of the health care systems in different nations.

MAJOR SOCIOECONOMIC AND POLITICAL DEVELOPMENTS

World circumstances in 1900 were the outcome of events and trends of the previous century. Each of the developments in the twentieth century, therefore, can be traced back to earlier history. With that in mind, one can identify 12 major socioeconomic developments in the twentieth century.

This chapter is an adapted and substantially revised version of "A World Perspective on Health Care in the Twentieth Century," *Journal of Public Health Policy,* 1(December 1980): 370-78, that was based on an address given at the University of Washington (Seattle) in June 1979.

Science and Technology. Mankind's knowledge of the structure and processes of nature has grown at a bewildering pace. The several scientific disciplines have contributed to each other's knowledge and together have produced what appears to be an endlessly expanding technology. It is hard to say whether the splitting of the atom and the mobilizing of nuclear power are matched by our understanding of the organic cell, but developments in genetics, biochemistry, physiology and other fields have led to enormous advances in the biomedical sciences and their applications.

Population Growth. The survival of the young and, to a lesser extent, of the middle-aged and elderly has been made possible through massive public health applications of the biomedical and environmental sciences. As a result, the world population has grown enormously— more in the twentieth century than in all previous centuries together.

Economic Crises and Wars. Capitalism, the dominant economic system throughout the world by 1900, continued to mature. The dynamics of market economies—partly free, partly monopolistic— evolved to the point of periodic breakdowns. Most prominent among these were the rivalry among capitalist nation-states that gave rise to World War I and the subsequent global economic collapse of the 1930s that lead to World War II.

Rise of Socialism. From each of these world wars came a revolution that gave rise to a socialist economy and a major socialist political state—the Soviet Union from the first war and the People's Republic of China from the second. Along with these two giants, there emerged several other, smaller socialist states. Together these constituted a growing political threat to the still dominant capitalist nations of the world.

Liberation of Colonies. The less economically developed lands of Africa, Asia, and Latin America, which had largely been taken over as colonies of industrialized European powers in the eighteenth and nineteenth centuries, became liberated in the twentieth century. Hence there arose scores of new, independent (politically, if not economically) nation-states. These came to be characterized first as "underdeveloped" and then as "developing" nations. To hasten their development, all of these new nations became engaged in various degrees of systematic economic and social planning.

Migration and Urbanization. With the continued development of industry and commerce in almost all nations, millions of people left the rural areas for urban areas in their country or in other countries. This resulted in the formation of huge cities with many millions of people and in hundreds of other cities of 50,000 people or more.

Mass Education. Urbanization resulted in increased exchange of ideas among people and in the extension of education to the masses as a function of the state. With mass education has come a much greater understanding of the dynamics of society, including greater political consciousness. This consciousness has stimulated liberation or equalization movements among social classes, among racial, ethnic, and religious groups, and between the sexes.

Dictatorships and Repression. In response to many demands for equalized standards of living, there naturally arose resistance among power elites to maintain their privileges. Most often this resistance has been expressed in military dictatorships to suppress forces for social change. Even such dictatorships (which came to characterize the majority of developing nations) had to allow some continuation of the movement toward equalization (along with their violent repression of open political minorities), if only to maintain social stability.

International Organizations. Other outcomes of the two devastating world wars were international organizations devoted to the attainment of peace—first the League of Nations and then the United Nations. Several specialized international agencies were formed as satellites of these bodies. These were devoted to the spread among nations of ideas in agriculture, education, welfare, health, and other fields — without ulterior motives. Such diffusion of ideas has been principally from the more socioeconomically developed nations to the less developed nations, a movement that previously depended on imperialism, which exacted a price in colonial exploitation of natural resources and people.

Growth of Wealth. In spite of the persistence of unequal standards of living between social classes in virtually every nation, the application of technology has led to continuing increases in global wealth. That is, more and more of the world's earthly goods have been mobilized for the benefit of mankind. With this increase in global wealth per capita, proportionately more resources could be devoted to services, such as education and health care, rather than to the necessities for survival, such as food and shelter.

Recognition of Resource Limits. As socioeconomic planning became widespread in developing nations—and, indeed, in most other nations—people and their leaders came increasingly to recognize the limits of the world's physical resources. Along with this came recognition of the finite capacity of the earth's physical environment to absorb the waste products of industrial processes and of human existence itself. Appreciation of these limits accelerated further the movement for social planning to conserve resources and protect the environment.

Collective Action. The extension of social planning, mass education, urbanization, and most of the other major developments of the twentieth century heightened people's understanding of the necessity of collective action for survival and for gaining various ends economically and politically. More and more, therefore, group activities were undertaken to protect or provide benefits for each individual.

There are doubtless omissions from this list. An engineer or theologian or lawyer would see the world from a different perspective. With the biases and priorities of a person in health science, however, I now consider the significant trends within health care; virtually all of them are outgrowths of the larger developments in world affairs.

MAJOR DEVELOPMENTS AND TRENDS IN HEALTH CARE

With further oversimplification, one may identify 15 major world developments in the field of health care. These are drawn somewhat less from reading about the world and more from direct observation of the health care sector of society in a number of countries over the last 30 years.

Health Manpower Growth. As science's potential for curing the sick and preventing disease has expanded in the twentieth century, larger and larger numbers of people have become devoted to the provision of health services. Since the various applications of the health sciences to human needs require specific knowledge and skills, thousands of schools and programs of training have been established to produce medical and associated personnel. This worldwide growth of health manpower has occurred much more rapidly than the growth of population. Although there are, of course, great differences among countries, the ratios to population of scientifically trained health workers have increased in almost all countries. The most rapid growth has occurred in the socialist countries, but growth has also occurred in the welfare states of Western Europe, in the transitional developing countries of Latin America, and even in the most underdeveloped countries of Africa.

Specialization. With the growing complexity of science and technology, along with urbanization and heightened demands for skilled services, health manpower and equipment have become more and more specialized. Specialization has expanded not only within the medical profession, where there are now some 50 or 60 specialty and sub-specialty fields, but also among nurses, dental personnel, technicians, pharmacists, rehabilitation therapists, mental health personnel, medical assistants, and others. The more this division of labor has characterized the health services, the greater the need has been for coordination among the many types of health workers.

Organization for Teamwork. In order to enable the diverse types of personnel to work together efficiently, many frameworks have evolved for allowing them to relate to the patient and to each other in a systematic manner. This organization of health care teams has been most effectively achieved in hospitals, where the greatest variety of skills are brought together to deal with complex diagnosis and treatment of the sick. Organization has also occurred increasingly in the construction and use of health centers for the ambulatory patient, to whom both treatment and preventive health services are provided. In rural areas of developing countries, the health center has become the standard mechanism for delivery of ambulatory care. Health centers and group practice clinics have come to play an increasing part in the cities of all types of countries.

Geographic Regionalization. Coordination of health personnel and facilities has been stimulated by specialization and urbanization on a geographic level as well. Thus, the provision of health services to the populations of large regions has increasingly been through pyramidal systems of facilities, staffed by clusters of personnel. These regionalized networks are intended to provide rural populations with access to the health care resources located in the cities.

Population Control. The rapid growth of the world's population has led to many strategies for birth control. Many of these strategies are social and economic, designed to influence reproductive behavior, but important among them is the spread of various contraceptive methods. Family-planning techniques are disseminated in a variety of ways but they are increasingly integrated with the general delivery of health services.

Geriatrics and Rehabilitation. Survival of the young, along with lowered birthrates, has resulted in higher proportions of aged persons in the populations of all industrialized countries and of many developing countries. As a result, the perceived need for treatment of the chronic disorders of later life has risen almost everywhere. Objectives have steadily broadened from curing the disease to rehabilitating the patient. These objectives, in turn, generate a need for more personnel and greater expenditures on health care. Virtually all industrialized nations have provided public support for such expenditures; in Australia and the United States, support for the aged has come even *before* such support for the young.

Environmental Sanitation. The concentration of people in cities and the growth of industry have created enormous problems in disposing of human and industrial wastes. Various engineering strategies for waste disposal have been developed, first in the larger cities but, as the century has advanced, in rural areas as well. Particularly important to public health have been the provision of safe water supply systems and the reduction or elimination of insects and other vectors of disease.

Health Care Planning. Liberation of the colonies and their transformation into independent nations have given rise to many focuses of national pride. Eager to accelerate their socioeconomic development, the new nations have undertaken systematic planning efforts, including the planning of health services. While the achievement of planning objectives in health care has often been compromised by the perpetuation of a substantial private medical market—not easily influenced by planning efforts—an enlarging proportion of health care expenditures is becoming subject to deliberate planning, principally by central governments. Much of this planning is devoted to strategies for assuring improved health services for low-income rural populations.

Socialized Health Care Systems. Successful social revolutions, which have transformed capitalist into socialist political economies, have given rise to fully planned and socialized health care systems. In these systems, the distribution of health services has been converted from a function of private enterprise, small or large, to a responsibility of government. The delivery of preventive and treatment services has been administratively and technically integrated.

Greater Expenditures on Health Care. As per capita wealth has increased, the portion of that wealth available for services has also increased. Hence, the share of almost every nation's per capita wealth (gross national product, or GNP) spent on health care has enlarged. In the most affluent countries this share now approaches 10 percent of the

GNP, but even in less developed countries it appears to be rising from 2 or 3 percent in the early part of the century to 4 or 5 percent today. This means that, even adjusting for inflation, more money is being devoted to the health services. Expenditures on support functions, such as health personnel training, facility construction, and medical research, have also increased.

More Collectivized Financing. In order to assure the availability of funds for the health care needed and desired by their populations, nations are raising an increasing share of health monies by collective strategies. While general government revenues are the most frequently used method, social insurance or voluntary insurance is being increasingly applied. Urbanization and industrialization facilitate the use of social insurance. For the effective raising of funds visibly earmarked for health purposes and visibly derived from workers and employers, social insurance has the great advantage of stability over the years; it is immune to the demands of other sectors of government financed through general revenues. It has been adapted by almost all industrial capitalist countries and by an increasing number of developing countries. Even though a social insurance program may start with protection of only a small fraction of the population, the share of population covered and the scope of benefits have tended to expand in every country employing this collective financing mechanism.

Quality Protection. The increasingly social financing of health services has stimulated greater popular and political concern that the money be wisely spent, particularly in the face of rising overall expenditures. As a result, the health services are becoming subjected to increasing regulation by both governmental and nongovernmental mechanisms. Various ways of certifying the qualifications of health personnel have been developed, as have various means of monitoring their performance. The manufacture of drugs, which in all nonsocialist countries has been closely linked to corporate enterprise, has been found to be particularly liable to abuses and economic waste in the pursuit of profits. Therefore, a large body of legal regulation over drug production, marketing, and distribution has evolved—most rigorous in the capitalist economies where drug manufacturing is most extensive.

Primary Care and Prevention. The enormous growth of science and specialization in the first two-thirds of the twentieth century has induced a reaction against advanced technology in the last third. Throughout the world people have come to recognize that highly specialized and sophisticated health services can be excessive, wasteful, and sometimes even harmful. Therefore a fresh interest has developed everywhere in the provision of "appropriate technology" and effective primary care, including personal prevention in the spheres of diet, exercise, and life-style. In order to attract more physicians to general medical practice, the field has been converted into a higher status and more lucrative specialty in a score of countries. New types of middle-level personnel are being trained in order to extend primary care more rapidly to rural populations; China's "barefoot doctor" is the best known of many such types. This extension of minimal health services to rural populations coincides with the objective of improving rural living conditions, if only to weaken the guerrilla movements that have arisen in the hinterlands of many developing countries.

Medical Humanism. Closely linked to the fresh emphasis on primary care, and in reaction to excessive technology, has been an affirmative concern for the feelings of the patient. Tender loving care has become an integral part of the objectives of health care systems in affluent countries and in at least the urban centers of less developed countries. Consumerism and the protection of patient rights have become widespread. The impersonality of large medical bureaucracies is being lessened by the appointment of ombudsmen, the establishment of grievance procedures for patients, and the creation of various citizen advisory committees. The large hospital ward is everywhere being replaced by smaller quarters sensitive to patient privacy.

Internationalism in Health. In order to spread knowledge about these developments in health care, the World Health Organization (WHO) and numerous nongovernmental international agencies have increased their scope of activity. Whereas in the early years of the century they were concerned mainly with halting the spread of communicable diseases across national borders (especially from the impoverished colonies to the affluent European nations), in the last decades of the century their goals have turned completely around. "Health for *all* by the year 2000" became the slogan of WHO, and that agency's director-general has not hesitated to call for political commitment in all countries to attain this goal. As a step toward this objective, WHO and UNICEF in 1978 held a world Conference on Primary Care at Alma Ata, in the Soviet Union. Practical measures for implementing the Declaration of Alma Ata are underway in countries on every continent.

HEALTH AS A RIGHT

In its 1948 Universal Declaration of Human Rights, the United Nations stated: "Everyone has the right to a standard of living ade-

quate for health and well-being of himself and of his family, including
. . . medical care . . . and the right to security in the event of sickness."[1]

In the same year, the WHO defined health as a state of "complete
physical, mental, and social well-being and not merely the absence of
disease or infirmity." Although both of these statements are affirma-
tions of inspirational goals, the paths to which are long and rugged,
there is no question that the world in the second half of the twentieth
century has been profoundly influenced by them. Whether an economy
is capitalist or socialist, whether the political structure is a parliamentary democracy or a military dictatorship, men and women are inspired
and motivated by the concept that universal access to health care is and
should be a basic human right.

The methods of implementing this concept vary in a thousand
ways among different nations at different times. The rate of approach
toward this goal varies greatly among nations and among social classes
and other population groups within nations, but there can be no question about the trends of the first four-fifths of this century. Forecasting
on the basis of these trends suggests a movement toward systems of
health care with those attributes briefly summarized above. One may
doubt whether mankind will ever achieve the ideal of "complete physical, mental, and social well-being . . . for all"—not so much because we
lack the knowledge or even the resources, but because the dimensions
of our ideal will become endlessly greater. It is this very feature of
human aspirations, in fact, that gives grounds for optimism about the
future.

NOTE

1. United Nations, *Universal Declaration of Human Rights* (New York: U.N.
Office of Public Information), 1948.

2

Financing the Health Sector:
Historical Development

*A crucial determinant of health care organization is its
means of economic support. In most countries, diverse methods of financing health care activities operate side by side.
The mix of these methods does much to shape a nation's
health care system, and each method has evolved from a special historical background.*

To draw a general picture of methods of financing the health
sector, one might first trace how different methods arose. One might
then analyze the several components of the modern health sector. Next,
one might describe what methods of financing have taken shape to
support each component. Finally, one might consider the mix of financing methods in any given country.

HISTORICAL DEVELOPMENT

The evolution of the numerous methods of financing health services and related activities—now definable as "the health sector"—
may be traced through eight major historical periods.

This chapter is an adapted and substantially revised version of "Financing the Health
Sector—A Global Vista" in Financing of Health Services: Proceedings of a World Health
Organization Inter-Regional Workshop, Mexico, November 26–30, 1979 (SHS/SPM/80.3),
31–39, that was based on an address given at the Workshop in Mexico City.

Primitive Medicine. The earliest form of health care was that undertaken in primitive communities to cope with disease. Based on mystical, religious, or magical concepts, healing procedures were applied by various village personalities. Chiefs, priests, and others provided healing services at first, but gradually healing became a separate occupation. Eventually healers discovered empirical treatments—heat and cold, herbs and potions—to complement procedures that involved supernatural forces to drive out the evil spirits believed to cause sickness.

Initially, payment for healing services was not expected, but gifts were given. When payment became customary, it was by barter. After its development in connection with commerce in the cities, money was used; eventually money became the medium of exchange in rural areas also.

Ancient Medicine. Three distinct types of healers developed in ancient Egypt: (1) priests, (2) magicians or sorcerers, and (3) physicians, who used empirical measures. In the main, physicians gave their patients drugs, which were made from plants, parts of animals, or minerals. Physicians served primarily royalty and the rich, while magicians and priests served the poor. These distinctions were not absolute, however, and an ordinary person afflicted with a grave illness might be treated by a physician. There was no money in ancient Egypt, so physicians were paid in various other ways. Those attached to a royal court or wealthy household received free lodging and food—the equivalent of a salary. For the treatment of persons outside the sponsoring family, the physician received gifts—the equivalent of fees.

In Babylonia there were two types of physicians—those who used drugs, and those who cut, or surgeons. Money had developed, and physicians were paid monetary fees. When a slave was treated, payment was made by the master. Surgeons were subject to punishment if their treatments were unsuccessful. A surgeon was required to pay a monetary fine, for example, if a slave died after an operation. If a nobleman did not recover after treatment, the surgeon might be made to suffer physical punishment or even death.

Greek and Roman Medicine (500 B.C.–600 A.D.). In classical Greece, there arose more systematic theories of disease. Disease was seen as a result of natural causes, with treatment being based on a rational response to the specific cause. Young men were trained by older physicians, the best known of whom was Hippocrates. The physician trained in the School of Hippocrates would treat both freemen and slaves, using principally drugs and little surgery. His fees were typically paid with money.

As city-states developed in Greece, they collected taxes for various civic purposes. Among these was medical care of impoverished freemen. Doctors were engaged on salaries for this work. This was, in effect, the beginning of tax support for health service. Medical treatment for slaves, on the other hand, was paid for by their owners.

During the Roman Empire, Greek doctors were often imported to Rome as servants, or even slaves, in the households of large landowners. They were provided food and shelter, the equivalent of low salaries. Public taxes were used in Rome for the construction of sewers to drain off dirty water from the streets. This was, in a sense, the beginning of tax support for environmental sanitation.

Medieval Health Care (600–1300). In the Middle Ages, feudal estates engaged doctors, who were attached to the manor of the landowner. These doctors received not only lodging but also a monetary salary. For this, they would treat both the landlord's family and the families of serfs.

As towns grew up, artisan doctors, who learned their skills by apprenticeship, set up private practice and were paid for their services by personal fees. Fees were also paid for surgery, which was done by barbers. Some artisans developed special skills, such as setting broken bones, extracting painful teeth, treating fevers, or using drugs for many disorders. Specialists in the concoction and dispensing of drugs became apothecaries, who were consulted mainly by the poor; they charged generally lower fees than doctors.

As universities arose, around the tenth century, the first school of medicine was founded in Salerno, Italy. Exactly how this medical school was financed is not clear, but some claim it was started by the Christian church, hence through charity. It was also supported by tuition payments from the students. In the northern cities of Europe, additional universities were established, and in them medical schools. Financial support came generally from a combination of local taxes and students' tuitions.

Hospitals were first founded by the Christian church in the eleventh century for the care of the poor, the disabled, and the destitute. They were an expression of mercy for those in misery, as well as a strategy for saving souls through penitence and prayer. Hospitals were thus financed not by payments from their patients, but by charitable donations to the church, donations from both wealthy and ordinary churchgoers. In the Moslem world, around the Mediterranean Sea, an equivalent pattern arose in the thirteenth century to provide merciful care to the destitute. Connected with large mosques were shelters for bed care of gravely ill worshippers.

As hospitals became larger and more firmly established in the main cities, the costs of operating them (food, bedding, fuel, drugs, and so on) increased, and funds were contributed from city tax revenues. Salaries for personnel were not required, for the nurses were Catholic nuns whose only pay was their food and lodging. Doctors also gave care as a Christian service without payment; their earnings came from fees paid by patients outside the hospital.

Renaissance and Reformation (1300–1600). With the continued growth of cities and various artisans in them, guilds of carpenters, coppersmiths, shoemakers, and other skilled craftsmen were formed. The guilds set standards for training and entry into different fields, but they also assumed certain fraternal functions. To help a member in distress, or his widow if he died, the guild would raise money through collecting regular contributions from its members. This was, in effect, the beginning of insurance against misfortunes like sickness or death. Later, guilds used their pooled money to pay selected physicians for treating sick members. The doctors might be paid by fees for each case or by a flat annual salary. Payment could also be made from the fund for drugs, but not for care in hospitals, which were unlikely to be used by guild members. To maintain hospitals, there were gradual increases in the grants from local public revenues.

As greater numbers of poor people accumulated in the towns and cities and strained the capacity of hospitals to care for them, local tax revenues were used to pay small salaries to "poor doctors"—that is, to doctors who treated the poor in their homes.

In the late 1500's, a merchant class began to take shape. This class looked upon the guilds as limiting competition and elevating prices. Therefore, steps were taken by the crown (that is, the government) to regulate the guilds. A successful artisan, on the other hand, might hire additional skilled craftsmen for wages—the beginnings of a working class and capitalist enterprise. The entrepreneur would then have to pay a tax to the crown for permission to operate this business.

Rise of Industry (1600–1750). As businesses grew, and with them factories, there arose a class of wageworkers (as distinct from independent artisans). By the 1700's, workers began to form cooperatives to protect their interests and to help each other. From these cooperatives (as in the earlier guilds), there evolved mutual sickness assistance funds—or, as we would now say, voluntary health insurance programs.

In this period, universities grew as centers of learning and as schools for training physicians and pharmacists. They were financed increasingly by local government, supplemented by gifts from wealthy philanthropists. Hospitals also became increasingly dependent on support from local government revenues; many became separated from the Christian churches, except for the retention of their saintly names. Finally, some completely nonreligious and even nongovernmental hospitals were built, through gifts of land and money from private individuals, hence the rise of the nonsectarian, nonprofit voluntary hospital.

This was the period of the flowering of science. Galileo, born in 1564, did his astronomical work from 1600 to 1642. Isaac Newton, 1642–1727, formulated general laws of nature. Leeuwenhoek, 1632–1723, studied biological matter and discovered the microscope. All this basic research led eventually to medical research, clarifying the causes of disease and leading to rational therapy. This early scientific and medical research was supported by rich patrons, by the universities, and by the scientists themselves, from their personal wealth as landowners or inheritors of fortunes. It was not supported by the Christian churches, which regarded science as a threat to religion, nor by government.

Industrial Revolution (1750–1900). As industry expanded at an increasing pace, several new social movements developed, and these influenced the economic support of health services.

The growing working class formed unions and eventually Socialist political parties. The first Socialist International organization took shape in Europe, issuing the *Communist Manifesto* in 1847. Naturally this stimulated a conservative opposition. One expression of this was a strategy by German chancellor Otto von Bismarck to win over working people from the Socialists. He piloted through the Reichstag in 1883 a law mandating that all workers with low wages *must* be protected by a sickness fund. These funds were subject to standards and regulation by the central government. This was the birth of social security as a method of financing medical care, and it eventually spread throughout Europe.

After about 1840, there developed in most European cities slum areas, where low-income working-class families lived. The crowded, miserable slum housing was a breeding ground for typhoid fever, tuberculosis, and other infectious diseases, and it gave rise to a reform movement for improved environmental sanitation. This was the origin of the public health movement, which was financed by local tax revenues; it is noteworthy that this occurred before the discovery of bacteria as a cause of disease.

With the discovery of pathogenic microorganisms around 1870, the entire nature of hospitals changed. They gradually became regarded less as places for the poor and destitute and more as facilities for the skillful treatment of serious disease in persons of all social classes. Affluent individuals began to pay personally for hospital care, which was provided in private rooms rather than in large, crowded wards. Thus, hospitals came to be financed from several sources: philanthropy (religious or other), local tax funds, and private patient fees.

As hospitals improved in quality and as social security (or social insurance) funds became stronger, insured workers were also admitted to hospitals. Not being paupers, they had access to private or semiprivate rooms, which were paid for by the insurance fund. This was a fourth source of financing for hospitals, and it contributed much to their further expansion. To acquire better staff for taking care of patients, hospitals organized formal training for nurses after 1870. The cost of these training schools was borne by all of the sources of financing mentioned above.

Modern Health Care (1900–1980). After 1900, there was continued rapid growth of industry and national wealth. Representative government became stronger, and taxation increased to support social services, including health protection.

In 1917, the first Socialist revolution occurred, in Czarist Russia. For the first time, health services became a right of citizenship;—hence they were financed from the general revenues of the nation rather than solely from local governments. The example of a Socialist state became both a threat and a stimulus to other nations of the world.

Everywhere, the scope of national taxation increased, gradually becoming more important than local taxation for the support of health and health-related services. National revenues in most industrialized countries became a major source of financing for (1) the universities, where physicians, pharmacists, and various health technologists were trained; (2) public health services, for the prevention of disease through public sanitation; (3) construction of hospitals and facilities for ambulatory care; (4) medical research; and (5) medical care of selected population groups, such as the very poor, military personnel, veterans, handicapped persons, the mentally ill, and others.

Another source of health care financing that arose in the twentieth century was industrial management. In response to laws regarding compensation for industrial injuries, employers developed in-plant medical services for workers, as well as safety measures. The scope of these industry-financed medical services varied with the type and size of the firm. Larger factories usually provided broader services—sometimes complete medical care.

Central ministries of health took shape in the twentieth century in order to supervise general public health services and other health activities financed from national revenues. Other branches of the central government, however, also supported and supervised certain types of services: (1) ministries of education usually financed the university training of health personnel, as well as health services for school children; (2) ministries of welfare often financed custodial care for the aged and chronically ill; (3) the health care of military personnel and veterans typically came under another ministry; and (4) health services for rural people might be financed by ministries of agriculture or special programs for community development.

Social insurance, or social security, also spread rapidly in the twentieth century. After 1920, it was extended outside Europe—first to Japan and Chile, then to many other countries on all the continents. Health care benefits under social security in developing countries usually started with industrial workers, even though they were typically only a small fraction of the population. The trend almost everywhere, however, has been toward expanded coverage, both of population and of services. Today about 75 countries use social insurance to finance health services to part or all of their populations.

Meanwhile, private family financing of health care has by no means disappeared; it has continued in various forms. In the most industrialized countries, it usually supplements the financial support provided by social security and tax funds. In most of the developing countries, private financing has become even more important as an urban middle class has grown up. Private financing—especially for drugs and traditional healers—also remains strong in rural areas of developing countries, where governmental programs are often weak.

Voluntary charity is still a source of financing for health facility construction and services in all types of countries, although it is declining in importance as a share of total expenditures on health care. A special form of charitable donation has arisen in many countries: donated labor in rural villages, for example to build water systems or health centers. In cities, voluntary agencies, such as the Red Cross for emergency services, attract the unpaid services of local citizens.

Finally, a new form of financing health sector activities arose after World War II—aid from the more developed to the less developed nations. We prefer now to speak of "technical collaboration" rather than "foreign aid." In economic terms, the financial exchange constitutes a return to the developing countries of some of the great profits earned in them by multinational corporations from the industrialized countries. Foreign financial support is mediated mainly through governments, although some comes from voluntary bodies such as churches. Governmental monetary transfers take two principal forms: (1) bilateral, such as those from the U.S. Agency for International Development (USAID), and (2) multilateral, through international organizations such as WHO or UNICEF (the United Nations International Children's Emergency Fund).

COMPOSITION OF THE HEALTH SECTOR

From this historical review, one can see how the composition of the health sector has become increasingly complex. Starting with the healing services of individual village practitioners, it has evolved to encompass a vast range of technical activities. These may be classified into five major types.

Medical Treatment Services. These services, which are the oldest, now consist of the services of physicians of numerous specialties; hospitalization (involving the care of nurses, technicians, and many others); drugs (both prescribed and nonprescribed); dental care; the services of traditional healers of many varieties; the services of special practitioners such as midwives, optometrists, podiatrists, psychologists, and others; numerous diagnostic procedures; diverse rehabilitation services; long-term patient care; and other types of treatment services.

Organized Preventive Services. Broadly speaking, the main categories are environmental sanitation, including safety measures to reduce accidents; personal prevention, including immunizations, preventive maternal and child health services, early case detection, and much more; health education on all aspects of healthful living; and the protection of workers' and school children's health.

Production of Resources. This consists principally of the training of all types of skilled personnel; the construction of hospitals, ambulatory care units, and other facilities; and the manufacture of drugs, medical supplies, and equipment.

Extension of Scientific Knowledge. This includes research and the dissemination of knowledge about health and health services through journals, conferences, and other means.

Regulation and Planning. The increased complexity of all the above components of the health sector has necessitated social regulation to control the quality and costs of services. The demand for meeting human health care needs has necessitated health planning rather than simple reliance on the mechanisms of the free market.

This description of the five main components of the health sector may be somewhat oversimplified, but it should convey the range and complexity of the field. Many other social factors contribute to health, of course, such as food, shelter, and transportation. To permit meaningful analysis, however, both national and international, the costs of these broad activities should not be counted within the health sector. One can think also of various borderline activities, such as custodial care of the aged, nutritional supplements, elementary education, basic scientific research (preceding medical research), and the construction of water or sewage systems. To achieve international comparability, however, it is best not to include these activities in an analysis of the costs of the health sector.

Even by the most conservative definition, the health sector now absorbs between 3 and 10 percent of the GNP in various nations. The health component of the GNP tends to be higher in the more affluent countries and lower in the developing countries.

HEALTH SECTOR FINANCING

The complexity of *sources* of financial support for health care parallels the complexity of the health sector itself. As new forms of financing (increasingly social, public, or collective) have evolved, the old forms have not died out: they have continued side by side with the new forms. The relative importance of different sources of financing, of course, continually changes, and the strength of different sources varies greatly among countries.

Thus, almost all countries make use of many sources of financing for the various components of their health sectors, although in very different proportions. Again oversimplifying one may group these sources into seven classifications.

Personal Households, or Families. This is the oldest source, and it still exists to varying extents everywhere. Payments from such personal sources are usually in money, but they may be by barter. If medical costs are high, a family may even have to borrow money and pay interest on the debt. This source most often supports curative services (including drugs) rendered to individual patients, usually for ambulatory medical care. Even in countries with highly collectivized systems of health care financing, some degree of personal financing usually persists.

Charitable Donations. These may come from a few wealthy individuals in large amounts, or from many persons in small amounts. They may be mediated through churches or other organizations. One variation of this source is voluntary labor. Another is money derived from lotteries, which may be conducted by charitable organizations. Charitable sources of health financing often support the construction of facilities. In more affluent countries, charity may support medical research. In developing countries, it may support health services for the poor—such as services offered through religious missions.

Voluntary Health Insurance. On a global level, this source of financing is not as important now as it was in the early nineteenth century. In a few affluent countries, however—such as the United States, Australia, and South Africa—it remains prominent. In many other countries, voluntary health insurance finances medical care for a small population of middle-class families. It usually pays for physician and hospital care in private settings.

Israel is unique in having an extensive system of voluntary, or nongovernmental insurance, that finances general medical care for about 85 percent of the population. This *Kupat Holim* program (operated by the Jewish Labor Federation) engages its own doctors on salary and operates its own hospitals and polyclinics.

Voluntary insurance may be developed to replace for some people the use of a governmental system of medical care, as in modern Great Britain; there, middle-class families purchase voluntary insurance in order to gain access to private doctors, rather than waiting their turn in the somewhat overburdened national health service. On the other hand, voluntary insurance may be integrated with a governmental system, as in the People's Republic of China. There, voluntary cooperatives in the agricultural communes support the costs of the barefoot doctors and other forms of health care. In the main, however, voluntary health insurance has evolved over the years into mandatory social security. The historical sequence noted earlier in Germany has characterized most countries in Europe and many in Latin America.

Social Security. Social security, or compulsory insurance for health care, is typically administered within the structure of national governments, but the funds are maintained separately from the general treasury of the nation. Hence, social security systems tend to be somewhat autonomous. The money is generally immune from political manipulation and has great stability over time. The funds are ear-marked for a specific purpose—namely, health service to a defined population.

It is sometimes argued that social security, by favoring urban workers with steady employment, aggravates discrepancies in health resources between urban and the more marginal rural populations. The evidence indicates, however, that social security financing basi-cally mobilizes for the health sector money that would otherwise not be spent for health services at all or, if it were so spent, would be used less efficiently, for purely private medical care. There is no evidence, as sometimes claimed, that social security health expenditures compete with and reduce support for government programs serving total popu-lations, including those in rural areas. On the contrary, social security systems enlarge the total national resources of the health sector and promote a more rational use of them. The fact is that the social security mechanism is being used increasingly by both industrialized and de-veloping countries. The proportions of national populations covered by these systems are also steadily expanding.

Industry. Monies used by various industrial enterprises for health service to workers are derived basically from the sale of their products. The services are most often for the care of work-related inju-ries, but they may also include prevention and the care of on-the-job illness. In some countries, enterprises may finance general medical care for workers and their families; this is particularly true in large enterprises, those with 1,000 workers or more. (This source should not, however, be confused with wage deductions or even payroll contribu-tions for health insurance or social security.)

General Government Revenues. Public revenues, or taxes, may be raised at several levels of government—local, provincial, or national. Taxes at any level may be of several types: levies on land, on the sale of commodities, on individual incomes, on corporate earnings, on im-ports, and so on. At each political level, revenues from these various sources are usually consolidated; then the government—whether par-liamentary or not—makes allocations for various purposes.

This source of health sector financing has probably been enlarg-ing more than any other. It has also come to be derived proportionately more from higher political levels—that is, nationally more than lo-cally. These trends reflect the advancing concept of health care as a social right.

The uses of general tax funds in the health sector are diverse. They support organized preventive services in all countries, even those with the most individualistic ideology. They are used for the medical care of selected populations, such as the poor, both in cities and in rural areas. Tax funds are used for the construction of health facilities, for the training of health personnel, for scientific research, and for the overall planning and regulation of health services. Tax expenditures for these purposes are made principally by ministries of health, but they may also be handled by other branches of government, such as ministries of education, agriculture, labor, or military affairs.

Most countries levy relatively higher taxes on families with higher incomes, although to differing degrees. There are also differences among countries in the rigor of tax collection. Nevertheless, the use of tax funds for health purposes generally tends to promote "redistributional justice" and to improve the accessibility of people to health services on the basis of need rather than individual wealth.

Foreign Aid. This last source of health sector financing is through international cooperation, typically between the more affluent and less affluent countries. As a proportion of a nation's total health expenditures, however, this source is usually very small, even in the least economically developed countries. This support, however, may be given to crucial components of the health sector, such as primary care in rural areas. Such external financing may help to launch new ideas in health care delivery, ideas that advance equity.

Sometimes, to simplify this overall analysis of health sector financing, these seven sources are grouped into two main types: (1) the private sources, consisting of personal households, charity, voluntary insurance, and industry and (2) the public sources, consisting of social security, general revenues, and foreign aid.

CONCLUSION

One can see how in each country the pattern of health sector financing can be understood best by grouping financial data according to: (1) the purpose or type of health activity for which expenditures are made and (2) the sources from which the financing is derived.

A simplified schema of such an economic analysis of the health sector in a hypothetical country is illustrated in table 2.1. Dollar figures have been provided to indicate the rough proportions among the amounts for various purposes and from various sources that one might expect to find in many countries. Determining the actual expenditures in each category for a specific country ordinarily requires complex data collection and analysis.

Table 2.1   Annual Health Expenditures in a Hypothetical Country, by
Source and Purpose, 1980

Source of Money	Medical Treatment	Organized Prevention	Resource Production	Medical Research	Regulation and Planning	Total
Purpose of Expenditure ($U.S.)						
Personal household	4,100	—	—	—	—	4,100
Charitable donations	100	—	300	100	—	500
Voluntary insurance	3,000	—	—	—	—	3,000
Industry	100	100	—	100	—	300
Social security	5,200	100	—	—	100	5,400
Government revenues	4,000	600	700	700	400	6,400
Foreign aid	100	—	200	—	—	300
Total	16,600	800	1,200	900	500	20,000

It is evident that this type of analysis can tell us a great deal about the social policies of a country in its health sector. Thus, in the hypothetical country of table 2.1, public sources (social security, government revenues, and foreign support) account for 60.5 percent of the total, and private sources for 39.5 percent. In general, the more health expenditures come from private sources, the more they are likely to vary with wealth rather than need; greater proportions from public sources are likely to yield greater health equity. Many other social and political factors, of course, are involved, but on the whole this generalization would be valid for most countries.

Table 2.1 also permits one to conclude that only 4 percent of total health expenditures support organized prevention, while 83 percent support medical treatment. The relative contributions of charity (2.5 percent) and of foreign support (1.5 percent) are very small, in spite of much publicity about these sources; in fact, where they have been studied, these hypothetical proportions correspond quite well with the realities.

Analysis of health sector financing along these two dimensions, then, is an essential task if one is to understand the dynamics of a country's total health system. The precise categories of "source" and, particularly, of "purpose" may well have to differ from those used here because of the recordkeeping practices in a particular country. Some such analysis, however, is clearly necessary if a nation is to engage in reasonable and comprehensive health planning in order to promote the health of its people most effectively and equitably.

3

The Structure and Types of
Health Service Systems

As a result of historical developments and countless current political, economic, and social influences, every country has a national health service system. In order to understand and compare these systems, it is helpful to analyze them in terms of a uniform framework of components. The world's approximately 160 national health service systems can be better understood by classifying them into nine major types.

In every country there is a system of health services, just as there are systems of education, agriculture, transportation, and other social activities. The health service system is devoted *primarily* to protecting and improving the health of the population by providing a great variety of preventive and therapeutic services. The system also has many secondary purposes, such as providing employment or generating profits, which I will not discuss here.

Based on an address given at the North Atlantic Treaty Organization's Advanced Research Institute on Health Services Systems, The Hague, Netherlands, 29 August–3 September 1982.

THE SCOPE OF HEALTH SERVICE SYSTEMS

To define health service systems as social activities for the provision of health services is not at all to imply that health services are the only or even the major determinant of an individual's or a population's health. Socially oriented physicians and others have recognized for centuries that the health of people is influenced by the food they eat, the work they do, the knowledge they acquire, and much more. Further, nutrition, occupation, education, and other physical and social factors are mediated in their influence on health by the biological traits of individuals. Hence a model on the *determinants* of health would look something like figure 3.1. I have not tried to show the relative magnitude of the various influences, because this is really not known in any generalized sense. Modern epidemiologists are struggling with this problem, mainly on a disease-by-disease basis.

My focus, then, is on the block in figure 3.1 identified as "health services". Whatever influence health services have actually had on the health of people, men and women everywhere and throughout human history have behaved as though they believed that these services were an important determinant of health. Every known society has taken actions to cope with disease or injury, to regain health, and, in more recent times, to prevent disease and promote health.

The precise ways in which societies have done this differ enormously. In the current era of nation-states, the complex of health-seeking activities in each nation has resulted in a national health service system. With the different economic, political, cultural, geographic, and social settings of nations, their health service systems are naturally diverse. They vary enormously in the details of their structure and function, and hence in their overall complexity. However complex, and however efficient, coherent, or purposeful in providing health services, a nation's activities devoted primarily to achieving health may be defined as a national health service system.

EVOLUTION OF HEALTH SERVICE SYSTEMS

The current contours of health service systems have inevitably been influenced by the major historical developments of science and of society. The steady extension of mankind's knowledge of and control over nature has obviously been a major force in determining not only medical science and clinical medicine, but also many aspects of health service systems. Consider, for example, the importance of bacteriology to the development of preventive public health programs or the impor-

Figure 3.1   Determinants of Health

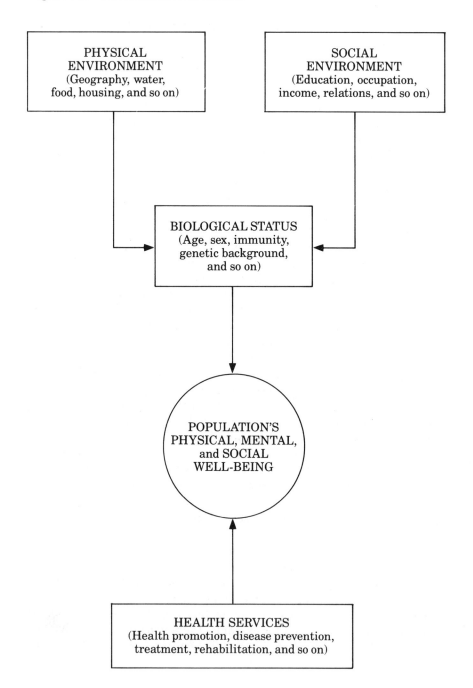

tance of organ pathology and surgery to the development of hospitals. The evolution of economic orders, or methods of exchange of goods and services, has had as great an impact on the shape of health service systems in the world today as the natural sciences have. I refer principally to the rise of capitalist and entrepreneurial economic orders over the last two or three centuries.

With the decline of feudalism and the rise of free trade, medical care became one of many commodities and services sold in the market. This process of exchange initially had distinct benefits in many settings. By providing physicians, apothecaries, and others with a source of income, it attracted many gifted persons into these callings and gave them incentives to work diligently. It also provided health services for many people in the newly developed cities—people who lacked the protection of a feudal lord. The growth of science and universities also led to the great expansion of knowledge and skills among practitioners of the healing arts.

As industry grew, however, and with it democratic and parliamentary forms of government, the concept of health service as a civic or public responsibility developed. This conception led to consequences in the domain of health services that were quite different from those associated with the process of free trade. Instead of expecting health services to be bought and sold in a marketplace, mechanisms were developed to provide health care to people on the basis of their human needs and in the interests of general community welfare. These trends were implemented through the founding and operation of hospitals for the poor (later for everyone), the rise of the public health movement, the organization of health insurance programs, and many other strategies for extending health services to general populations.

Over the last century, these two concepts of health services have developed side by side, although the conflict between health care as a market commodity and health care as a social service or even a basic human right has become more and more manifest. With the birth of the World Health Organization and the rise of many equivalent movements in almost all countries, the concept of health care as a right has gained ascendency. Accordingly, the complete dependence of health care on market transactions in the private sector is now widely regarded as leading to social inequities and serious deficiencies in health service systems. Therefore, most countries have intervened in the marketplace and have developed various kinds of collective financing and regulated provision of health service. The extent of this intervention has increased generally over time almost everywhere, but the manner and details of its application have varied greatly. These variations have influenced all components of health service systems and, in large part, determine the characteristics of the national systems.

COMPONENTS OF NATIONAL HEALTH SERVICE SYSTEMS

What, then, are the components of health service systems? Simply, they are the many activities that lie behind, that support, and that arrange for the delivery of health services to people. Exactly what is a health service? Bed care in a hospital is clearly a health service, but what about care of an elderly person in a custodial institution? Vitamin therapy of a child with rickets is surely a health service, but what about a subsidized lunch program for all school children? The custodial institution for the aged and the school lunch program obviously influence the health of people, but, unlike hospital care, health is not their *primary* purpose. A health service, therefore, can be best defined as an activity whose primary objective is health—its maintenance, its improvement, or, if lost, its recovery.

Even with this restricted definition, health service systems are complex affairs. In simplified form, their components consist of (1) development of resources, (2) organization of programs, (3) economic support, (4) management, and (5) delivery of services. The principal relationships among these components are shown in figure 3.2. If one proceeded no further than this model, I believe that one would still understand correctly the basic health service system of every country in the world. Within each of the components, however, there are many structures and processes—or, if you prefer, subsystems and sub-subsystems—that define the system in each nation. The highlights of each of the five components may be briefly considered.

Development of Resources

Essential for the provision of health services are numerous types of human and physical resources. In their simplest forms, these consist of manpower, facilities, commodities, and knowledge. The production or development of these resources requires inputs from various other social systems—education, construction, manufacturing, and so on— that I will not explore here. It may be noted that financing is not

Figure 3.2 A Health Services System—Structure, Relationships, and Function

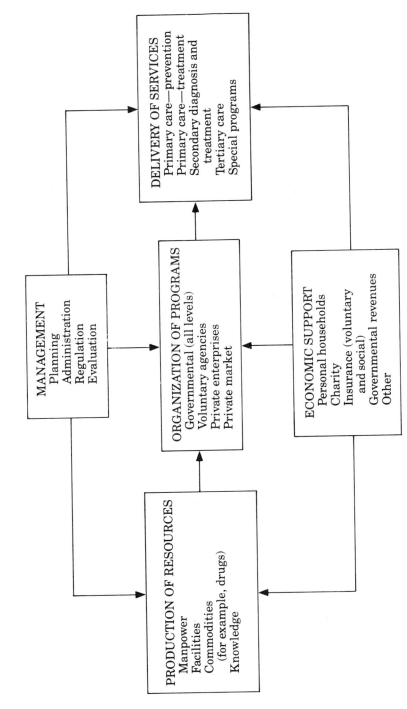

MANAGEMENT
Planning
Administration
Regulation
Evaluation

DELIVERY OF SERVICES
Primary care—prevention
Primary care—treatment
Secondary diagnosis and
treatment
Tertiary care
Special programs

ORGANIZATION OF PROGRAMS
Governmental (all levels)
Voluntary agencies
Private enterprises
Private market

ECONOMIC SUPPORT
Personal households
Charity
Insurance (voluntary
and social)
Governmental revenues
Other

PRODUCTION OF RESOURCES
Manpower
Facilities
Commodities
(for example, drugs)
Knowledge

regarded as a resource; rather, it is a medium of exchange convertible into resources and services, as noted below.

Health manpower includes physicians, healers, and a variety of other personnel in all countries. Their formal or informal training, their precise functions, their work settings, their interrelationships, and their regulation differ widely among health service systems. Their numbers and ratios to population, their geographic distribution, and their qualitative level of performance influence substantially the effectiveness of the health service systems of their countries.

Health facilities also take many forms. The oldest of these are hospitals for the diagnosis and treatment of the seriously ill. Aside from general hospitals for most short-term illnesses and injuries, there are special hospitals for long-term illnesses such as mental illness, cancer, and tuberculosis, as well as hospitals for childbirth or the care of children. Of increasing importance in recent decades are facilities for the organized provision of ambulatory care—health centers, polyclinics, health posts, and so on. Pharmacies, laboratories, and even private medical quarters must be counted among a system's health care facilities.

Health commodities are growing in importance with advances in technology. Best known are drugs and other therapeutic or even preventive substances, behind which stand worldwide industrial establishments. Over the centuries, drugs, whether found in nature or synthetically produced, have multiplied enormously and have become objects of international trade involving virtually all countries. Their production, distribution, and consumption involve all five components of health service systems. Similar dynamics apply to other commodities, such as diagnostic and therapeutic equipment, prosthetic devices, eyeglasses, wheelchairs, laboratory reagents, bandages, and much more.

Knowledge may not be conventionally regarded as a resource, but it is obviously basic to the operation of every health service system. Scientific knowledge is produced both by observation and experimental research, behind which are further human and technological requirements. Knowledge leads to technology; like the other three types of resources, it must be applied in various ways to result in health services.

Organization of Programs

The organization of resources into various functional relationships, or programs, oriented toward certain ends constitutes the second main component of health service systems. The sponsorship of programs may be governmental, voluntary nonprofit, or entrepreneurial, and the proportions among these types are crucial determinants of the general nature of a health service system.

In the realm of government, health service programs come under numerous agencies, best known of which is the ministry of health. Organized preventive health services are always a responsibility of the ministry, and the scope of their other functions is widening in many countries. In most countries, other governmental agencies are responsible for social insurance programs that finance medical care. Numerous other ministries may be involved in other aspects of the health service system, such as education of personnel, construction of health facilities, environmental controls, and so on. Depending on the size of a country (both in population and geography), each ministry may have organized peripheral units at regional, provincial, and local levels, and these units may operate with varying degrees of autonomy.

Nongovernmental and nonprofit (often charitable) organizations in most countries develop and operate health programs that tackle certain diseases (such as tuberculosis or cancer) or serve certain populations (such as children or the aged). Voluntary agencies may also operate health insurance programs. Associations of health professionals monitor their members' behavior and often represent their members in negotiations with government.

The entire private establishment for providing health services must be considered part of this component of health service systems. While not organized in the usual sense, it functions through a market in which the services are bought and sold at certain prices. The sellers include physicians, hospitals, pharmacists, and so on, and they relate to buyers (patients) with varying degrees of competition or cooperation. Health services provided to workers by private industrial enterprises must also be considered in this private sector.

Economic Support

Every health service system must have various sources of financing for the development and organization of health resources into programs. In every country there is more than one source of financing, and the proportion of money derived from each source determines many characteristics of the system.

In every country, private individuals or families are a source of economic support for health services, typically for treatment of personal disease. Donations to charity are another source, and these may take the form of donated labor as well as money. Nongovernmental or voluntary health insurance is another source of great importance in certain countries.

General taxation is a source of support for resource development and health services in every nation. The exact types of taxes (on land, income, purchases, and so on) and the political levels at which they are collected vary widely, but everywhere tax funds are used for general prevention and for medical treatment of at least part of the population. Mandatory or social insurance is a special form of governmental taxation, in which the funds are earmarked for a specified purpose—such as medical care—and they are used only for the benefit of the persons contributing to the insurance fund (and usually their families). In many developing countries, foreign aid or overseas charity may help support the health service system.

The mix, or proportions, of these several sources of economic support leads to policies that influence the nature of a health service system more decisively than any other system component. It is obvious that support derived from private individuals channels resources and services to those who have the money to spend, while support derived from general revenues can be used for services to others. The dynamics of economic support are, of course, very complex, but they obviously have great implications for health care equity. On a world scale, the proportion (not the amount) of health-related funds derived from private sources has been declining, while the proportion from public sources has been increasing.

Management

Management is another form of support for the operation of a health service system. Management includes various types of social control, including planning, administration, regulation, and evaluation. Each of the processes may be carried out with various degrees of informality or rigor. Likewise, all four of the elements of management may be in either the public or private sector.

Planning may be done at the central or local level of the health service system, or it may be done at various combinations of these levels. Its scope may vary with the types of health activity affected, in relation to unplanned or free market operations. Administration includes several activities in system operations, such as the exercise of authority, delegation of responsibility, communications, coordination, and so on. Regulation is usually governmental, but not always: it includes various legal and nonlegal forms of surveillance intended to assure that system activities are in accord with certain standards.

Most regulation has been established in response to abuses identified in the free market of health services and, to a lesser extent, in the public arena.

Evaluation is a difficult process in any health service system, because it depends on a flow of information that may be difficult to arrange. This information should concern the development of resources, the organization of programs, and the delivery of services. Arriving at sound judgments about the success or effectiveness of all these activities usually requires statistical data, which may be examined in relation to standards or objectives. In the absence of such data, evaluation may be based simply on general impressions of certain informed observers. By either method, evaluation provides feedback to the administration in a health service system, pointing to needed changes in organization.

Delivery of Services

The operation of the four components described in a health service system leads to the final component: delivery of services to people. These include all forms of health service: preventive, therapeutic, and rehabilitative. In terms of the complexity of the delivery process, the services are primary, secondary, and tertiary, or they may involve special programs.

The types of personnel, facilities, and work setting for delivery of these services differ substantially among health service systems, particularly between industrialized and developing countries. The differences are also great between the less organized and more organized types of systems, the latter having health personnel in much more deliberately organized teams for both hospital and ambulatory care. Within any one type of system, there may be several different patterns of health care delivery, particularly for selected population groups or diseases. Health services for military establishments or for the mentally ill, for example, are delivered through highly organized arrangements in all countries. One pattern of delivery, however, is bound to predominate within each system type. The extent of planned relationships between and among primary, secondary, and tertiary care, or regionalization, will also vary in different systems.

DETERMINANTS AND TYPES OF HEALTH SERVICE SYSTEMS

The combined characteristics of all five health service system components define the type of system found in each country. In the

Figure 3.3   Health Service Systems, by National Economic Level and
Health Care Policy

Economic Level	Health Care Policy		
	Permissive (laissez-faire)	*Cooperative (welfare)*	*Socialist (centrally planned)*
Affluent (industrialized)	1. United States Australia	2. Norway Great Britain	3. Soviet Union Czechoslovakia
Moderate (developing)	4. Thailand Philippines	5. Peru Malaysia	6. Cuba North Korea
Poor (underdeveloped)	7. Ghana Nepal	8. Tanzania Sri Lanka	9. China Mozambique

approximately 160 countries of the world, no two systems are exactly
alike, but one can understand the systems better by clustering them
into certain major types. To do this, one must consider the basic determinants of the character of national health service systems.

My own observations suggest that the major influences are economic and political. In addition, there are always several other influences, which one may group under the heading of cultural.

The economic development of countries can be quite readily
scaled in terms of their per capita GNP. Although this index tells
nothing about the distribution of income in the country, it does describe
national wealth. Countries with relatively high per capita GNPs are
mainly industrialized; those with low per capita GNPs are mainly
agricultural. Deviations from those tendencies are seen in several pe-
troleum-exporting countries, which have relatively high GNPs without
being industrialized.

The political characteristics of a country are not so easily identified and scaled. Although I have been searching United Nations and
other international statistics for a clear indicator of political ideology—
extent of centralized organization and control or extent of governmental versus private control of social affairs, or both—I have not yet found
one for many countries. In the absence of such an indicator, therefore, I
am proposing to scale national health service systems along a con-
tinuum describing the extent of organization of the systems themselves. With these two dimensions, each scaled into just three levels, I
derive a matrix of health service systems, as shown in figure 3.3.

Cultural influences could be added to the analysis by adding a
third dimension to the matrix—or even fourth and fifth dimensions,

which could be shown by multiple matrixes. One must consider under the rubric of culture a country's general technological development, as well as its religions, community structures, family customs, and languages. With sufficiently detailed consideration of all these influences, the world's 160 nations would probably yield 160 different types of health service systems.

With the relatively simple classification shown in figure 3.3, the nine concepts are probably sufficiently refined to provide useful understanding of how the main types of health service systems work. In each of the nine types, the names of two countries have been inserted as examples, although some systems are more prevalent than others. My impression is that the most frequent types today are probably 2, 5, and 8. With respect to economic levels, the countries in the top row (1, 2, and 3) have annual per capita GNPs of $3,000 or more; in the middle row, this figure is between $400 and $3,000 (with the greatest clustering around $1,500); in the bottom row the annual per capita GNPs are under $400 (and usually under $300).

Space does not permit even a brief synopsis of each type of health service system in figure 3.3, but a few remarks may be made about the characteristics of the systems under each kind of health care policy. In the permissive systems (1, 4, and 7), the private sector for delivery of ambulatory health care is quite strong. Expenditures for health services come predominantly from private families, rather than government. The resources (manpower, facilities, commodities, and knowledge), of course, are much lower in 4 than in 1, and they are lowest in 7. Most health care is delivered by individual practitioners (physicians, health auxiliaries, and traditional healers), rather than teams of personnel.

In the cooperative systems (2, 5, and 8), a major proportion of the costs of health services has been collectivized through governmental mechanisms, including social insurance. The great majority of hospital resources are in governmental facilities, and in most of these the doctors, along with other personnel, work on full-time salaries. In 5, the proportions of populations protected by social insurance are much smaller than in 2, but they are expanding. Central governments play a large role in health program management, but a substantial role is played also by local governments and local communities.

Socialist health service systems (3, 6, and 9) are almost entirely governmental. Virtually all resources are within the government and health service is theoretically available to all residents without cost (except for small charges made in 9). In 3, the central government exercises controls over all aspects of the system, with somewhat more local participation in 6 and 9. Preventive services are emphasized in all these systems, and their delivery is integrated with the treatment services.

These highlights of the nine types of health service systems are simplifications, but they may suggest some aspects for differentiation. If any action is to be taken to improve the health services of a country—in quantity, quality, or equity—it is obvious that it will have to differ in all nine types. Moreover, one would have to take account of not only the economic level and the degree of organization, but also religions, community structures, and other cultural features.

TRENDS

In a very general way, with some notable exceptions, national health service systems are evolving toward greater organization—that is, from the left to the right hand side of figure 3.3. This is seen in trends with respect to collectivized economic support, health care delivery patterns, policies of management, and, in fact, all components of health systems. To a lesser degree, the trend is to move from the bottom to the top row of the figure, as many (but certainly not all) countries undergo economic development. This development is reflected most concretely in health service systems by steady enlargement of health resources—ratios of health personnel to population, supply of hospital beds, and availability of health centers. The impacts of these trends are clearly reflected in worldwide improvements in life expectancy, infant mortality, and other indexes of health. In the years between 1955 and 1975, the life expectancy at birth in the developed regions of the world increased from 64.3 to 70.3 years. Even in the much poorer, developing regions it increased from 42.5 to 53.2 years. The rates of these improvements are not the same in all countries, but the overall trend is still favorable. Changes in physical and social environments contribute to these trends, but health services must play a substantial part as well.

The health status of populations depends on many influences beyond health services. Improvements in health, therefore, require progress in many sectors of society. One need not wait, however, for enormous changes in a total society to expect significant gains in health. More effective and equitable health service systems can achieve better "health for all" as WHO puts it, in a relatively short time.

Part Two

Developing Countries

4

Health and Distribution of Income in Developing Countries

The relationship of poverty to disease is well recognized in all countries. Measurements of national health, however, relate only marginally to indexes of national wealth. An explanation may be partially found in the uneven distribution of wealth within countries and the related disparities in health care expenditures. These imbalances are particularly great in developing countries.

The relation of health to economic level both in families and in nations has long been appreciated. In 1790, Johann Peter Frank spoke of "the people's misery as the mother of disease."[1] The modern public health movement in Europe stemmed from the observation that disease was much more prevalent among the poor.[2] Well before foreign aid programs, the health status of entire nations was recognized to be related largely to their levels of wealth.[3]

HEALTH AND ECONOMIC LEVEL

In more recent years, the interdependence of health and the economic development of countries has been explored in greater detail. The sickness, disability, and premature death of people have come to be recognized as factors retarding their productivity and economic devel-

Based on a working paper prepared for the Office of International Health, Department of Health, Education, and Welfare, 1978.

opment, just as the poverty of nations has become understood as a major—and probably the most crucial—determinant of the morbidity and mortality of their populations.[4]

Yet, as more has been learned about how social and environmental factors influence the health of populations, the relationships between health and wealth have come to be considered far more complex than simple linkage. The most widely used measure of a nation's economic level is its GNP per capita per year. Thus, the 1973 per capita GNP in U.S. dollars of Ethiopia was $83, of Brazil was $750, and of the United States was $6,155.[5] The corresponding infant mortality rates (deaths per 1,000 live births in the first year of life) in these three countries were 162, 110, and 19.[6]

Thus, while the general relationship between per capita GNP and infant mortality is clearly inverse (the poorer the country, the more of its babies die before their first birthdays), it is also clearly not linear. Wealth (as reflected in per capita GNP) in the United States, for example, is 74 times greater than in Ethiopia, and in Brazil is about 9 times greater than in Ethiopia. The infant mortality rate in Ethiopia, however, is only about 8 times higher than that in the United States and not twice as high as that in Brazil. The same sort of irregular relationship applies to life expectancy and other available indexes of health status.

It is not necessary for two sets of measurements of different phenomena to be completely consistent in order for a statistical correlation to be very high. However, the striking fact is that exploration of the correlations between health measurements and the per capita GNP of countries yields many extreme deviations from a linear, or consistent, trend. This is shown in table 4.1, in which 20 countries with per capita GNPs between $100 and about $1,000 are listed in rank order, along with their reported average life expectancies at birth. The data are derived from a report of the World Bank. The countries, while all considered less developed, were selected to represent a wide range of economic levels, yet to have reasonably reliable statistical data.[7]

More impressive than the generally positive correlation between wealth and health are the numerous deviations from a linear relationship. These deviations are graphically illustrated in figure 4.1, which is based on the same data shown in table 4.1. The diagonal line has been determined by the least squares technique and shows the incline that would describe a perfectly linear relationship between per capita GNP and life expectancy (the numbers next to each point in the figure correspond to the numbers assigned to each country in table 4.1).

Why should life expectancy in Sri Lanka (1) be so much above the regression line, while that in India (2) is so much below the line? Both

Table 4.1 National Wealth and Life Expectancy at Birth in 20 Countries, about 1973

Country	GNP Per Capita ($U.S.)	Life Expectancy (years)
1. Sri Lanka	100	67.8
2. India	110	49.2
3. Ivory Coast	330	43.5
4. Turkey	340	56.4
5. Colombia	370	60.9
6. Zambia	380	44.5
7. Malaysia	400	59.4
8. Taiwan	430	61.6
9. Iran	450	51.0
10. Brazil	460	61.4
11. Albania	480	68.6
12. Peru	480	55.7
13. Cuba	510	72.3
14. Costa Rica	590	68.2
15. Mexico	700	63.2
16. Jamaica	720	69.5
17. Yugoslavia	730	67.5
18. Chile	760	64.3
19. Bulgaria	820	71.8
20. Venezuela	1060	64.7

countries have approximately the same per capita GNP and are in the same general geographic region of Asia. Likewise, why should Mexico (15) have a higher per capita GNP than Cuba (13), when both are in the same region and have a similar cultural heritage?

THE ROLE OF INCOME DISTRIBUTION

It is obvious that factors not reflected in per capita GNP are playing a large part. The number of factors potentially exerting an influence on health status must be very great, but I hypothesize that an important and measurable indicator of many of those factors is the *distribution* of wealth among a nation's population. Overall national wealth remains important: one need not go so far as to dethrone GNP entirely because of its inadequacies.[8] Ways should be found, however, to adjust the basic information provided by GNP for at least some of the many other determinants of a people's level of living, including their health.

Fortunately, economists have long been aware of the problem and have developed measurements of income distribution. One of the best

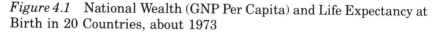

Figure 4.1   National Wealth (GNP Per Capita) and Life Expectancy at Birth in 20 Countries, about 1973

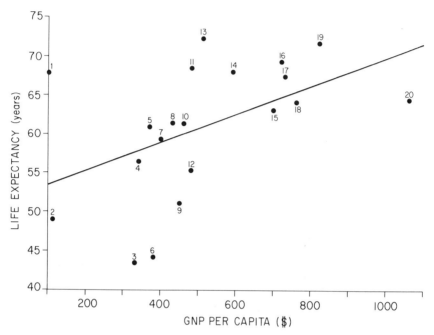

established is the Gini coefficient, formulated by an Italian scholar to reflect the degree of equality or inequality in the distribution of income among various sectors (percentiles) of the population. Thus, in a population characterized by perfect equality, where each tenth of the population received exactly one-tenth of the national income, the Gini coefficient would be 0. In a highly inequitable setting, where the upper tenth of the population received all the income while the other nine-tenths received none, the Gini coefficient would be 1.0. Of course, every country falls somewhere between these two extremes, and the lower the coefficient, the greater the equality of income distribution.

The World Bank staff has calculated, from a variety of sources, Gini coefficients for 79 countries, including 18 of those shown in table 4.1.[9] In order to attempt to adjust the per capita GNP data in this table for each country's income distribution, the data may be multiplied by the reciprocal of the Gini coefficient; thus, the adjusted per capita GNP of more equitable countries would be raised and that of less equitable countries would be lowered. The results of these calculations, along with data on life expectancy and infant mortality rates, are presented in table 4.2.

On the basis of the data presented in tables 4.1 and 4.2, we may

Table 4.2 National Wealth Adjusted for Its Distribution and Health
Status Measurements, about 1973

Country	Gini Coefficient	Gini-adjusted GNP ($U.S.)	Life Expectancy (years)	Infant Mortality Rate
1. Sri Lanka	.358	279	67.8	50.3
2. India	.461	239	49.2	139.0
3. Ivory Coast	.516	640	43.5	138.0
4. Turkey	.544	625	56.4	153.0
5. Colombia	.546	678	60.9	67.9
6. Zambia	.488	779	44.5	150.0*
7. Malaysia	.497	805	59.4	38.5
8. Taiwan	.317	1356	61.6	18.0
9. Iran	.473	951	51.0	160.0
10. Brazil	.553	832	61.4	110.0
11. Albania	.242†	1984	68.6	87.0
12. Peru	.571	841	55.7	53.6
13. Cuba	.242†	2107	72.3	28.7
14. Costa Rica	.429	1375	68.2	68.2
15. Mexico	.558	1254	63.2	60.9
16. Jamaica	.558	1290	69.5	27.0
17. Yugoslavia	.333	2192	67.5	44.0
18. Chile	.487	1561	64.3	71.0
19. Bulgaria	.206	3981	71.8	26.0
20. Venezuela	.591	1794	64.7	52.0

*Estimated on the basis of infant mortality rates reported by several other similar African countries; data from Zambia for the 1970's are not available.

†Estimated by calculating the average of Gini coefficients reported for five other Socialist countries: Bulgaria (.206), Czechoslovakia (.183), Hungary (.235), Poland (.253), and Yugoslavia (.333).

test the hypothesis offered above. That is, does the per capita GNP of a country adjusted for income distribution yield a higher correlation with measurements of health status than does the per capita GNP alone?

HEALTH AND WEALTH ADJUSTED
FOR INCOME DISTRIBUTION

The coefficient of correlation between per capita GNP and average life expectancy for the 20 countries in table 4.1 is positive at .495. Thus, despite the deviations from linearity noted above, the general relationship between national wealth and life expectancy is positive, though weakly so. When the same life expectancy figures are correlated with the Gini-adjusted per capita GNP data, as shown in table 4.2, the positive coefficient of correlation rises to .624, an increase of 26 percent. It is evident, therefore, that adjustment of the per capita GNP of a country by its income distribution appreciably strengthens the positive correlation to its population's life expectancy.*

An equivalent dynamic characterizes the relationship between per capita GNP and infant mortality rate (IMR) in the 20 countries. The coefficient of correlation between the average per capita GNP and the IMR is negative, as would be expected, at .454. When the Gini-adjusted per capita income is related to the IMR, the negative coefficient of correlation increases to .509, a rise of 11 percent. (The somewhat lesser differential than for the life expectancy data probably reflects the less complete reporting of infant deaths in developing countries than of deaths at older ages; deathrates at all ages are the basis for calculating life expectancy figures.)

In 1979, G. B. Rodgers of the International Labour Organization analyzed life expectancies in 56 countries, in relation to their income distributions, as reflected by the Gini coefficients. He concluded:

> The results for life expectancy at birth suggest that the difference in average life expectancy between a relatively egalitarian and a relatively inegalitarian country is likely to be as much as five to ten years. The distribution of income may not be the only factor operating of course— inequality in income distribution is likely to be associated with inequality in access to health and social services, in education, and in a number of other aspects of society relevant to mortality.[10]

Besides noting statistical evidence of the influence of income distribution on health status indicators, one may note some of the social conditions behind the numbers. The per capita GNPs of Sri Lanka (1) and India (2), as noted, are almost the same, but in Sri Lanka the life expectancy is considerably longer and the IMR much lower. Both countries have the heritage of the British colonial medical services, which were frugal but relatively systematic, and both were strengthened after national independence; further, there is no reason to suspect any differences in the reliability of the vital statistics. It may be noted also that back in 1938, when both countries were under British rule, the infant mortality rates (IMR) were almost the same—167 per 1,000 live births in India (British provinces) and 161 per 1,000 in Ceylon (Sri Lanka today).[11] By 1973 the Indian IMR had declined to 139 per 1,000, while Sri Lankan IMR descended much farther to 50.3 per 1,000.

---

*If the adjustment of per capita GNP for income distribution were made by multiplying it by the reciprocal of the Gini coefficient *squared*, the positive correlation coefficient with life expectancy would be strengthened even further. However, the effect of the simple adjustment applied here should be enough to confirm the basic argument.

In 1973, the Gini coefficient for Sri Lanka (.358) reflects a much more equitable distribution of the available income than in India (.461). In both countries, the average income level is extremely low, there is great unemployment, and the prevailing standard of living is very poor. However, since about 1960 Sri Lanka has been mainly under the control of semisocialist coalition governments; it has nationalized the plantations growing its principal export, tea, and has introduced various other social reforms. Among these has been a government policy of extending basic education to virtually all children and distributing each week one free pound of rice to 90 percent of the population, plus one pound at one-third of the market price.[12] Such equalizing programs have been much weaker in India, and the difference is doubtless reflected in the data on infant mortality and life expectancy.

Another illustrative comparison, as is clear from figure 4.1, may be drawn between Mexico (15) and Cuba (13). Mexico's per capita GNP ($700) is appreciably higher than Cuba's ($510), but the distribution of wealth is very different. The Gini coefficient for Cuba (.242) suggests an equalization of income distribution more than twice as great as that for Mexico (.558). Both countries have developed rather strong health service systems in their main cities, but in the rural areas, where most of the populations live, Cuba's improvements over the last 20 years have won worldwide attention.[13] The substantially longer life expectancy and lower IMR in Cuba, compared with Mexico—as well as with other Latin American countries of similar or greater per capita GNP— are doubtless related to the equalization of income distribution achieved after the revolution.

It may be pointed out that Cuba's life expectancy was greater than Mexico's even in 1950–55, before its revolution. One must not forget, however, the enormous difficulties faced by Cuba after the Castro government came to power—flight of its doctors, blockade and embargo of trade (including medical supplies), physical invasion at the Bay of Pigs, and so on. In these very years, Mexico was acquiring great national wealth through its discovery of large reserves of petroleum. In Costa Rica, moreover, with higher per capita GNP than Cuba, the male life expectancy in 1950–55 was 56.0 years—only slightly lower than Cuba's 56.7 years; by 1970–75, the Costa Rican life expectancy at birth had risen to 67.5 years, while in Cuba the attainment was 70.2 years.[14]

These phenomena need not be attributed solely to the semisocialist or communist ideologies found in Sri Lanka and Cuba; however, the influence of these political systems on income distribution and therefore on health status would seem to be clear. The data from Taiwan (8) and Iran (9) illustrate the effects of income distribution in two countries of very similar political complexion (both being widely recognized as conservative). The per capita GNPs of these two countries are quite similar: Iran, $450; Taiwan, $430. Iranian wealth is largely due to its oil production, the earnings of which are concentrated in relatively few hands. Compared with Taiwan, Iran's income distribution is noticeably inequitable, as reflected in its Gini coefficient of .473 versus Taiwan's .317. The greater economic equity in Taiwan would surely help explain that country's much greater life expectancy and very much lower infant mortality.

In spite of this general confirmation of the importance of income distribution to health status, over and above the per capita GNP in a country, it is apparent from the data cited that income distribution is not the whole story. Even with per capita GNPs adjusted by the Gini coefficients, the relationships to health status, while strengthened, obviously do not approach 1.0, or a perfect correlation. In none of the 20 countries examined is income distribution found to be completely equitable, as reflected by the Gini coefficients. Moreover, other factors in a population's living conditions and health service system must surely be exerting substantial influences on health status.

In recent years, social scientists have been exploring the relationship of mortality rates (or life expectancies) to various "noneconomic" measures of social well-being. Preston and others have emphasized the concrete benefits of basic public health programs (insect control, health education, and so on), even when economic development has been weak.[15] Multivariate analyses of numerous social variables have shown the very great influence of educational levels or literacy on health indexes, particularly the infant mortality rates.[16] Basic education is, of course, dependent mainly on actions by government in all nations. Even more than health service, education is a public sector activity. Put the other way around, the equitable distribution of health services requires even greater governmental assumption of responsibility than the provision of widespread public education.

EQUITY AND THE PUBLIC SECTOR
OF HEALTH SERVICES

The issue of equity in health care systems may be considered along other lines. Most important, how equitably are health services distributed in relation to a population's need for care? Unfortunately, there are few countries on which such distributional data are available. One may answer this question in approximate terms by examining the *sources* of a nation's health expenditures. Insofar as equity of health care distribution is to be achieved, the funds must generally be derived from

Table 4.3   Health Expenditures in Four Developing Countries: Percent of GNP and Percent Derived from Public Sources, about 1965

Country	Percent of GNP Spent for Health	Percent from Public Sources
Chile	5.6	42.1
Sri Lanka	3.7	59.8
Kenya	3.6	42.0
Tanganyika	2.5	66.6

public rather than private sources. Private expenditures are typically for the benefit of the individual or family that makes them, and the amounts vary with affluence much more than with health needs. For health services to be provided in equitable relation to needs, especially in developing countries, they must ordinarily be financed through public (usually governmental) sources.

The sources of health care expenditures are available for the United States and some of the more affluent industrialized countries, where national statistics are well maintained. The U. S. government, for example, reports that in 1976 the population spent about $140 billion for health purposes ($638 per capita), or 8.6 percent of the GNP.[17] Of this amount, 42 percent was derived from governmental sources. Equivalent data on developing countries are seldom available, but some data come from a 1961 WHO study.[18] Four developing countries were included in the study, with findings as shown in table 4.3. It would appear from these data that, even in the developing countries, an appreciable proportion of health spending in 1961 must have come from nonpublic sources (ranging from 33.4 percent in Tanganyika to 58 percent in Kenya), in spite of the very low income levels of the vast majority of the people in these countries.

PRIVATE SECTOR IMPLICATIONS FOR HEALTH IN DEVELOPING COUNTRIES

Although data on the sources of health care expenditures are scarce, a few recent observations indicate relationships that should cause serious concern. An investigation in Colombia, for example, found somewhat over 7 billion pesos devoted to health services in 1970–71; of this amount, about 51 percent was derived from private

Figure 4.2   Health Expenditures: Proportions for Affluent and Poor People in One Developing Country, about 1975

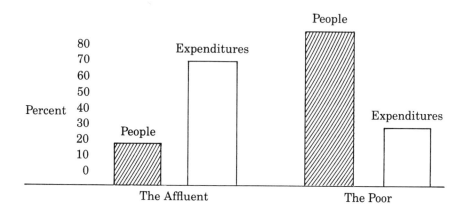

sources and 49 percent from public sources.[19] I was able recently to make some rough estimates of health service expenditures, by source, in another developing country of Latin America.[20] In brief, I found that public sector sources accounted for 47.5 percent of health expenditures, of which more than 40 percent was concentrated on employed urban workers (under a social security program) (see chapter 5). The private sector was the source of 52.5 percent of health expenditures. A sociological study of the same country reported the distribution of social classes as follows: landowners, large merchants, and so on, 1 percent; steadily employed workers, civil servants, and so on, 17 percent; peasants, laborers, and indigent persons, 82 percent.[21] If these data on social class are related to the findings on national health expenditures, one can estimate that about 18 percent (17 plus 1) of the population receives health services costing about 70 percent of the money spent, while the impoverished 82 percent of the population receives services costing 30 percent of the health money. Figure 4.2 shows the relationship in the form of a graph.

The imbalance illustrated in figure 4.2 is based upon estimates from one Latin American country, but the basic type of relationship would probably apply to most developing countries. It is a relationship that not only spells extreme inequity, but also obstructs health planning, since planning is very difficult in the private sector. This imbalance cannot be adjusted within the boundaries of the health services alone—it involves the overall social and political policy with respect to taxation and other means of allocating a nation's resources.

APPROACHING HEALTH EQUITY

As a practical matter, more equitable distribution of resources is not likely to succeed through legal prohibitions on private spending. Even in socialist countries born out of social revolution, private medical practice has not usually been prohibited.[22] Instead, the equalization of resources in relation to need has been approached by strengthening the public sector. This has also been the strategy in Great Britain and other welfare states. If public services are made effective enough, fewer and fewer people will purchase private ones. One need not be concerned about an extremely small elite—1 or 2 percent of the population—who will seek and pay for private health care under any circumstances. If the health needs of 98 percent of a population can be reached by a public system of health service, a small fraction of inequity may be tolerated as a safety valve to avoid pressures in the system.

The attainment of fully equitable income distribution is a social goal of stupendous proportions. Income distributions approaching Gini coefficients of 0 are improbable. However, the attainment of equity in health service distribution, through reasonable strengthening of the public sector of health care as a basic human right, is well within the reach of any nation that is committed to this goal.

NOTES

1. H. E. Sigerist, *Landmarks in the History of Hygiene* (London: Oxford University Press, 1956), 47.
2. E. Chadwick, *Report on the Sanitary Conditions of the Laboring Population of Great Britain*, 1842. Edited with an introduction by M. W. Flinn (Edinburgh: University Press, 1965).
3. C.-E. A. Winslow, *The Cost of Sickness and the Price of Health* (Geneva: World Health Organization, 1951), 75–84.
4. G. Myrdal, *Asian Drama: An Inquiry into the Poverty of Nations*, vol. 3 of *Health* (New York: Pantheon, 1968), 1553–1619.
5. United Nations Conference on Trade and Development, *Handbook of International Trade and Development Statistics* (Geneva, 1976), 333–38.
6. World Bank, *Health: Sector Policy Paper* (Washington, D.C., 1975), 72–73.
7. Ibid.
8. O. Gish, "Health by the People: An Historical Exploration," unpublished paper, 1976.
9. S. Jain, *Size Distribution of Income: Compilation of Data*, staff working paper no. 190 (Washington, D.C.: World Bank, 1974).
10. G. B. Rodgers, "Income and Inequality as Determinants of Mortality: An International Cross-section Analysis," *Population Studies* (July 1979): 343–51.
11. League of Nations, Health Organization, "Annual Epidemiological Report" (Geneva, 1941).

12. R. Shaplen, "Letter from Sri Lanka," *New Yorker* (13 September 1976): 131–51.
13. M. I. Roemer, *Cuban Health Services and Resources* (Washington, D.C.: Pan American Health Organization, 1976).
14. United Nations, Department of International Economic and Social Affairs, *World Population Trends and Prospects by Country, 1950–2000* (New York, 1982).
15. S. H. Preston, *Mortality Patterns in National Populations* (New York: Academic Press, 1976), 62–88.
16. R. N. Grosse and B. H. Perry, "Correlates of Life Expectancy in Less Developed Countries," *Health Policy and Education* (March 1982): 275–304.
17. R. M. Gibson and M. S. Mueller, "National Health Expenditures, Fiscal Year 1976," *Social Security Bulletin* 40(4) (April 1977): 3–22.
18. B. Abel-Smith, *An International Study of Health Expenditure and Its Relevance for Health Planning*, public health paper no. 32 (Geneva: World Health Organization, 1967).
19. D. K. Zschock, R. L. Robertson, and J. A. Daly, *Health Sector Financing in Latin America: Conceptual Framework and Case Studies* (Washington, D.C.: U.S. Dept. of Health, Education, and Welfare; Office of International Health, December 1976, Processed).
20. M. I. Roemer, "Increasing the Efficiency of the Guatemalan Health Service System" (Guatemala City: U.S. Agency for International Development, 1977). See chapter 5 in this book.
21. M. Monteforte T., excerpted in Melville, 1971. Reported in USAID/Guatemala document SWA-1/16/74, rev. 2.
22. M. G. Field, *Soviet Socialized Medicine: An Introduction* (New York: The Free Press, 1967), 43–46.

5

Guatemalan Health Services: Structure, Performance, and Costs

In Guatemala, the health care system is complicated by the operation of several virtually autonomous subsystems. The efficiency and costs of the Guatemalan system are adversely affected by the lack of coordination among these components. A similar diversity of arrangements for health care is found in most of the other 20 Latin American countries.

The "efficiency" of a system refers to the ratio of its output to its input. In health service systems, the input consists of many types of personnel, facilities, equipment, and other resources. The output is the change in health status (an improvement, it is hoped) of a population. In general, however, it is very difficult to attribute to health services alone any improvements occurring in the health status of a population, since so many other influences—food, employment, housing, education, and so on—are also involved. Therefore it is customary to measure the output of a health care system at an intermediate point, namely the types and quantities of health services provided (or produced). In other words, what services are produced in relation to the resources made available?

The efficiency of a health care system must be distinguished from its effectiveness. Effectiveness refers to benefits—the results achieved—without respect to costs (which reflect the input of re-

Based on a field study done in 1977 as part of a health sector assessment sponsored by the Guatemalan Academy of Medical, Physical, and Natural Sciences in cooperation with USAID.

sources). A program could be very effective yet inefficient, if it yielded good results at an extremely high cost. Efficiency, on the other hand, refers to costs (inputs) as well as results (outputs). It has an economic dimension as well as an evaluative one. My concern in this chapter is with the efficiency of the Guatemalan health care system.

There seems to be widespread consensus in Guatemala that the health care system is operating at a relatively low level of efficiency. In the first place, it is widely believed that the resources available to the health services are inadequate to meet the health care needs of the population, even if these resources were optimally used. Secondly, and probably more important, those resources that are available are not being efficiently applied.

THE CURRENT HEALTH CARE SYSTEM AND ITS SUBSYSTEMS

As in all countries, the health care system in Guatemala has evolved along several paths over the years. Each component has separate origins, indicating that the current scene is not the result of a logical or rational plan. Each subsystem is identified with a relatively distinct pattern of economic support and mode of delivery. These subsystems include:

1. Ministry of Public Health and Social Assistance (MOH)
2. Guatemalan Institute of Social Security (IGSS)
3. Other governmental health programs
4. Organized private, voluntary health organizations (PVOs)
5. Industrial and agricultural enterprises
6. The private health care sector, both traditional and modern

The main features of each of these subsystems are briefly described.

Ministry of Public Health and Social Assistance

Since its establishment in 1944, MOH has gradually expanded its resources and programs throughout Guatemala. Its strongest aspects have been in the national capital, Guatemala City, and the *departamento* in which it is located, but since about 1970 increasing attention has been given to building up services in the rural areas. The services provided are both preventive and therapeutic, and they are furnished through a network of health posts, health centers, and hospitals.

Administrative direction of the MOH program is highly centralized in the national headquarters. Some years ago, the nation was divided into eight health regions, each of which contained two to four local *departamentos*,[1] but now the regional offices have been abandoned. Instead, the country is divided into 24 health areas, which report directly to the national headquarters. Each health area has a health chief, only a few of whom have had public health training. The chief is theoretically responsible for all MOH activities in his area—both preventive and curative—except for certain "vertical programs" administered directly from the top. The major vertical programs at this time are tuberculosis and malaria control, although the intention is to decentralize these eventually.

Most of the MOH services are provided through facilities for ambulatory service, bed care, or both. Starting with the most rural and peripheral units, there were 510 health posts, 71 type B health centers, 11 type A health centers, 29 departmental hospitals, and 10 metropolitan hospitals in 1975.[2]

Health posts are located in rural municipalities with a population of at least 2,000. They are staffed essentially by allied health personnel, mainly briefly trained auxiliary nurses. In recent years, some health post staffs have been strengthened with the addition of more thoroughly trained *tecnicos de salud rural* (rural health technicians), numbering 212 in 1976.[3] The type B health centers are staffed by one physician plus allied health personnel, sometimes *tecnicos de salud rural*. The type A health centers have two physicians and a larger number of nurses and other allied health workers; they also usually have a small number of beds for maternity patients, trauma cases, or other patients under observation pending possible transfer to a hospital. The total number of beds in all health centers is only 161.

In the 39 hospitals of the MOH there are 9,407 beds of all types.[4] More than 1,000 of these are in a psychiatric hospital, and more than 500 are in a tuberculosis sanatorium (although many persons with tuberculosis are put in general hospitals). This amounts to a ratio of 1.6 hospital beds per 1,000 population—or, if the mental and tuberculosis institutions are excluded, 1.4 beds per 1,000. These ratios are, of course, very low.

The staffing of these hospitals varies with their size: the larger facilities have several doctors and professional nurses, while the smaller ones may have only a few. Even though most of the hospital beds outside the metropolitan capital are in MOH facilities, about 60 percent of MOH beds are in the capital *departamento,* where about 25 percent of the national population lives. The overall staffing of nonmetropolitan hospitals, moreover, is much weaker than that in capital

Table 5.1   Ratio of Personnel to Beds in Two Large and Two Small Hospitals

Hospital	Beds (No.)	Personnel (No.)	Personnel Per Bed
San Juan de Dios	1081	1436	1.3
Roosevelt	829	1301	1.6
San Benito	92	50	0.5
Huehuetenango	72	30	0.4

city hospitals. Comparing the nation's two largest general hospitals with two randomly selected small ones, the staffing ratios are found to be as shown in table 5.1. Compared with hospital staffing ratios in more developed countries, those in even the large Guatemalan hospitals are low; in the small peripheral hospitals they are extremely low. One must ordinarily expect higher staff-to-patient ratios in large institutions serving more complex cases, but the extreme understaffing in Guatemala's peripheral MOH hospitals has a substantial bearing on the efficiency of these units.

Institute of Social Security

Since 1946, Guatemala—like virtually all other Latin American countries—has developed a special program of health services for steadily employed public and private workers and, to a limited extent, their dependents. In several respects, however, the population covered and the medical benefits provided by the IGSS are more restricted than are those in most other countries of the hemisphere. Social security in Guatemala is financed by earmarked contributions, or quotas, from employers and workers; these quotas are derived from a percentage of wages. Since the government is also a large employer, it pays quotas on behalf of governmental employees; in addition, the law requires it to pay a special allotment drawn from general revenues (unfortunately, the latter has not been paid regularly). All monies are kept in a social security fund separate from the national treasury, and they may only be used for medical and other social benefits decided upon by the social security directors. While these operations come under the general surveillance of the ministry of labor, the independence of the social security fund yields a high degree of autonomy in policy decisions.

General medical care is provided only for workers in the metropolitan *Departamento de Guatemala*. Health services for dependents of these workers are limited to maternity service and general health care of children until their second birthday. Outside the metropolitan *departamento*, services to workers are restricted to the treatment of accident cases, although these include nonoccupational as well as work-related injuries; dependents of these workers have no benefits. On the other hand, workers in Guatemala's agricultural enterprises, unlike agricultural workers in most other Latin American countries, receive these benefits as long as the farm, or *finca*, employs five or more workers.

As of 1975, the number of persons served in any way by this health program was 741,000, or 13.2 percent of the national population (5.6 million in 1975).[5] With respect to complete medical care—that is, the benefits available to workers in the metropolitan center—the persons served numbered 278,770, or just 5 percent of the national population. The other 8 percent were entitled only to traumatological services and, in the capital area, to some maternity and infant care.

These services are provided principally through IGSS's own facilities. These consist of 31 hospitals, with 2,098 beds, and 39 ambulatory care units. The seven hospitals in the metropolitan center have 60 percent of the beds, while the remaining 24 hospitals are much smaller and have only 40 percent of the beds. Similarly, IGSS operates 11 relatively large ambulatory care clinics in Guatemala City and 28 small such units (many simply first-aid stations) in the rest of the country. These distributions reflect the relatively comprehensive range of services available to insured workers in the national capital and the limited services to which other workers are entitled.

Insured persons under IGSS receive much more health care than the rest of the population does. The quality of services is also probably better. Social security funds per person served are clearly greater than MOH funds. The IGSS facilities are better equipped, and personnel get higher salaries. Small wonder that there is a sense of rivalry rather than cooperation between these two major health agencies.

Other Governmental Agencies

Several other governmental agencies in Guatemala provide health services or are related to health care in some manner. These include the following:

1. The military forces in Guatemala, as in almost all countries, have a well-developed health care program with their own personnel and facilities. The national police likewise have their own health care program.

2. In the Office of the President (under the direction of the president's wife) there is a separate social welfare program

(Bienestar Social) devoted mainly to nutritional and related health services for impoverished children.

3. Below the level of the *departamentos* there are 327 local *municipios*; many of them, especially the larger ones, take responsibility for water supply, refuse disposal, and other aspects of environmental sanitation. It is also common for municipalities to construct health posts, which are then staffed and operated by the MOH. In the metropolitan *departamento*, a few small dispensaries are operated directly by municipalities.

4. The Ministry of Public Works is responsible for the construction of most hospitals, health centers, and environmental sanitation resources, although architectual plans and financial support come from the MOH or other sources.

5. The University of San Carlos is semi-autonomous but is linked to the Ministry of Education and is financed almost entirely by the central government. It is a large institution with a long tradition and great prestige. Guatemala's only school of medicine, as well as its schools of dentistry and pharmacy, are in this university. There is an open admission policy in these professional schools, so any secondary school graduate may be admitted, although the great majority flunk out after a year or two, and only a small fraction are graduated. Directly relevant to the health care system is a university requirement that, before earning the academic degree, every medical student must work for six months at a rural health post.

Private, Voluntary Organizations

A great variety of PVOs, largely although not entirely under religious auspices, offers health services throughout Guatemala. A recent study estimates that 150 of these PVOs are health-related.[6] While the ultimate objectives of most of these organizations may be religious, they provide at the same time a significant amount of health service.

Private Enterprises

Private enterprise—industrial and agricultural—provides a limited amount of health service in Guatemala. At a few large factories in the metropolitan area, there are in-plant health services; these services are concerned largely with industrial injuries or occupational diseases.[7]

A great share of Guatemala's agricultural output is provided by large *fincas* with scores or hundreds of workers. The living conditions of the great majority of farm workers are extremely poor; they are most deleterious for the migratory workers (an estimated 80 percent of the 500,000 farm workers). Nevertheless, two associations of Guatemalan coffee growers have taken the initiative to provide limited ambulatory medical services to migratory workers.[8] These services are provided through two clinics that are staffed by full-time doctors and serve several thousand workers and their families. Although the main support comes from the *finca* owners, patients must also pay a small fee for each service.

The Private Health Care Sector

The nonorganized, private health care sector in Guatemala is very large. While its full extent is not clear, one may draw certain inferences from the data available from various sources.

Most ubiquitous are undoubtedly the health services provided by *curanderos*, or traditional healers, in Guatemala's several thousand small villages, especially in the central highlands, which are inhabited almost wholly by pure-blooded Indians. Along with the *curandero*, who is usually male, is the *comadrona*, or midwife, who attends the great majority of Guatemalan childbirths.

The number of traditional healers can only be guessed. Of the nearly 6 million people in Guatemala, about 4.5 million live outside the metropolitan center. Assuming about one *curandero* for each 500 persons, one arrives at an estimate of 9,000 *curanderos*. Most of these, however, do not work fulltime at their healing activities, but make their living principally in agriculture or other pursuits. The same applies to village midwives, on whom there are more definite data. The law requires that midwives be registered in their municipality, and a 1975 survey of these registers yielded a count of about 16,000.[9] Considering that midwives probably work less regularly than *curanderos*, the estimate of 9,000 for the latter may not be very far off the mark. Even if one estimates that there are only 3,000 full-time-equivalent *curanderos*, the number would still exceed substantially the number of trained physicians in Guatemala.

While both healers and midwives are essentially part of the private health care sector, the charges made for their services are highly variable. They are often paid by barter, and the amount varies with the affluence of the patient and the severity of the case. As in conventional medicine, charges are also greater if the practitioner has acquired a reputation for many cures or good service.

Trained physicians are registered with the Colegio Médico de Guatemala, where in 1976 they numbered 2,560.[10] It is known, however, that this registry includes the names of many physicians not in the country, or not even alive. In 1973 there were 1,270 physicians employed by the two major public agencies, MOH and IGSS. Together these programs have increased their medical staffs by about 100 physicians per year; thus the 1976 total would be about 1,570, leaving a balance of about 1,000 other physicians on the registry. Assuming that about half of these other physicians are not actively working in Guatemala, the total of active physicians in 1976 would be about 2,000, or a physician-population ratio of about 1 to 3,000.

Virtually all Guatemalan physicians, whether employed by an organization or not, engage in private practice. Most of the approximately 600 doctors employed by IGSS are paid for four hours' work per day; the balance of their time is devoted mainly to private practice.[11] Of approximately 900 physicians attached to the MOH, most are theoretically employed full-time, but it is widely recognized that nearly all engage in a significant amount of private practice to supplement their modest salaries. A study by the Colegio Médico in 1972 found that only 8 percent of Guatemalan doctors (160 persons) were in private practice exclusively.[12] Thus, some 340 physicians would be engaged in the military services, in the university, in PVOs, or in other organized settings. Virtually all of the 92 percent of doctors with salaried employment, it must be emphasized, engage in some private practice, the income from which typically rises with the doctor's age.

Another component of the private sector in Guatemala is the private hospital. There are 59 of these, containing about 1,200 beds; more than two-thirds of them are in the capital city. Those in the peripheral departments are mainly for private maternity cases.

Guatemalan dentists devote more of their time to private practice than do physicians, since the development of systematically organized dental programs is very weak. In 1973, 115 dentists were engaged by MOH and IGSS; there were 376 dentists in the nation.[13] As in most developing countries, dental care is principally a luxury for a small, affluent minority.

Local pharmacies are still another component of the private health care sector, and a very important one at that. In Guatemala, as throughout Latin America, a great proportion of the population goes directly to pharmacies for medication to cope with their symptoms; since a doctor's prescription is seldom demanded, the patient thereby avoids a doctor bill. In addition, of course, thousands of drugs are prescribed by doctors. There are 224 pharmacists in Guatemala, but fewer than 20 are employed by the two major public programs. Thus, around 200 are engaged in retail pharmaceutical practice or work for pharmaceutical firms. In addition, in the smaller towns drugs are frequently dispensed at general stores, without benefit of pharmacist. Privately purchased medications play a substantial part in the health care system of Guatemala.

There are a few other providers of private health services in Guatemala—opticians, prosthetic shops, and so on. Even though most of the data offered above are approximations, it is clear that the private health care sector in Guatemala is substantial.

FUNCTIONING AND EFFICIENCY OF CURRENT HEALTH SERVICES

Having reviewed the general structure of the Guatemalan health care system and its several subsystems, I now examine its outputs and their approximate costs. The information available on services provided, or utilization rates, and the expenditures involved is fragmentary and incomplete; much of it, furthermore, is not disaggregated into categories that permit meaningful analysis. Nevertheless, some rough impressions may be gathered from the data available.

The operations of the Guatemalan health care system may be analyzed in terms of the types of services provided. It will then be possible to present estimates on the aggregate expenditures for all these services from different sources.

Traditional Medicine

Expenditures for traditional healing and village midwifery, as noted, are part of the private economic sector. Judging by the previous estimates of 9,000 *curanderos* and 16,000 *comadronas*, most of whom work only part-time, the volume of services must be relatively great. Undoubtedly some patients are helped, whether because of the healer's empirical knowledge or because of the patient's psychological responses attributable to the healer, but we do not know how much. Even though expenditures are relatively low—most services probably require payment in kind or cash payments of less than 1 *quetzal* (1 quetzal—$1U.S.) the efficiency in this subsystem is probably low. The actual rates of utilization and expenditures for traditional medicine in Guatemala, as well as the therapeutic results, warrant quantified study.

Ambulatory Medical Services

The principal data on ambulatory medical services are those produced by the MOH. These services are financed by general revenues of

Table 5.2   Consultations at Guatemala's Ministry of Health Facilities, by Type of Patient, 1975

Type of Patient	Health Centers	Health Posts	Total
Maternity	115,492	54,329	169,821
Children	205,849	122,841	328,690
General adults	470,389	674,972	1,145,361
All patients	791,730	852,142	1,643,872

the central government, which are derived from income taxes, import tariffs, excise taxes, and so on.

A report furnished by MOH for 1975 gives information on various ambulatory services provided by health centers and health posts in the nation's 24 health areas.[14] Combining figures from several tables in that report yields the data in table 5.2. These data combine consultations with physicians and consultations with paramedical personnel. The figures indicate, however, that the great majority of patients (about two-thirds) at the health centers are seen by physicians. At the health posts, as one would expect, services by paramedical personnel greatly predominate—about three-fourths of the total.

Recalling that in 1975 the MOH operated 82 health centers (both type A and type B) and 510 health posts, one may calculate the approximate volume of services per day provided by these basic ambulatory care facilities. Regarding the 82 health centers, the aggregate number of consultations of all types comes to 9,655 per center per year. Assuming, conservatively, 250 working days per year, this amounts to 38 consultations per day.

Similar calculations regarding the 510 health posts yield an average of 1,359 consultations per post per year. Assuming only 200 working days per year for the posts, since on many days the auxiliary health worker would be away in the community, leaving the post unattended, they would average 6.8 consultations per day.

In addition to providing maternal, pediatric, and general adult consultations, health centers and posts provide other services, such as immunizations, medications, certain laboratory tests, and so on. Nevertheless, one must conclude that these average numbers of patients served per day—38 by the health centers and 6.8 by the health posts—appear extremely low. Moreover, relating the grand total of 1,643,872 consultations to a national Guatemalan population of about 5.6 million in 1975, one derives an average of only about 0.30 consultation per person per year provided by MOH ambulatory care facilities.

These statistical calculations and estimates serve to confirm the observations reported by many physicians, both in the MOH and elsewhere. The consensus is that both the MOH health centers and health posts are greatly underutilized, in relation both to their staffing and to their general capacities. The problem is reported to be much more serious in the rural areas than in the national capital and the few other peripheral cities. Possible reasons for this and corrective actions that might be feasible require exploration.

Certain similar calculations may be offered regarding the ambulatory services provided in the IGSS program. In the metropolitan area, general medical care is offered to insured workers, along with maternity care for wives and general care for children up to the age of two years. The IGSS annual report for 1975 indicates a total of 475,698 consultations of all types provided to these persons. Because of the three components of this insured population (workers, mothers, and children), it is difficult to compute an aggregate average rate. For the primary workers, however, there was in 1975 a national total of 251,718 consultations of all types at an IGSS health station, polyclinic, or hospital outpatient department. This averages 0.91 ambulatory service per insured worker. While this rate is rather low compared to that in other Latin American social security programs, it is three times as high as the national average for ambulatory services in the MOH program (0.30).

The rate of ambulatory services provided by the IGSS program outside the national capital, where the benefits are limited to accident cases, is obviously much lower. In 1975, there were 107,494 consultations for trauma among the 271,392 insured workers in the nonmetropolitan areas. This amounts to a rate of 0.40 ambulatory contact per insured worker per year. These services were provided at 28 nonmetropolitan ambulatory care units, an average of 3,821 services per unit per year. Assuming 250 working days per year, the average output would amount to 15.3 trauma services per unit per day. Although much higher than the consultation output of the MOH health posts (6.8 per day), which are similarly staffed with one or two auxiliary personnel, the rate of service still appears very low. In an eight-hour working day, this would mean fewer than two patients seen per hour.

It may also be noted that, among all the trauma cases getting care, about two-thirds are reported to be work-related. Yet we know epidemiologically that, in general, nonwork accidents are more numerous than work-related accidents. One may infer, therefore, that in most non-work-related accident cases involving insured workers, workers are not even seeking medical care at IGSS facilities.

A third source of data on ambulatory services is the clinic program of the two Associations of Guatemalan Coffee Growers. The first such clinic, established in southeastern Guatemala, averages 617 consultations per month for a population of about 20,000 persons entitled to service. On an annual basis, this would yield about 0.37 consultation per person per year—again, apparently quite low. Calculated another way, this clinic is served by a full-time doctor plus two auxiliary nurses, who see about 29 patients per day (assuming 250 working days per year). If one assumes that half of these patients are seen by the nurses and half by the physician, in an eight-hour day the physician would see about two patients per hour—many fewer than is considered efficient in organized medical care programs.

Finally, one must recognize the output of private physicians. At present, only the crudest estimates may be offered. One may recall the earlier estimate of about 2,000 physicians in Guatemala in 1976 and the fact that about three-quarters of them are employed in some type of organized program, predominantly part-time. A conservative estimate would suggest that Guatemalan physicians on the whole average about three hours (some estimate four hours) of private practice per day, or about 6,000 medical hours per day in the aggregate. In private practice, physicians often work on weekends, holidays, and so on, so one may assume 300 working days per year, or a total of 1.8 million medical hours per year. Some physicians obviously are busier than others, but, blending estimates from several observers, one may assume that private physicians average three to four ambulatory cases per hour, or about 6 million consultations per year.

These cases are undoubtedly concentrated in the small (perhaps 5 to 10 percent) affluent fraction of the population, especially families in the capital city. On a national basis, nevertheless, private practice would contribute about one ambulatory service per person per year in the Guatemalan population of around 6 million. On the other hand, if we relate these privately financed services to a more realistic high- or moderate-income population base of 600,000 (10 percent of the national population), the rate would be ten ambulatory services per affluent person per year—a figure twice that of the United States (about five per person per year). In terms of equity, this estimate of ambulatory medical services for the most affluent section of the population may be compared with the rate of 0.30 furnished to the mass of the low-income population by the MOH programs—a ratio of 33 to 1.

Hospital Services

Data on hospitalization in Guatemala, like data on ambulatory care, are available from both the MOH and the IGSS programs. For purely private hospitals, one may make some estimates.

In the MOH hospitals, the ministry reports for 1973 a total of 154,878 admissions (or discharges), including both short-term general and other hospitals.[15] For a population in that year of some 5.5 million, the rate of hospitalization would come to about 28 per 1,000 population per year—very low in comparison with that of other Latin American countries. The average length of stay in the general hospitals (excluding long-term institutions) was 18 days, although in 1976 it was reported lowered to 14 days. While this figure represents long stays, it is not unusual for developing countries on all continents. Long average patient stays are associated with low ratios of hospital staff and with the poor general health of patients, which requires longer periods for recovery. Long stays also suggest that patients are hospitalized in a relatively advanced stage of their disease, when recovery takes more time.

The occupancy rate of MOH general hospitals in 1973 was also excessively high, reported at 102.5 percent. In other words, on the average day there were more patients occupying hospital beds than the hospital could properly accommodate. This fact is clearly related to the very low ratio of general hospital beds noted earlier (1.4 beds per 1,000 population).

Hospitalization experience in the IGSS programs is very different. The 2,098 beds in IGSS hospitals in 1973 include those throughout the country. Beds in the capital *departamento*, where general medical care is a benefit, numbered 1,257. For the 278,773 insured workers there, this would mean a ratio of 4.5 beds per 1,000 workers. Even allowing for the fact that wives of workers are entitled to maternity care and children under age two may receive general hospital and medical care, this bed supply is still far higher than that in the MOH program. Moreover, judging from the situation in social security hospitals of other countries of Latin America, the ratio of IGSS hospital personnel per bed is doubtless higher than the ratios reported for MOH hospitals.

Combining hospitalizations of both adult workers and children under two years, there were in 1975 14,042 patients admitted. Of these, 8,278 were adults, or a rate of 29 admissions per 1,000 insured workers per year. While this rate is almost identical with the MOH rate (28 admissions per 1,000 per year) for the entire country, the exclusion of maternity and child admissions—which are quite numerous in Guatemala nationally—means that for working adults alone the IGSS hospital admission rate must be substantially higher than that in MOH facilities. The average length of stay for general sickness in the IGSS hospitals is 11.6 days, much shorter than that in MOH hospitals. The occupancy levels are also lower than in the MOH hospitals, at

72.3 percent in the adult wards and 84.6 percent in the children's wards.

The above hospital utilization data apply to the IGSS program for general medical care. For the trauma program, which is nationwide, the facts are very different. Outside the capital area, the IGSS program maintains 841 beds, of which 510 are in its own relatively small hospitals, and 331 are under contract in MOH facilities but reserved for IGSS accident cases.[16] From the data provided by IGSS it is not possible to calculate the occupancy rate of these nonmetropolitan IGSS hospital facilities, but many observers state that it is usually very low. With admissions limited to trauma cases, there is a tendency to serve patients with even minor injuries and to keep them hospitalized much longer than necessary, merely to maximize the occupancy level. In 1975, there were 27,286 trauma patients admitted throughout Guatemala (including the capital and the surrounding *departamentos*). This constituted about one in five accidents receiving health care, the total number of such cases in 1975 being reported as 132,222.

It would appear, in summary, that the IGSS hospital program in the capital *departamento* is operating quite efficiently. The average length of stay of patients and the occupancy levels appear reasonable. Outside the metropolitan center there is evidently extravagance in the provision of hospital facilities that only serve accident cases.

Finally, one should note the 1,208 beds in 59 Guatemalan hospitals under other auspices, predominantly private. While there are no statistical data on these, it is apparent that their average size is only about 20 beds—much smaller than the 240-bed average in MOH facilities. In fact, if one considers separately the four principal private hospitals in the national capital, each with about 60 to 80 beds, the remainder must average under 17 beds each. The four principal metropolitan private hospitals are relatively well staffed and equipped, but they serve only the small fraction of affluent people who can afford the costs—about $20 per day for the basic room, board, and nursing care, plus additional charges for drugs, tests, operating room use, and so on. The smaller, private hospitals are less well staffed, less expensive, and largely devoted to maternity cases.

Pharmaceutical Services

Drugs and related pharmaceutical products are largely imported. Even when foreign corporations establish plants for drug packaging and distribution in a country like Guatemala, the raw chemicals from which most drugs are compounded are ordinarily imported. As a result, drugs are a relatively expensive component of health service in most Latin American countries. Moreover, direct purchase of drugs, without prescriptions, is very common; it is a presumably less costly form of relief from symptoms than consultation with a physician, and buying drugs is usually less bothersome than going to a hospital outpatient department or a health center.

In the health care subsystems of both the MOH and IGSS, drugs are included in the overall health services provided, both at ambulatory care facilities and in hospitals. Although data on the amounts of drugs so dispensed were not obtained from these agencies, it may be assumed that, being purchased in large quantities, they cost less than in retail pharmacy trade. Drug costs are, in any event, included within the overall figures for MOH and IGSS medical care programs reported later.

One frequently hears comments on the inefficiencies of drug dispensing by the MOH network of health centers and health posts. The policy evidently is to maintain a central supply depot in the national capital, and to dispense batches of drugs and supplies to all MOH facilities each month. The content of these shipments is evidently based on standard central lists, and the amounts are related to the population theoretically served by each local unit. Shipments are not based on any arrangement for periodic orders or requests submitted by each local health center or health post. As a result, one hears many accounts in Guatemala about inappropriate shipments—too little of one type of drug locally required or too much of another. Even when a local health center doctor or other health worker makes a specific request for certain drugs, supplies, or equipment, there are apparently long delays before they are received and frequent errors in the items sent. Somewhat similar inefficiencies are said to apply to non-metropolitan MOH hospitals. The resultant inadequate supply of locally needed drugs is blamed by many for the low utilization rates at most MOH ambulatory care units; patients who cannot be given the medications they need, it is claimed, are naturally disappointed and do not return. The whole reputation of the local health unit is then spoiled in the surrounding community.

In the IGSS program, proper drug availability is not as serious a problem, because the great bulk of drug usage occurs in the metropolitan center. In Guatemala, as in other Latin American countries, however, the drug problem in the social security program is principally abuse by patients. Since privately purchased drugs are relatively costly, some insured patients seek and obtain drugs that they do not take themselves but resell to noninsured patients, or even to local merchants. This practice, to the extent that it exists in Guatemala, is wasteful for IGSS and potentially harmful to both the insured patient and to the person who takes a drug without medical advice.

The most serious problems in pharmaceutical services, however, are in retail trade. As noted earlier, private purchase of drugs in retail pharmacies, or even in general stores, with or without medical prescription, is very frequent in Guatemala. Some idea of the extent of the problem is conveyed by the results of a marketing survey of 100 retail pharmacies conducted in 1976 by a Swiss firm.[17] The survey indicates that retail sales of drugs in Guatemala probably exceed $40 million (U.S.) per year. These sales do not include expenditures for drugs by the MOH, the IGSS, or other organized health care subsystems, which generally do not purchase drugs from retail pharmacies. The dimensions of this component of the total Guatemalan health care system will be evident below.

Preventive Services

There is worldwide consensus that prevention should be emphasized in all health care systems. In Guatemala, however, as elsewhere, the trend over the last 50 years or so has been toward proportionately greater expenditures on hospital services and technology for diagnosis and treatment of disease. There is difficulty, of course, in defining the exact scope of preventive service and in drawing a clear line between prevention and treatment. An immunization is unquestionably a preventive procedure, but what about a medical examination made in response to a symptom, during which some other, unsuspected disease is detected at an early stage? Much ordinary ambulatory health care of this sort is also preventive. Prevention also depends on many factors not usually considered "health services," such as aspects of environmental control (for example, motor vehicle safety regulations), nutritional practices, habits of life, housing, and working conditions.

In the MOH program, of course, prevention is expected to receive special emphasis. The 1976 expenditures of the ministry, in fact, identify 12.3 percent (about $4.9 million out of $39.9 million) for preventive services. Exactly what this proportion means is not clear, and it may be too low in light of the comments above. The expenditure statement of the IGSS program, on the other hand, does not identify funds for prevention, but many of its ambulatory services, especially to mothers and children, are clearly preventive in purpose.

The old adage that an ounce of prevention is worth a pound of cure is doubtless true for most infectious diseases and for malnutrition, both of which abound in Guatemala. One must, nevertheless, not jump to the conclusion that greater expenditures for prevention, or even for the prompt ambulatory care of disease to prevent its advance, will necessarily reduce the need for expenditures on medical treatment. The fact is that prevention, which is most effective in the younger years of life and can substantially increase life expectancy, keeps people alive so that they may later acquire diseases that demand treatment. In the more highly developed countries, where prevention of infectious diseases and malnutrition has been quite effective, the expenditures for medical care have not declined. Instead, they have risen absolutely and relatively, both to overall health care costs, and to total costs of living.

The value of greater emphasis on preventive services, therefore, must be calculated on the basis of their effects in extending the length and the quality of life, not on the hope of financial savings from the provision of less medical care.

These comments on preventive services also apply to other subsystems of health care in Guatemala—the voluntary health organizations, the private medical and dental sectors, and so on. The *Bienestar Social* program in the Office of the President, which had a budget of $4.3 million in 1976, is almost entirely devoted to preventive services for mothers and children.

Administrative Functions

Administrative functions, and their costs, are difficult to define. To some extent, every organized or even individual setting for health care involves administration, as well as the direct provision of services. The 1976 financial statements of the two principal governmental health agencies of Guatemala specifically identify certain expenditures as administrative, but the lack of such identification in other components of the health care system should not lead one to believe that corresponding administrative expenses do not exist.

The MOH accounts for 1976 specify a cost of $7,742,300, or 19.4 percent of the total, for administration. Similarly, the IGSS 1976 accounting specifies $7,886,100, or 18.5 percent, for administration. These proportions undoubtedly seem high in relation to those of comprehensive medical care programs, such as the Kaiser-Permanente Health Services in California, which are reported to devote less than 10 percent of their income to administrative functions. Without knowing exactly how these different figures are derived, such comparisons may not be justified; it is likely, however, that government agencies—in Guatemala or elsewhere—would be inclined to understate, rather than overstate, their administrative expenditures.

In the discussion of PVOs providing health services, it was noted that about 150 such entities exist. Many or most of these raise funds through campaigns for charitable donations, which invariably entail significant administrative expenses. Moreover, the very existence of so many different and typically small organizations, each with its own administrative tasks, entails significant overhead expenses, which could be reduced by coordinating or consolidating efforts. Substantial administrative expenses are also hidden in the large expenditures for privately purchased drugs. A U. S. Senate investigation of the major pharmaceutical companies in the 1960's disclosed that 26 percent of the wholesale price of drugs was attributable to advertising and other marketing costs, which are only one element in administration. To a lesser extent, but nevertheless a part of all private medical, dental, and hospital care, there is administrative overhead.

In general, consolidation of multiple health functions achieves economies of scale in administrative expenses. While this may appear most obvious for the nearly 20 percent of total expenditures going to administration in the major MOH and IGSS programs, it is doubtless also applicable in some degree to most other components of pluralistic health care systems.

Estimated Aggregate Expenditures

Before considering ways to improve the efficiency of the Guatemalan health care system, it would be helpful to attempt to summarize the costs of its several components and to observe the relative contributions of each. This is most practical in terms of the subsystem sponsorships reviewed above, particularly in light of some of the comments on their functioning and efficiency. Much of the data for this summary are derived from the USAID Robertson report;[17] for the missing components, estimates are based on information or inferences from other sources.

The basic tabulation is offered in table 5.3. Each item is numbered to permit explanation of how the expenditure has been estimated.

1. The 1976 MOH expenditures are reported as $39.9 million. Of this amount, however, 12.3 percent was for transfer payments to the social security program, on behalf of all governmental employees.

   (MOH acts as a conduit for the contributions of all central government agencies.) This proportion of MOH expenditures must be subtracted in order to avoid counting it twice; $34.98 million remain.

2. The IGSS expenditures for 1976 were reported as $42,637,000. Of this amount, however, 25.7 percent was referrable to cash disability benefits. Subtracting this proportion

Table 5.3   Estimated Expenditures for Health Services in Guatemala, 1975 or 1976

Agency or Health Care Component	Expenditure ($U.S.)	Percent
Public		
1. Ministry of Health (adjusted)	34,980,000	
2. Social Security-IGSS (adjusted)	31,677,000	
3. Presidency (*Bienestar Social*)	4,305,000	
4. Municipal health expenditures	1,000,000	
Total public	(71,962,000)	47.5
Private		
5. Voluntary organizations	4,500,000	
6. Drug purchases	40,000,000	
7. Physician's care	24,000,000	
8. Hospitals	5,400,000	
9. Dental care	4,500,000	
10. Private enterprise and miscellaneous	1,000,000	
Total private	(79,400,000)	52.5
Grand total	151,362,000	100.0

leaves adjusted expenditures for medical purposes of $31,677,000.

3. This expenditure by the *Bienestar Social* program for maternal and child health services is given in the Robertson report.

4. This estimate of $1 million spent by the municipalities is somewhat arbitrary, but one can be confident that the amount is relatively small.

5. The figure of $4.5 million for PVO health-related activities is estimated by Keaty and Keaty in their recent USAID study of these 150 private organizations.[6]

6. The estimated $40 million for private drug purchases has been derived from the Swiss marketing study of 100 community pharmacies. Robertson considers this figure more likely to be an underestimation than an overestimation.

7. The estimated expenditure of $21 million on care from private physicians has been derived from two estimates, which were arrived at by different methods. One method was to combine the estimates of two knowledgeable physicians about the average monthly gross income of sets of Guatemalan doctors in four different brackets of earnings. This method yielded a figure of $25.2 million. The second method was based on the estimate offered earlier that private physicians give 6 million

ambulatory consultations per year; at an average of $3 each (to be conservative) this would yield total payments of $18 million for ambulatory medical service. In addition, the supply of about 1,200 private hospital beds—assuming an occupancy rate of 300 days per bed per year (about 82 percent) with an average stay of six days—would yield roughly 60,000 private inpatient cases per year. At a conservative average of $50 per case, this would yield gross medical income of $6 million. Added to the estimated earnings for ambulatory care, the sum is $24 million—remarkably close to the estimate of $25.2 million derived by the first method. The lower figure in the table ($24 million) is used simply in the interests of conservatism.

8. The figure of $5.4 million for private hospital care is derived from an estimate of 360,000 days of care in the 1,208 private hospital beds, at an overall charge of $15 per day. In the larger metropolitan private hospitals, daily charges are well over $20, but in the many smaller, maternity-focused hospitals the charges are less, leading to the estimated average of $15 per patient-day.

9. Private dental costs are based on the official registry of 376 dentists in Guatemala and an estimate from two observers that their average private gross earnings are $1,000 per month, yielding an annual figure of $4.5 million.

10. Finally, the estimate of $1 million spent by private enterprises for medical care and for miscellaneous other purposes (eyeglasses, prosthetic appliances and so on) is somewhat arbitrary, but conservative in the light of deficient information.

Altogether, this analytical exercise yields an estimated expenditure for health purposes in Guatemala of about $151,362,000 in 1976. No allowance has been made for traditional healing, which, while relatively inexpensive, would doubtless raise the private sector figure higher if it were included. Nor have the health care expenditures for the military forces or police been considered in the public sector. The expenses of constructing water and sewerage systems have also been omitted because they are only indirectly related to health, and the university training of health personnel is not counted because it has customarily been attributed to the education sector.

Of the total, somewhat over half is found to be in the private sector and therefore less amenable to planning than the smaller share in the public sector. It is important to recognize, furthermore, that

MOH expenditures account for only 23.1 percent of the total. Thus, if a substantial improvement is to be achieved in the efficiency of Guatemalan health services, attention must be given to far more than the performance of the MOH program.

Exploration of the basic causes of the manifest inefficiencies in Guatemalan health services were beyond the scope of this 1977 investigation. The deficiencies undoubtedly reflect, however, the low priority accorded to the health sector in national government planning and policy. The salaries paid to physicians and other health personnel in MOH facilities are low, leading to weak motivation of these personnel. Funding of drugs and other supplies is inadequate, so that health centers and posts are frequently faced with shortages of key items. As a result, people bypass the health posts and centers, going directly to the better staffed hospitals, which are therefore crowded both in their outpatient and inpatient departments—yielding perfunctory care. It is small wonder, therefore, that the governmental health services as a whole account for less than half of health expenditures in the Guatemalan economy, while the private sector, with its many inequities, absorbs more than half. Improvement undoubtedly will require substantial strengthening of the public sector in health service, as well as coordination of its several components.

NOTES

1. World Health Organization, "Guatemala," in *Fifth Report of the World Health Situation* (Geneva, 1975), 106–8.
2. Ministerio de Salud Pública y Asistencia Social, *Proyecto: Aumento de Cobertura de Servicios de Salud, Red de Servicios Por Areas de Salud* (Guatemala City, 1975), cuadro 24.
3. National Economic Planning Council, unpublished data, 1976.
4. Ministerio de Salud Pública y Asistencia Social, *República de Guatemala Recursos Humanos y Distribución de Camas en Instituciones de Salud Pública* (Guatemala City, 1975), 166–67.
5. Instituto Guatemalteco de Seguridad Social, *Informe Anual de Labores 1975* (Guatemala City, 1976).
6. C. A. Keaty and G. A. Keaty, "A Study of Private Voluntary Organizations in Guatemala," U.S. Agency for International Development, May 1977.
7. W. Ascoli of Guatemala City, personal communication.
8. G. D. Brown, *Extension of Health Services to Farm Workers in Guatemala*, (Washington, D.C.: U.S. Agency for International Development, 1977).
9. P. Harrison, "Maternal-Child Health Study," U.S. Agency for International Development, May 1977.
10. A. Viau, personal communication.
11. J. Aguja, Director of Medical Services, IGSS, personal communication.

12. Colegio de Médicos y Cirujanos de Guatemala, *La Expectaria de Quehacer Médico Guatemalteco* (Guatemala City, 1972).
13. H. Figueroa of the National Economic Planning Council, personal communication.
14. Dirección General de Servicios de Salud, *Memoria Anual de Actividades de Areas de Salud 1975* (Guatemala City, 1976).
15. República de Guatemala, Ministerio de Salud Pública y Asistencia Social, *Diagnóstico de la Situación de Salud a 1973* (Guatemala City, 1974).
16. Derived from data in M. I. Roemer and A. Ormosa, *Health Service Coordination in Guatemala* (Washington, D.C.: American Public Health Association and U.S. Agency for International Development, 1975).
17. R. L. Robertson et al., "Financing the Health Sector of Guatemala," U.S. Agency for International Development, June 1977, 13–14.

6

Planning Primary Health Care
in Barbados

*Barbados is an attractive island nation in the eastern Carib-
bean Sea. In 1978 it undertook to launch a national health
service, in which every resident would be entitled to complete
health care. The first phase would provide primary health
care for everyone, and this chapter describes the process of
planning for attaining that objective.*

One of the many former colonies emancipated in recent years is
the Caribbean island of Barbados. After three centuries under British
rule, Barbados became a sovereign nation in 1966. In 1976, national
elections brought to power the Barbados Labor Party, which, in its
campaign, called for establishment of a national health service (NHS).
Even though the population of this small island was only about
260,000, setting up a program in which everyone would receive comprehensive health care required a great deal of careful planning.

With a grant from the Inter-American Development Bank, Barbados engaged Kaiser Foundation International to carry out this planning, particularly the first phase, which was to develop a system
making primary health care available to everyone.

Based on a field study done in 1979 as a consultant for Kaiser Foundation International
and under the sponsorship of the Inter-American Development Bank.

EXISTING HEALTH STRUCTURE

Like so many other newly independent countries, Barbados started with the heritage from its colonial period. As a relatively favored colony, with an economy built on sugar production and tourism, this heritage was not insignificant. The level of education of the people was remarkably high, with close to 100 percent literacy. Although the population is overwhelmingly black—descended from former slaves from Africa—health resources had been developed far more than in any African colony. Shortly before emancipation, an impressive new general hospital of 534 beds, named after Queen Elizabeth, had been constructed. Some 200 physicians (including those in training at the hospital) served the population—a ratio of 1 doctor to 1,300 people. In 6 of the 11 parishes into which the island was divided, there were small district hospitals, which cared for aged and chronically ill patients; these hospitals had a total of 818 beds.

The Barbadian health care system could be described in terms of the classical pyramidal model of primary, secondary, and tertiary medical care. At the base of the pyramid were several components of primary care which, as the focus of this account, will be analyzed below. Secondary care included ambulatory specialist services in the scheduled outpatient clinics of the Queen Elizabeth Hospital (QEH). There were also many specialists in private practice, principally the salaried hospital consultants who were free to practice in their private quarters after their hospital hours. The long-term patient care available in the district hospitals could also be regarded as part of secondary services. Tertiary care was available on the inpatient wards of QEH.

Based on long tradition, almost all services at QEH were without charge. Except for a small number of private beds, this applied to both inpatient and outpatient care. Since the island is only 21 miles long and travel time to the hospital from any point is seldom more than an hour, much of the day-to-day primary care for minor illness was provided by the casualty service of the QEH outpatient department. The full range of sources for primary care requires greater elaboration.

THE SPECTRUM OF PRIMARY HEALTH CARE

The major source of primary care in Barbados was a complement of some 52 physicians in private general practice. Their fees were modest, and most of them were fairly busy. These doctors could not easily serve as continuous or permanent sources of primary care, however, because of the several other channels for such care open to all or most of their patients.

Much of the QEH casualty service's care was for minor conditions. In addition, virtually all the privately practicing specialists saw many patients whose conditions were quite appropriate for the attention of a general practitioner (GP). Another primary care resource was a network of 11 clinics for indigent patients, located at or near the district hospitals. These were staffed by the private GPs for a few hours each week.

Finally, an important component of primary care was the preventive service offered at six public health centers located around the island. Staffed by Ministry of Health physicians, nurses, and other health personnel, these units offered traditional, preventively oriented maternal and child health services, venereal disease and tuberculosis control services, health education, and so on. The record of child immunizations was especially good. Sanitary inspections were done by personnel based at the health centers.

The challenge for planning an effective system of primary health care, covering everyone, was quite clear. The resources previously offering primary care through five separate channels had to be mobilized and integrated. The crucial question was whether the existing resources, if properly organized, were capable of meeting the needs of all 260,000 Barbadian people? If so, how much would it cost and how could the money be raised?

Health planning is often defined as a process of identifying problems and then formulating various options for their solution. The task in Barbados, however, was easier, insofar as the government had decided in advance that, for effective primary care, it wished to emulate the British pattern of general practice, with a panel of patients linked (by their own choice) to each GP. The primary care physician would be paid for integrated treatment and preventive services by monthly capitation allowances. The planning question could be reduced, therefore, to a simpler form: How many GPs would be needed to provide the quantity of primary care that one could expect would be demanded? The cost, in turn, would depend on the average gross income that a GP in Barbados should probably earn. The answers to these questions required some quantification of health care utilization and incomes from medical practice.

PAST PRIMARY CARE UTILIZATION AND A FORECAST

Anticipating NHS developments, a few farsighted GPs in Barbados had conducted a study of ten private general practices over a 12-

month period in 1977–78. Adjusting for certain characteristics of their sample, and applying the findings to all GPs on the island, one could estimate that in a recent year all Barbados GPs had provided a total of 278,000 patient visits, or attendances. Data on the other four channels of primary care utilization were available from different sources.

The QEH outpatient department had records of patient attendances for various purposes. Leaving aside the services of scheduled specialty clinics, patient visits essentially for primary care of nonurgent conditions numbered 55,000 during a recent year. Records of the 11 district clinics showed 23,000 visits from indigent patients in 1978. For preventive purposes, the six public health centers gave 84,000 patient services in the last year of record. Most difficult to determine was the volume of primary care attendances in the private practices of specialists. Based on discussions with several doctors, a figure of 33,000 was estimated.

The aggregate of primary care services from all five sources, therefore, came to 473,000. An estimated 5 percent of these, however, was believed to be for the care of tourists, so the total services to Barbadian citizens amounted to about 450,000. The population in 1977 was 254,000, so there were an average of 1.77 primary care attendances per person per year. This rate was rounded off to 1.8 attendances because it was assumed that there was some underreporting.

One could anticipate that, under conditions of freely accessible primary health care for everyone, utilization of medical services would increase: the question was, How much? Under the proposed capitation pattern of remuneration (in contrast to fee-for-service), much of the incentive for physicians to maximize repeat patient visits would be altered. Various studies in the United States and Canada—where utilization of ambulatory care under changing organizational schemes had been quantified—showed that, under conditions similar to the sequence planned for Barbados, utilization rates rose, but not very rapidly. One important study in Montreal, Canada, showed that, after statutory health insurance was initiated, the rate of medical attendances for different income groups shifted (the poor got more care and the affluent got slightly less) but the overall rate remained virtually the same.

It was hypothesized, therefore, that, in the first year of the Barbadian NHS, the rate of attendances for primary care would rise by no more than about 25 percent. Hence the previous aggregate utilization rate for primary care of 1.8 attendances per person per year would increase to 2.25. For a population of 260,000 in 1980, this would mean 525,000 patient-doctor encounters. How much medical manpower would this require?

To answer this question, one had to estimate the average duration of a general physician visit in Barbados. Three GPs were interviewed, and it was concluded that, in an average practice, a GP saw four to five patients per hour. It was further assumed that, under Barbadian conditions, the average practitioner would see patients for 40 hours per week and would work for about 48 weeks per year. This meant that for each GP in Barbados between 7,680 and 9,600 attendances could be provided in a year. Averaging these two figures, the required number of attendances would be 8,640 per GP per year. Precisely how should these ambulatory services be provided?

PRIMARY CARE TEAMS

Keeping in mind that the pattern of health care delivery being planned would combine therapeutic and preventive services, and that efficient use should be made of the physician's time, it was realized that many medical functions did not require a highly trained practitioner. Such activities as injections, observation of normal babies, and blood pressure and temperature determinations could be done perfectly well by a registered nurse under medical supervision. It was planned, therefore, that each GP should serve as the head of a primary care team, the other members of which would include a nurse for clinical functions, a clerk-receptionist, and a nurse for home visits and other community outreach functions.

With such primary care teams, the physician would not be obligated to spend the full 40 hours seeing patients each week. Several hours could be spent—as normally expected in medical practice—in reading medical literature, writing patient records, doing some travel to patient homes, and so on. The 40-hour week for 48 weeks per year (1,920 hours) would, in effect, represent the available time of each primary care team.

Accordingly, how many primary care teams would be required to meet the expected demand? The estimate of 8,640 patient attendances per doctor (or team) meant that the total demand of 585,000 attendances in the country would necessitate 67.7 primary care teams. Could this number of health personnel be expected by 1980? To answer this question, it was necessary to take stock of the medical and allied health personnel available in Barbados.

HEALTH MANPOWER RESOURCES

An official registry of all physicians is maintained in the Barbados Ministry of Health. Since the island is small, the registration officer or other officials had some information about virtually all doctors on the list. As of February 1979, a name-by-name review led to identification of 206 registered physicians: active GPs 52; in-hospital consultants (specialists), 36; specialists outside the hospital, 11; public health physicians, 12; young doctors in training at QEH, 78; and physicians who were retired or abroad, 17.

With the pattern of integrated primary care contemplated and the assurance of agreeable conditions for medical practice, certain assumptions could be made about the future availability of GPs. All of the 52 active practitioners could be expected to enter the NHS. Of the 11 out-of-hospital specialists (including gynecologists and internists), it was estimated that three would enter NHS general practice. Of the 12 public health doctors, it was estimated that three—engaged then in essentially clinical (not administrative) work—would become GPs. It was forecast that the new program would attract about 12 of the 78 interns and residents at QEH into general practice. This yielded an estimated total of 70 GPs. If this total were not achieved, the remaining GPs could be taken from the waiting list of GPs seeking to immigrate to Barbados.

Hence, it was concluded that the estimated 67.7 GPs needed to staff primary care teams could be met by the supply of doctors in Barbados in 1980.

It was then necessary to determine how many of the other personnel needed for the primary care teams were available. The registry of nurses in the Ministry of Health contained 438 names, and many of these nurses were actually seeking employment; 67 to 70 nurses were considered easily available to do clinical work in the primary care teams. The supply of trained public health nurses, however, was only 35; another 32 nurses would have to be trained for community health work in the 67 primary care teams. A telephone survey of the 52 active general practices showed that 21 medical clerk-receptionists were currently working. An additional 46 or so could be acquired and trained quite easily from Barbados high school graduates.

Thus it was realistic to expect that the health manpower requirements of all 67 to 70 primary care teams could be met in 1980 and subsequent years. If 100 percent of the population took advantage of the NHS, each primary care team would, on the average, serve about 3,700 persons (men, women, and children). Since not everyone would be likely to enroll immediately, this average in 1980 might be 3,500.

ADMINISTRATIVE REQUIREMENTS

A health care system involving some 70 primary care teams with a panel of 3,500 persons for each would not operate automatically.

Administrative management would be needed. The organizational and administrative requirements would involve such tasks as:

— Assuring physical facilities for the 70 primary care teams

— Arranging for recruitment of allied health personnel to work agreeably with the 70 GPs

— Maintaining the list of members on each team's panel, in order to assure availability of health care and proper remuneration of the health personnel

— Assuring equipment at each site for simple laboratory tests, refrigeration of materials for immunization, maintenance of records, and so on

— Supervising or consulting with the teams to assure that proper preventive services (formerly offered at public health centers) are offered regularly

— Arranging for the education of the people in the general operations of the NHS

— Making appropriate payments to each primary care team

— Offering a channel to receive and act upon any complaints from either patients or providers

— Carrying out other administrative duties

To carry out these functions, it was proposed that Barbados should be divided into three regions, averaging 85,000 persons each. A regional administrative staff would consist of the personnel needed not only to monitor the services of 20 to 25 primary care teams, but also to conduct health education, continue with environmental sanitation work, assure the maintenance of both medical and administrative records, and so on. This administrative staff would include, therefore, a public health administrative director, a senior public health nurse, a health educator, clerical personnel, and others.

Certain activities to promote quality would also have to be carried out. These would include operation of programs of continuing education for physicians and other personnel, assuring the patient's right to change affiliations with a team if dissatisfied, distribution of proper laboratory and related supplies, and so on. Financial processes would include management of certain incentive payments to primary care teams, such as capitation supplements for (1) improved physical premises, (2) aged or other high-risk members on a panel, (3) grouping of two or three primary care teams in urban health centers (or polyclinics), and (4) recognition of seniority and merit.

COST ESTIMATES

The next planning question, of course, was how much would this entire program cost? The lion's share of costs would be the capitation and other payments to the 70 primary care teams; additional outlays would be necessary, however, for the performance of laboratory tests, for regional administration, for start-up activities, and so on.

Among the operating costs of primary care teams, the salaries to be paid to nurses and other personnel were well known (on the basis of previous customs), and their aggregate amount could be easily estimated. The capitation payments to be offered to physicians presented a more difficult problem.

On the basis of other countries' experience in establishing national health insurance programs, it was decided that winning the cooperation of members of the medical profession would require assurance that their annual incomes would be equivalent to or higher than previous levels. How could these levels be determined? Through discussions with various physicians, both in private practice and in public service, estimates were made of the range and probable average of gross GP incomes (derived, of course, from professional work). Then the figures were increased by 25 percent, because doctors would be working harder under the NHS than previously, and because general inflation had to be taken into account. The resulting figures were then tested at a meeting with the medical association.

When average annual GP income estimates were finalized, these were divided by the average panel size of 3,500 to derive the basic capitation amount. This came to about B $1.70 per panel member per month ($1.00 Barbadian equals $.50 U.S.). Calculations could then be made of incentive supplements for various purposes. It was decided that these monthly payments should cover the cost of medical practice overhead (rentals or equivalent, public utilities, supplies), but not the salaries of other primary care team personnel. The latter would be paid directly by the governmental authority, in order to assure that every primary care team included the necessary and appropriate staff. The traveling expenses of community health nurses would also be covered directly by the regional administrative offices.

To give a sense of proportion about the entire program, the estimated total cost for the first year of operation came to approximately B $9 million. This total consisted of: B$4.4 million in basic capitation payments to GPs; B$800,000 in incentive payments; B$2 million for nurses and allied personnel; B$750,000 for regional administration; B$350,000 in start-up costs; and B$700,000 for other costs.

These outlays would not be entirely new; instead, they would partially replace previous Ministry of Health expenditures for the provision of preventive services and certain other functions to be performed by the new primary care teams. Altogether, the savings involved would amount to about B$3 million—leaving a balance of B$6 million to be raised for new public expenditures in the NHS.

The new *public* expenditures would not constitute totally new economic burdens for the Barbadian people: previous *personal* expenditures on private GP services had amounted to an estimated B$4.5 million. This amount would essentially be transferred from private to public sector spending. Only the net balance of B$1.5 million would constitute totally new health expenditures for supporting the primary care phase of the national health service.

SOURCE OF FUNDS

How would the overall costs of B$9 million for primary health care be raised? In general, national health *service,* as distinguished from national health *insurance,* implies that financial support is derived nearly or entirely from general government revenues. (Government support of the British national health service has been some 85 percent.) In Barbados, however, the government had made a policy decision that the bulk of NHS costs would not be derived from general public revenues.

The obvious alternative was to derive funds from a social insurance system, principally for old-age pensions, that had been in operation since Barbados' independence in 1966. This program covered an estimated 80,000 to 90,000 workers. There was no information in the insurance files, however, to indicate the number of dependents of each covered worker. If major funding were to be derived from an increase in the social insurance contributions (really, earmarked taxes), then one would have to know the number of dependents to be covered by the contributions collected from each primary worker and his or her employer.

To acquire this information, a special questionnaire was sent to a random sample of 1,000 workers from the old-age insurance files. Some 400 questionnaires were returned, and these indicated that each worker had an additional 1.35 dependents in the household. A small sample of the nonrespondents was then selected for household interviews, and it was discovered that these persons usually had more than 1.35 dependents. It seemed reasonable, therefore, to raise the estimate of dependents to 1.50 per covered worker.

On the basis of 85,000 workers in the old-age insurance program, this would mean a total of 127,500 dependents and an overall coverage of 212,500 persons. This constituted 82 percent of the Barbadian population. Hence, it was proposed that the social insurance tax be elevated by the amount necessary to yield 82 percent of the B$9 million NHS cost, or B$7.38 million.

Taxable wages in Barbados—the basis of contributions to the old-age pension fund—were about B$460 million. Hence, to yield the required B$7.38 million, the established insurance tax would have to be raised by 1.6 percent. Dividing that equally between worker and employer would require additional contributions from each of 0.8 percent. Such an increase—in return for the primary care benefits and the elimination of out-of-pocket expenditures—was considered politically acceptable by the prime minister and his cabinet.

The balance of 18 percent of NHS costs, or B$1.62 million, would then be drawn from general revenues. This figure, in fact, was less than the B$3 million that would be saved from the Ministry of Health budget (because preventive and other services by NHS primary care teams would take the place of public health centers). With the net saving of B$1.38 million, the ministry could expand its services in other fields, such as environmental sanitation, long-term care of patients in the district hospitals, or mental health.

Thus, the planning of the primary care phase of the Barbados NHS concluded: (1) health manpower and other resources would be adequate to meet the anticipated demands for service; (2) the net additional costs for the proposed NHS primary care delivery system, taking into account the saving of previous public sector expenditures and private out-of-pocket spending, would be surprisingly small; and (3) more than four-fifths of the costs of primary care could be derived from a small incremental contribution to the established old-age insurance system, with the balance coming from the regular budget of the Barbados Ministry of Health.

RAMIFICATIONS AND SEQUELS

The above planning proposals would presumably yield an improved system of integrated primary health care for the entire population of Barbados. Further actions would be needed, however, if a *comprehensive* NHS were to be achieved. These would require further planning and expenditures.

General hospital care was already available for nearly everyone in Barbados at government expense. For tourists or affluent patients who preferred care in a private setting, there were a small number of private beds in QEH, as well as in two private facilities (with a total of 123 beds in the three). These facilities would continue to operate.

If specialist services were to be included in the NHS, additional arrangements and expenditures would be necessary. For inpatient care, a full range of specialists (plus interns and residents) was already on salary at the QEH. To reduce the inequities associated with private specialty practice and fee-for-service remuneration, however, the hospital-based specialists would have to be paid higher salaries to assure their full-time dedication to the NHS. If some specialty service were to be covered in private offices, this could conceivably be included as a NHS benefit, with some copayment required from the patient.

Further planning would be necessary for coverage of prescribed drugs. As imported products, drugs tend to be quite expensive in Barbados. Special strategies would be required to achieve bulk purchasing of certain essential drugs, emphasis on generic compounds, and efficient methods of distribution. If private pharmacies were to play a continuing role, a negotiated schedule of prescription prices would have to be developed.

To include dental care in NHS, additional manpower would be required. The small supply of professional dentists in Barbados could not possibly meet the demand, and a training program for New Zealand–type dental nurses would have to be launched. Fluoridation of the water supply would also be advisable for prevention of dental caries. The NHS benefits for corrective eyeglasses and other prosthetic appliances would also require further planning.

Finally, to assure good rehabilitative service to long-term patients, including the mentally ill and retarded, additional actions would be required. The care of such patients was already under public auspices, through facilities of the Ministry of Health. Besides the six district hospitals mentioned, there is also a large, 658-bed mental institution. Upgrading the physical plant of these facilities and improving their staffing would naturally require further public expenditures. Such investments, however, would come at a later stage of the NHS, depending on general economic conditions in Barbados.

The planning of the primary care phase of the Barbadian NHS was finished in early 1979. As one would expect, the preliminary announcement of the plan attracted clear support from labor unions and other consumer organizations and opposition from professional groups.

In the medical profession, some GPs supported the plan enthusiastically, since it would strengthen their role as primary care providers and would also assure them of good incomes. Other GPs, however, opposed the plan because they feared they would lose their "freedom" under a system regulated by government.

Most of the specialists opposed the plan from the outset. Since every Barbadian would become entitled to general care from a primary care team, many of the patients formerly consulting specialists privately would switch to GPs. Specialists would be dependent mainly on GPs for referral of patients. A compensatory increase in their salaries for hospital-based work would help, but the lucrative opportunities of private office practice would decline.

A third source of opposition was certain of the senior medical personnel in the Ministry of Health itself. These officials, who had worked for years building up the maternal and child health program (including immunizations) in a network of public health centers (three major ones and six satellite units), viewed the plan with apprehension. They feared that the GPs in the primary care teams could not be trusted to carry out the preventive program, and they were not sure that the community nurses would work as conscientiously in the primary care teams as they had done under direct supervision of the ministry.

In the light of this controversy, the government decided in late 1979 to delay NHS implementation, which had been planned for 1980. In 1981 there would be another general election, and the governing Barbados Labor party did not wish to jeopardize its reelection by contention around the issue of "socialized medicine". The party remained committed to the NHS goal, however, and it won the 1981 election. In 1982, it began implementation of the primary care phase. Because of economic reverses (caused by a decline in tourism), however, the NHS was initiated with coverage only of Barbadian citizens over 65 years of age. It is planned that other age groups will be covered later.

7

The Structure of Health Services in Thailand

The developing countries of Asia vary greatly in their history, size, political policy, culture, and other attributes. Unlike Latin America or Africa, there is no "typical" Asian country. Thailand, with a per capita GNP of $420 (U.S.) in 1977 is not as poor as India ($150) or as economically developed as Malaysia ($930). Its political ideology is strongly oriented toward laissez-faire capitalism, and this is reflected in the pluralism of its health care system.

The health care system of Thailand, like that of virtually all countries, consists of many subsystems. Depending on one's focus of interest, one can define these subsystems in several different ways.[1]

HEALTH SERVICE SYSTEM

From the viewpoint of public health or social action, one can analyze the system according to (1) its individual, or free market, components and (2) its organized programs. A similar form of analysis can delineate the health care system into (1) the private sector and (2) the public, or governmental, sector. With respect to historical develop-

This chapter is an adapted and substantially revised version of chapter 1 in *The Health Care System of Thailand* (New Delhi: World Health Organization, Regional Office for South-East Asia, 1981), that was based on field work while a consultant for the World Health Organization in 1978, advising the faculty of public health at Mahidol University in Bangkok.

ments, the system may be analyzed according to subsystems of (1) traditional healing and (2) modern health care.

Considering the objectives of health services, the system components can be classified as (1) therapeutic or curative and (2) preventive. Geographically, the system may be divided into (1) urban and (2) rural subsystems. There are doubtless other ways in which the complex health care system may be analyzed.

These subsystems may be further analyzed into sub-subsystems. Thus, traditional healing may be of several different types; likewise, modern health service may be analyzed according to (1) ambulatory care, (2) hospital or institutional care, (3) medications or drugs, and (4) various other technical components.

My focus in this analysis is on the administration, or management, of the health care system for the purpose of improving its impact on the health of the population. An appropriate approach, therefore, is an analysis of its *organized* components. I will then consider the other aspects of the system—private and public sectors, traditional and modern service and so on—which may shed light on its overall structure and functions.

SOCIOPOLITICAL SETTING

Thailand is one of the few nations of Southeast Asia that has never been a colony. It was an absolute monarchy from its origins in the seventh century until 1932. In 1932, the king accepted a constitutional and representative form of government.[2] In 1957, central power was seized by a military group. Since then, except for short periods in 1974 and again in 1976, the ruling government of Thailand has been composed essentially of high military officers.[3]

In 1977, the national population was estimated at more than 44 million people living in four geographically definable regions, as shown in table 7.1.

The nation is divided into 71 provinces, one of which constitutes the national capital, Bangkok. Within the provinces are 124 municipalities, which carry certain local governmental responsibilities. The national capital has special status under the Bangkok Metropolitan Authority. Counting it and all 124 municipalities as urban, one finds the population to be about 15 percent urban and 85 percent rural. In the rural areas, there are about 600 "sanitary districts," which have not yet been upgraded to the status of municipalities.

For various administrative purposes, the provinces *(changwads)* are divided into districts *(amphoes)* and the districts into communes

Table 7.1 Geographical Distribution of the Population of Thailand, 1977

Region	Area (square miles)	Main Feature
Central	62,000	Plain and lowland
Northern	42,000	Mountainous
Northeast	66,000	Plateau
Southern	30,000	Peninsular

Table 7.2 Number and Typical Population of Governmental Jurisdictions

Jurisdiction	Number	Typical Population
Province	71	500,000
District	570	70,000
Commune	5,547	8,000
Village	48,847	600

(tambons). The smallest social unit is the village *(muban).* The number and typical population of each of these governmental jurisdictions are shown in table 7.2.

In 1977, the per capita GNP of the Thai population was about $420 per year, being generally higher in the cities and lower in the rural areas. Buddhism is the religion of over 90 percent of the population. Being predominantly agricultural, the economy is based largely on the growth, exchange, and export of rice, tapioca, corn, and rubber.

Each of the many subdivisions of the Thai health care system evolved from distinct historical roots. The basic structure of these subdivisions may be summarized, examining first those in the government, or public sector, and then those in the private sector.

MINISTRY OF PUBLIC HEALTH

The principal governmental agency responsible for health services—but by no means the only one—is the Ministry of Public Health (MPH).[4] It was established in 1942, in the midst of World War II, before which governmental authority for public health was vested in the Ministry of Interior (where many health functions still remain).

Central Administration

The MPH has undergone several reorganizations since its founding. In 1978, its responsibilities at the central level were divided among six departments or offices:

1. Office of the Under-Secretary of State for Public Health
2. Department of Medical Services
3. Department of Communicable Disease Control
4. Department of Health
5. Department of Medical Sciences
6. Office of Food and Drugs

The MPH has a network of provincial chief medical officers for health administration in the rural areas of the 71 provinces. Under each of these 71 officers are district health officers to staff the 570 districts.

The six departments or offices of the central MPH are organized into divisions, with a wide variety of functions. For example, the Office of the Under-Secretary of State for Public Health includes a personnel division, a health education division, a health planning division, and several more units.

The Department of Medical Services is essentially responsible for the management or supervision of large governmental hospitals. These include the mental hospitals operated directly by the MPH and the large general hospitals at the provincial level. The national cancer institute and the institute of pathology, which engage in both patient care and research, are also in this department. It should be noted, however, that there are numerous smaller district hospitals of the MPH that are not the responsibility of the Department of Medical Services. Furthermore, there are several hospitals under other ministries of the government and an increasing number of private hospitals (both non-profit and for-profit) that are not supervised by the Department of Medical Services.

The Department of Communicable Disease Control is responsible for nationwide campaigns against (certain) communicable diseases that are relatively prevalent in Thailand. These include malaria, tuberculosis, filariasis, venereal disease, and leprosy. The operation of these disease-control programs is mainly through a vertical flow of authority, from the central government to the provinces and municipalities. Although there has been, in recent years, a movement to decentralize health programs and to increase authority at the provincial level, these communicable disease control programs are still managed essentially from the top of the pyramidal structure of the MPH.

The Department of Health is responsible for supervising most of the other prevention-oriented programs of the MPH. These programs are in such fields as nutrition, family health, dental health, and environmental sanitation. Highly important has been the delegation to this department of responsibility for several innovative programs in primary health care, to be discussed below. Moreover, since most of the family health services (maternal and child health and family planning) are delivered through a nationwide network of facilities for ambulatory service (health centers, midwifery centers, and medical and health centers), the standards for operation of these facilities are promulgated and supervised by this department. Most of the medical and health centers are at the district level and contain a small number of beds (10 to 30) for minor illness or emergency care; these have recently come to be called district hospitals. In spite of the fact that these sn.all hospitals are mainly curative in nature, rather than preventive, technical supervision of them has remained with the Department of Health.

The Department of Medical Sciences is responsible for managing a variety of technical services that are performed mainly at the central government level. These include, for example, a radiation protection service division, an entomology division, and a virus research institute.

The national health laboratories project is exceptional in attempting to organize a network of clinical laboratory services throughout the country, as well as operating a major central laboratory in Bangkok.

The Office of Food and Drugs—the newest of the major administrative entities of the MPH—is responsible for protecting the population against hazards in the consumption of food and drugs and in the use of cosmetics. In Thailand, as in many other developing countries, drugs—both those that are prescribed and those bought over the counter—constitute a substantial share of all expenditures for health purposes in the nation. The establishment of this office signifies an effort by the MPH to introduce greater controls over this important health matter. Drug abuse is only one aspect of the larger pharmaceutical problem.

Under the general surveillance of the Office of Food and Drugs, but operating as a semi-autonomous government enterprise, is the government pharmaceutical organization. This entity was set up in 1939, originally under the Ministry of Economics, to prepare drugs for use in governmental facilities and to save on foreign exchange.[5] In 1942, when the MPH was formed, it was transferred there and was eventually combined with the division of medical depot of the Department of Medical Sciences. Currently, the government pharmaceutical organization produces 384 items, which, it is estimated, constitute nearly half of the drugs and vaccines distributed to governmental hospitals and health centers throughout Thailand.

Local MPH Administration

Traditionally, the functions of the MPH just summarized were carried out under highly centralized authority, but in recent years greater delegation of responsibility to the local level has been stressed.[6]

As noted earlier, each of the 71 provinces has an office of the provincial chief medical officer (PCMO). The PCMO is a public health physician who is responsible for supervising both the preventive and the curative functions of the MPH throughout his province. He oversees the general hospital in his province (there is at least one in each province and sometimes two, making a total of 88). These hospitals vary from 60 to as many as 800 beds. The PCMO is also responsible for the technical supervision of the work of the district health offices in the province. Each of these offices is headed by a district health officer, who is not a physician but typically a sanitarian with additional training in general public health administration.[7]

In some of the districts there are district hospitals of 10 to 30 beds, staffed by at least one physician along with nurses and other health personnel. Also, within some of the communes there are health centers staffed only by nurses and allied health personnel. In some of the villages, especially the larger ones, there are midwifery stations, staffed simply by trained midwives. Health centers and midwifery stations come under the general supervision of the district health officer; the district hospitals—being staffed with physicians—come under the direct technical and administrative responsibility of the PCMO.[8]

The PCMO in each province is appointed by the Under-Secretary of State for Public Health and is *technically* responsible to him. He may be advised and assisted on various technical problems, however, by specialists from the several other departments of the MPH. At the same time, the PCMO is *administratively* responsible to the governor of his province, who is appointed by the Department of Local Administration of the Ministry of Interior. Provincial governors are important officials in Thailand, and it is evident that the PCMO must show great discretion in combining his exercise of technical responsibilities under the MPH with his administrative responsibilities under the provincial governor.

In the same way, the district health officer, while technically responsible to the PCMO, is administratively responsible to the overall governmental district officer. The latter official, like the provincial governor, is part of the network of authority under the Ministry of Interior.

The most recent development in the network of local health services under the MPH is the program of training village health volunteers and health communicators in selected villages throughout the nation.[9] Starting with the movement to limit population growth through encouraging family planning, this program has broadened to encompass the provision of general primary health care. These village health workers are part-time, and depend for their livelihood on some other occupation. They are not considered part of the bureaucratic structure of the MPH or any other governmental agency. They are selected by local village leaders, and their functions are limited to certain aspects of primary health care, particularly the dispensing of contraceptive pills and of drugs for minor ailments.

Thus, it is evident that the MPH both centrally and at the several peripheral levels has a very wide range of functions. They embrace both preventive and curative services, and they involve liaisons with various officials of provincial and local governments within the nation-wide network of governance under the Ministry of Interior. Even so, there are numerous health activities under the direction of other ministries of government, under voluntary nonprofit auspices, and in the purely private sector. On the whole, the scope of MPH authority does not extend to these other activities; when it does, the relationship is indirect. Moreover, below the level of the provincial health offices, there are many gaps and personnel vacancies in the current structure.

MINISTRY OF INTERIOR

As noted earlier, public health responsibilities were carried out by the Ministry of Interior (MI) before the MPH was established in 1942. Since then, the MI has by no means abandoned all its health responsibilities; it continues to exercise some of them in various ways.

The Department of Local Administration in the MI was organized around 1911 and was responsible for establishing the nationwide structure of provinces, districts, communes, and villages. Among other things, the basic law entrusted to each commune (*tambon*) the protection of the population's health. This was implemented by getting the people to choose a responsible person—the *tambon* doctor. This official was, of course, not a physician, but usually a traditional healer whom the people knew. The *tambon* doctor was responsible to the general district officer, and it was his duty to oversee environmental sanitation, to encourage vaccinations (which might be given by district public health authorities), and to provide first aid or simple remedies to the injured or sick. The quality of performance of these *tambon* doctors was naturally extremely limited.[10]

In about 1950, brief training courses in elementary hygiene were given by the MPH to the *tambon* doctors and to traditional midwives, who were appointed to work with them. A supply of simple drugs was provided to the *tambon* doctor by the government pharmaceutical organization. Today, there are an estimated 5,000 *tambon* doctors serving under the MI throughout the nation. Most of them are farmers, and their health work is only part-time; some are "health assistants" who were formerly in the military forces. They receive a small stipend of 200 *baht* (1 *baht* equals $0.05 U.S.) per month from the government, but they may also collect payments for the drugs they dispense, and some engage in private practice. These *tambon* doctors are expected to work cooperatively with the network of health personnel of the MPH, but the extent to which this occurs is uncertain.

Another, quite separate, health function of the MI is the overall supervisory responsibility for public health services in the nation's municipalities. In 118 of the 126 municipalities of Thailand, there are municipal doctors designated by the MI. These are physicians who are paid about 3,000 *baht* per month by the ministry (through subsidies to the municipal governments) for supervising environmental sanitation and communicable disease control. In the larger municipalities, they are assisted by a staff of sanitarians and nurses paid entirely from municipal revenues. The municipal doctor may operate a small, public first-aid clinic, and he serves also as coroner to investigate suspicious deaths. Nearly always the municipal doctor is engaged in private medical practice, from which he earns his principal livelihood. He is administratively responsible to the elected mayor of the municipality, but he may seek technical advice from the PCMO.

Outside Bangkok, municipalities range in population from about 10,000 to 50,000. Municipalities are responsible for operating any public systems of water supply or sewage disposal. In constructing public water supplies, the smaller ones usually work with a state enterprise of the central government.

The Bangkok metropolitan authority (BMA), governing a population of more than 4 million, reports directly to the MI, but other municipal governments come under the supervision of their respective provincial governors. The entire public health program of the BMA is, of course, much more highly developed than that of the provincial municipalities.

Department of Public Welfare

Quite separate from the health activities of the MI's Department of Local Administration are those of its Department of Public Welfare. While the several divisions of this department are oriented toward general social assistance to disadvantaged persons, much of this work has implications for health service. Thus, the division of child and youth welfare operates 21 institutions for orphaned or abandoned children, with a total census in 1978 of about 12,000 persons under 18 years of age.[11] Included in this protective care is a certain amount of health care. Other programs with some health care content include disaster relief (which, for example, helped nearly 600,000 persons, mainly victims of floods or storms, in 1976); four homes for the destitute, with 2,000 residents; and a vocational rehabilitation program for the disabled.[12]

The Department of Public Welfare also operates six homes for the aged, with 1,200 residents. It conducts a program of rehabilitation for "socially handicapped women" (prostitutes), which includes three institutions with 2,000 residents. Several hundred thousand persons are isolated, illiterate members of hill tribes in northern Thailand; the department conducts a varied program for them, emphasizing agricultural and social development and including health protection. Opium addiction is a special problem in this tribal population.

Of special interest because of its possible long-term health care implications is a program of social security for employees of private industry being explored by the Public Welfare Department. This is still in an early planning stage, and implementation is not expected for some years.

Other Functions

Among the responsibilities of municipal, provincial, district, and other levels of local government is the operation of primary schools. Although secondary schools and some primary schools are the responsibility of the Ministry of Education, most primary schools, which offer instruction only for grades one to four, are operated by local authorities and supervised by the MI. These schools instruct the children on elementary principles of personal hygiene.

The Department of Public Works is another component of the MI. This agency provides consultation and standardized plans (engineering and architectural) for the construction of health centers and other health facilities. It does the direct construction of piped water systems in municipalities and sanitary districts with a population of more than 5,000. It may also participate in the drilling of deep wells in rural villages, in cooperation with the MI's Department of Local Administration and the MPH.

The Department of Labor inspects factories to determine if the workers are being protected from various hazards of accident or occupational disease. Since 1972, furthermore, Thailand has had an industrial injury compensation act for employees of firms in the Bangkok area that have 20 or more workers.[13] Recently, this industrial injury coverage was extended to such firms in 22 provinces. This program is administered by a compensation fund office in the Department of Labor. In addition to monetary benefits, an injured worker is entitled to medical and hospital services worth up to 20,000 *baht* per case; these services are usually rendered by private personnel and facilities, who are paid by the compensation fund.

HEALTH FUNCTIONS OF OTHER MINISTRIES

Besides the MPH and the MI, with its diverse departments, other ministries support numerous activities that contribute to health services of some type in Thailand. These may be noted briefly.

Ministry of Defense

As in nearly all countries, there is a well-established organization of military forces in Thailand. In order to assure the efficiency and good health of their personnel, the Thai army, navy, and air force operate a network of 18 hospitals.[14] These institutions serve not only the men on active military duty, but also, to some extent, their families. At all military posts there are military medical officers or trained auxiliary medical corpsmen for rendering day-to-day ambulatory medical care.

In addition, there is one hospital maintained by the Ministry of Defense for military veterans who have disabilities related to their military service. In Bangkok, an institute of pathology is operated by the Ministry of Defense to carry out research and to do tissue studies for patients in the military facilities.

Ministry of Education

As noted earlier, most primary schools (grades one to four), which come under the supervision of municipalities, are in part a responsibility of the Department of Local Administration of the MI. Financial support for these schools, however, and the full responsibility for primary schools in rural areas, come under the Ministry of Education. This ministry also finances and operates all secondary schools, certain technical training institutions, and some colleges and universities.[15]

In all of these schools, especially those at the secondary level, some instruction is offered in personal hygiene and other aspects of health education. The schools also provide a convenient setting for administering immunizations or special screening tests.

State University Office

Until recently, responsibility for the 11 universities in Thailand was vested in the Office of the Prime Minister. In 1976, the bureau with this function was removed and given separate authority as the state university office. The office includes six of the nation's seven medical schools, several other faculties for training health professionals, and the teaching hospitals affiliated with them. The cost of operating these health science schools, and especially the teaching hospitals, is a substantial portion of overall national expenditures for health services; yet the latter facilities are administratively separate from the nationwide network of hospitals supervised by MPH. The national research council, which, among other things, conducts and also subsidizes medical research, has remained in the Office of the Prime Minister.

Ministry of Agriculture and Cooperatives

Among its many surveillance responsibilities in agricultural production and marketing, this ministry is responsible for enforcing the law controlling pesticides that may be harmful for human consumption. It also vaccinates animals to prevent and control zoonotic diseases (that is, animal diseases that may be spread to human beings).

Office of the Prime Minister

Attached to this important central authority are several special offices that have some bearing on health services. The bureau of the budget exercises final authority over central government appropriations to the MPH. The civil service commission controls the establishment of all new categories of health personnel and determines the levels of all governmental salaries; thus, any efforts of the MPH, for example, to modify salary scales (which may be important for reaching health objectives) must be approved by this commission. (Approval usually depends on the relationship to salary levels in other ministries.)

The national statistical office, attached to the Office of the Prime Minister, conducts household surveys that elicit, among other things, information on health expenditures by families. It also has final responsibility for assembling information on births, deaths, and net changes in the population of Thailand. The national environmental board exercises surveillance over major projects that may modify the environment in ways that create hazards to health.

The all-important National Economic and Social Development Board is also within the Office of the Prime Minister. Among its many national planning responsibilities is the final approval of five-year plans for the health services, which are drafted initially in the MPH. Related to this planning is the Department of Technical and Economic Cooperation, which coordinates financial and technical support from various international sources; this support makes a substantial contribution to the development of the health services.

Ministry of Industry

The Ministry of Industry, which is concerned with the overall development of industrial enterprise in Thailand, has certain responsibilities involving the safety of industrial processes and the control of environmental pollution by factories. The Factory Acts of 1969 authorize this ministry to inspect and approve all factories that have seven or more workers or that utilize machinery of two or more horsepower.[16] Although there are thousands of small workshops below this size, an estimated 40,000 factories come under Ministry of Industry surveillance. The commonest type is rice mills, which are located throughout the nation; other types, concentrated in Bangkok and a few other cities, manufacture textiles or wood products, do printing, repair machinery, and produce various consumer goods. Factories of the specified size require licensure every three years, and this entails inspection by one of 120 inspectors of the factory control division. These inspections are expected to identify potential accident hazards; the division may enforce the safeguarding of workers by requiring the use of protective equipment (such as masks or earmuffs). Another common problem is stream pollution from industrial by-products. In 1977, for example, about 200 factories were temporarily closed down by the Ministry of Industry until pollution problems were corrected.

There seems to be some overlap between the factory inspection functions of the Ministry of Industry and the worker protection functions of the Department of Labor in the MI. The latter agency also has 88 inspectors for occupational safety and health. Labor legislation requires that firms with 500 to 1,000 workers maintain in the plant a clinic staffed by a nurse; if there are more than 1,000 workers, a physician is supposed to be within access at all times.[17] It is the Labor Department that is expected to enforce this legal requirement, as well as to identify hazards for accidents or occupational diseases and enforce preventive measures. The occupational health division of the MPH's Department of Health also makes special studies of occupational diseases when invited to do so.

Ministry of Finance and Other Ministries

Under the Ministry of Finance is the Bank of Thailand, the national tobacco monopoly, and numerous other state enterprises. These may be either wholly governmental operations or partnerships between government and private investors. Most public utilities, such as electricity, water, and telephone service, are of this nature. Some, such as the port authority, are under the Ministry of Communications or elsewhere in the government.[18]

Altogether, there are some 72 of these state enterprises, which tend to be large organizations with hundreds or even thousands of workers. Virtually all of these enterprises provide some type of health service to their employees. The port authority and the railroad system even operate special hospitals for their workers.

VOLUNTARY HEALTH ORGANIZATIONS

Outside the sphere of government are numerous private, non-profit organizations with various charitable functions, including health service. It is required that these organizations—many of which are linked to religious bodies—be registered with the Department of Religious Affairs in the Ministry of Education. An official of this agency estimates that there are as many as 6,000 charitable agencies officially registered and that about 100 of these are principally or entirely devoted to the provision of health services.[19]

The largest voluntary health organization is probably the Red Cross of Thailand. This organization collects donations of blood, operates blood banks, furnishes blood for transfusions to hospitals throughout the country, and operates an eye bank. The Red Cross also operates first-aid emergency clinics in Bangkok and a few other cities, as well as some ambulances. One of the largest hospitals in Thailand, the Chulalongkorn Hospital in Bangkok, was founded by the Red Cross and is still nominally owned by it, although it is financed almost entirely by the central government. In addition to the funds it raises from private philanthropy, the Red Cross receives regular subsidies from the national government.

Another important voluntary health agency is the Anti-Tuberculosis Association of Thailand. Most of the activities of this organization are conducted in Bangkok, where it operates a chest clinic and a 100-bed chest hospital.[20] The association also operates two mobile chest X-ray units, which screen persons in factories and schools in the Bangkok metropolitan area. It maintains a laboratory for sputum ex-

aminations and provides continuing education to doctors on tuberculosis and other chest diseases. It is noteworthy that, in spite of its
voluntary, nonprofit character, the Anti-Tuberculosis Association requires payments for most of its services. The hospital budget, for example, amounts to about 6 million *baht* per year, but only about 150,000
baht of this amount is contributed by the association from charitable
sources; the rest is derived from patient fees. A substantial proportion
of patients are government employees, whose care is paid for by their
ministries. A small charge is also made for chest Xrays—10 *baht*—to
cover the cost of the film. One of the services that is free of charge is
BCG vaccination against tuberculosis.

The worldwide movement to limit population growth has given
rise to several voluntary health agencies in Thailand. Perhaps the
most effective of these is the community-based Family Planning Society, which promotes contraceptive practices in thousands of villages
throughout the nation. This organization cooperates closely with MPH,
which coordinates Thailand's national family planning program.[21] As
was noted for the Anti-Tuberculosis Association, only a small portion of
the costs of the Family Planning Society is derived from charitable
contributions. Most of its funds come from grants given by international and national governmental bodies and from fees paid by patients
for contraceptive pills or other birth control supplies.

This is not a comprehensive study of the many voluntary health
agencies in Thailand, but certain general categories of sponsorship or
function can be mentioned. There are about 25 religious or semi-
religious missions from overseas (generally Europe and North America), that provide certain health services. Hospitals are operated by the
Baptist Mission, the Seventh-Day Adventists, the Church of Christ,
and other Christian sects. Some religious missions also operate clinics
for ambulatory care. The services of these facilities are supported principally by patient fees, but the salaries of several key medical personnel are paid by foreign philanthropy; some low-income patients are
treated without charge or for reduced fees. Overseas philanthropic
foundations, such as the Rockefeller Foundation, the Ford Foundation,
and the China Medical Board, have long contributed to the development of medical education and research in Thailand.

Within Thailand, there are numerous foundations supported by
charitable contributions from members of certain ethnic groups. Chinese merchants, for example, support the Kwong Soo Hospital Foundation, which maintains maternity homes for women of Chinese background. There are similar foundations supported by Japanese, Moslem,
and other groups. Buddhism, the predominant religion of Thailand, is
the basis of many charitable activities impinging on health. The Tran

Narmjai Foundation, for example, makes various expenditures, among which 53,000 *baht* were devoted to health activities in 1978.

There are associations involved with various diseases other than tuberculosis: leprosy, venereal disease, cancer, crippled children, and blindness are the objects of educational or other health activities supported by voluntary agencies. The Thai royal family solicits donations for certain health purposes.

PRIVATE INDUSTRIAL ENTERPRISES

Among the functions of government discussed above was the authority to inspect industrial enterprises. The actual medical services provided or financed by private companies for their workers must, however, be recognized as a subsystem within the health services of Thailand.

In-factory medical services are rare, except in establishments with hundreds of workers. Aside from the state enterprises discussed above, there are an estimated 300 private companies with 500 to 1,000 employees and another 150 or so with over 1,000 workers.[22] If the current labor legislation is being properly implemented, these 450 private companies should be providing a great deal of medical and nursing services to their workers and, sometimes, the workers' families. Some of the large companies go beyond the requirements of the labor law and support the costs of general medical care for their employees and, often, their families as well. These benefits are offered by firms to promote good labor-management relations and to maintain a healthy, efficient, and devoted work force. These managerial practices may be considered paternalistic—for the purpose of discouraging the organization of workers into labor unions.

Whatever the motives of these special health care programs for industrial employees, a frequent mechanism for conducting them is private group insurance. The American International Assurance Company, for example, carried 120 group insurance policies for various firms in 1974.[23] When an insured employee (or his dependent) is sick, he may seek care from any private physician or hospital, or both, with part or all of the expenses being indemnified by the insurance company. For example, one insurance plan offered by this company costs 19.60 *baht* per month per worker and indemnifies the patient up to 7,500 *baht* for surgical fees; another plan, costing 16 *baht* per worker per month indemnifies up to 6,000 *baht* for surgical fees. The monthly premium may be paid entirely by the employer or jointly with the employee. Sometimes employers will pay the full premium for employee coverage and require a deduction from the employee's wages for coverage of dependents.

Another pattern of private insurance has recently been started in Thailand. A small group of private physicians has organized a clinic known as Thailand Medical and Surgical Plan, Ltd. For a fixed per capita monthly premium, this clinic offers general medical care, including hospitalization, to the employees of enrolled firms.[24] Since the clinic physicians have no financial incentive (as under fee-for-service remuneration) to maximize the services provided, the premiums for this health care protection are probably lower than those of commercial insurance companies, such as the one described above. This program embodies the U.S. concept of health maintenance organizations; in fact, it is managed by a former administrator of the Kaiser-Permanente Health Program, the largest health maintenance organization in the United States.

This account of the medical services provided by private industry for its employees is obviously superficial. It is offered, however, mainly to identify the existence of this subsystem of the health services of Thailand.

PRIVATE, FOR-PROFIT HEALTH SERVICE

Finally, one must recognize the operation of a purely private, for-profit (proprietary) sector in the health care system of Thailand. Although this chapter has been devoted mainly to an analysis of organized health programs, under various governmental and nongovernmental sponsorship, the dimensions of the nonorganized, private health care sector are very large in Thailand and require special attention.

Traditional Healers and Related Resources

For centuries before Western medicine was introduced into Thailand in the early nineteenth century, healing services were rendered by Buddhist priests and by a variety of nonclerical healers. The latter employed various treatment methods, including both the invocation of supernatural forces through magic and empirical physical procedures, such as massage and various herbal remedies.[25]

Thousands of these traditional healers still render services to the sick in rural villages, and even to some extent in the towns. As more effective scientific services have become available, the relative importance of traditional healing has declined; but, as several anthropological studies have shown, it has by no means disappeared. In fact, many traditional healers have learned of the effectiveness of certain modern drugs, such as the antibiotics, and use them along with magic.

The treatment of the traditional healer—both in its magical and in its physical modalities—is a logical response to Thai theories about the causation of disease. On the other hand, some healers in the villages do not abide by any theoretical concepts; they simply give injections for any and all ailments. These "injectionists" are to be distinguished from classical healers, and it is understandable that Thai public health officials refer to them as quacks, or charlatans. They are sometimes former students who have failed out of a training program (for example, a school for sanitarians) or former medical corpsmen from the armed forces or simply unscrupulous persons who take advantage of the widespread belief among uneducated people that any injection into the body has healing powers.

Another type of private health practitioner is the untrained midwife, or traditional birth attendant. These are almost invariably older women who have given birth to many children of their own and who gradually acquire skills in helping with childbirths. Along with the delivery process, they often employ certain practices in maternity care which reflect long tradition, even though they may actually be harmful to the mother or infant. Many traditional midwives, on the other hand, have been given training by public health authorities and play roles within officially organized health programs.

Traditional healers of all types are seldom engaged full-time in their work. They may be farmers or storekeepers or housewives or something else. If they render service only rarely, they may not even expect payment, either in money or in kind, for what they do; but the majority charge fees for their services. In this sense, they are in private practice, even though their charges may be very low. Sometimes a traditional healer who has won a reputation for great effectiveness may charge as much as a trained physician.

Drug Sellers

Quite separate from traditional healers are various types of stores selling drugs—usually a combination of modern pharmaceutical and ancient traditional remedies. There are hundreds of licensed pharmacies devoted exclusively to the sale of drugs of both types. In addition, drugs may also be purchased in thousands of stores selling food or other merchandise in the towns and villages.

In the vast majority of cases, the patient simply goes to the store selling drugs and describes his or her symptoms. The proprietor or salesperson, who is seldom a trained pharmacist, selects a package of drugs or dispenses a quantity of some herbal remedy that he advises the patient to take in a certain way. Only rarely does the Thai patient present a doctor's prescription to be filled; physicians typically dispense prescribed drugs from their own supplies. Often the patient simply requests the compound he wants, based on his own past experience or the advice of others. This self-care with nonprescribed drugs or the purchase of drugs recommended by the seller probably is the commonest pattern of response to sickness in the rural population of Thailand.

Private Physicians and Dentists

Relatively few graduates of modern schools of medicine or dentistry in Thailand are exclusively devoted to private practice. On the other hand, almost all medical and dental practitioners who are employed in one of the governmental or other organized health programs spend part of their time in private practice. When they complete their duties in a hospital, health center, or other facility, they usually serve patients in private clinics. They charge patients on a fee-for-service basis and typically earn much more from this private work than from their salaried positions.

The numbers, distribution, specialty status, and other features of Thailand's medical and dental manpower are recorded in a registry at the MPH. Private services tend to be more heavily concentrated on city or town dwellers with high incomes. Low-income patients with illnesses causing them great anxiety may occasionally consult a physician or dentist privately, despite the relatively high charges.

Private Hospital Care

In Bangkok and other principal cities of Thailand (typically provincial capitals), there is an increasing number of private, proprietary hospitals. In these facilities, which are usually small, the patients are attended either by a selected staff of private physicians or by any private practitioner in the area. These hospitals are to be distinguished from voluntary (nongovernmental) and nonprofit hospitals, even though patients in the latter institutions must also pay private charges for their care.

Many governmental hospitals, especially the larger ones, maintain a small percentage of beds for private patients. The physicians serving these patients, unlike those in exclusively proprietary hospitals, must always be members of the salaried medical staff of the hospital. When a patient is served in a private room of a public hospital or in any bed of a private hospital, payment must usually be made separately for the hospital care and for the physician's services.

There are a relatively small number of private providers of other types of medical care in Thailand, such as private-duty nurses; sellers of eyeglasses, hearing aids, or other prosthetic devices; and physical therapists. All types of *private* health service combined—traditional, self-care, and modern—actually comprise the majority of all health services rendered to the Thai people. Thus, in the total health care system of Thailand—whether quantified by volume of services or expenditures for them—the private sector is substantially larger than the organized programs, both governmental and voluntary.

NOTES

1. M. I. Roemer, *Comparative National Policies on Health Care* (New York: Marcel Dekker Co., 1977).
2. Royal Thai Government and World Health Organization, Regional Office for South-East Asia, *Country Profile: Thailand* (Bangkok, 1977).
3. "Thailand: Politics and Social Affairs," in *Asia 1978 Yearbook* (Hong Kong: Far Eastern Economic Review, 1978), 321.
4. Ministry of Public Health, *Public Health in Thailand* (Bangkok, 1973).
5. Charoen Chittasombat, *Presentation of the Governmental Pharmaceutical Organization* (Bangkok: Conference on Health Economics, 1974).
6. Chalard Tirapat, *Medical Referral System in CBD Project* (Bangkok: Mahidol University public health faculty, 1977).
7. Samlee Plianbangchang, Director of the Technical Division, Department of Medical Services, MPH, personal communication, Bangkok, November 1978.
8. Uthai Sudsukh, Director of the Rural Health Division, Office of the Under-Secretary of State, MPH, personal communication, Bangkok, November 1978.
9. Debhanom Muangman, *New Approach to Rural Health Care in Thailand and Its Possible Application to Other Developing Countries* (New Delhi: World Health Organization, South-East Asia Regional Conference of Schools of Public Health, 1978).
10. Dumrong Soonthornsaratoon, Director General of the Department of Local Administration, Ministry of Interior, personal communication, Bangkok, November 1978.
11. Ministry of Interior, Department of Public Welfare, *Facts and Figures as of January 1978* (Bangkok, 1978).
12. _____, *Annual Report 1976* (Bangkok, 1977).
13. "Thailand," in *Social Security Programs Throughout the World* (Washington, D.C.: Social Security Administration, 1975), 220–21.
14. World Bank, *The National Family Planning Program—A Sector Report: Thailand,* report no. 724a-Th (Bangkok, 1975), 36.

15. Bureau of the Budget, *Thailand's Budget in Brief: Fiscal Year 1978* (Bangkok, 1978), 30.
16. Phisaln Khongsamran, Director of the Factory Control Division, Industrial Works Department, Ministry of Industry, personal communication, Bangkok, November 1978.
17. Vinat Montanan, Chief Occupational Health and Safety Inspector, Division of Labor Standards, Department of Labor, Ministry of Interior, personal communication, Bangkok, November 1978.
18. "Public Enterprises," *Siamraj Magazine* (5 November 1978).
19. Rangab Watanasing, Chief of the Cultural Division, Department of Religious Affairs, Ministry of Education, personal communication, Bangkok, November 1978.
20. Songkram Supcharoen, Secretary-General of the Anti-Tuberculosis Association of Thailand, personal communication, Bangkok, November 1978.
21. S. Burintratikul and M. C. Samaniego, *CBFPS: A Community-Based Approach to Family Planning* (Essex, Conn.: International Council for Educational Development, 1978).
22. Estimates made by Mr. Vinat (see note 17).
23. L. G. Ginnetti, *Private and Consumer Interests by American International Assurance Company* (Bangkok: Conference on Health Economics, 1974).
24. Information from J. Shepperd, M.D., World Health Organization consultant, Mahidol University, faculty of public health, personal communication, November 1978.
25. J. N. Riley and S. Sersi, *The Variegated Thai Medical System as a Context for Birth Control Services* (Bangkok: Mahidol University, Institute for Population and Social Research, 1974).

8

Health Care Policies
In Kenya

The countries of Africa, more than those of any other continent, have been under colonial domination by foreign powers until quite recently. After independence, there was great social turmoil in many of these countries, as different political groups contended for power. In Kenya, violence was prominent before national liberation, but after liberation, in 1963, a period of political stability lasted for nearly 20 years. Kenyan health policies are illustrative of others in African countries that are devoted to the socioeconomic ideology of free enterprise.

Kenya is one of several former British colonies on the coast of East Africa; it won its national independence in 1963, four years after the violent Mau Mau uprising led by Jomo Kenyatta, who became the new nation's first president. In 1981, Kenya had a population of 16 million and had acquired a reputation for political stability, in contrast to most African countries. This reputation was shaken in 1982, when young officers in the air force attempted a military coup, but they were soon subdued.

Based on a field study made in Kenya, August 1982.

SOCIOECONOMIC STRUCTURE

The economy of Kenya is mainly agricultural (coffee, tea, cereals, cottons), although significant shares of its income are derived from light industry, tourism, and mining. Production and trade are dominated by the ideology of free enterprise, and this is reflected clearly in Kenya's health care system. The nation's per capita GNP in 1979 was $380 (U.S.), which puts Kenya in the bottom third of the world's national economies.

As is true in most African countries, the people of Kenya are identified with many tribes. Kenya's 47 or so tribes no longer play an official role in governing social affairs, but they still influence relationships and loyalties. Most important among the tribes are the Kikuyu, who constitute about 20 percent of the population. Since the mid-nineteenth century, Christian missionaries (mainly from Europe) have had great influence; thus some 60 percent of the population are now Protestant or Roman Catholic. Mission medical services played a significant part in the conversion strategy. The literacy of the population has improved markedly since independence, and in the late 1970s was estimated at 65 percent for men and 35 percent for women, with 93 percent of children being enrolled in primary schools. More than 90 percent of the Kenyan population is of black African background, but the small balance, divided between Asians (mostly from India) and Europeans, earns a disproportionately high share of the national income.

Kenya is divided into seven provinces, plus the large capital city of Nairobi, which has a population of nearly 900,000. The provinces are further divided into 41 districts, which play an important part in the organization of health services. Governance of the provinces and districts, as in the colonial period, is not entrusted to the local people, but is in the hands of commissioners appointed by the central government. At independence, the major political party was the Kenya African National Union (KANU), and in 1981 it was declared by President Daniel Moi to be the only legal party. Thus, political power and influence are concentrated in the KANU leadership, which is based mainly in Nairobi and to a lesser extent in the nation's second city, Mombasa. Some 85 percent of Kenya's total population, however, lives in rural areas.

STRUCTURE OF THE HEALTH CARE SYSTEM

The free market ideology of the Kenyan economy permeates health care, as it does other sectors, but in the formal structure of the health care system a central Ministry of Health (MOH) plays the major role. This authority is responsible not only for all preventive, public health services in the traditional sense, but also for the establishment and operation of public hospitals, the registration of health practitioners, the training of many types of personnel, and various forms of environmental and pharmaceutical regulation.

Ministry of Health

The top technical officer of the MOH is the director of medical services, under whom are deputy directors in charge of hospitals, rural service development, training, medical research, administrative matters (financing and personnel), and other functions. The Minister of Health appoints a provincial medical officer for each of the seven provinces; this officer is assisted by administrative personnel, nurses, sanitary officers, and others. In Nairobi and three other cities, a medical officer is appointed by the Ministry of Local Government. Within each province are districts, each headed by a district medical officer of health (DMOH), also appointed centrally. In 1982, all 41 of the DMOH posts were staffed with a physician (a few being expatriates), who is theoretically responsible for all health activities (public and private) in this district.

The DMOH may be assisted by a nursing officer, a hospital secretary (administrator), a sanitarian, a health educator, a nutritionist, and others. Most districts, however, do not have full complements of such personnel as yet; they remain to be trained. Only a fraction of the DMOHs, furthermore, have had public health training, and it is not surprising that they spend most of their time giving clinical service in the district hospital or in rural health centers.

Below the level of the district, the MOH has been developing since 1972 a network of rural health units (RHUs) intended to provide general primary health care to the rural population. The plan calls for 254 RHUs, or about six per district, each serving about 54,000 people (varying from 10,000 to 100,000). The headquarters of a RHU would ordinarily be in a health center, around which there might be several small dispensaries or health posts. Each RHU is to be headed by a clinical officer, who is not a physician, but typically a young man who has had 12 years of basic schooling and 3 years of training in a hospital on elementary diagnosis and treatment. The RHU staff would also include "enrolled nurses," sanitary technicians, family health educators, and others. To learn cooperative teamwork for primary health care, all these persons receive a three-month training course at one of six rural health training centers established in six of the seven provinces.

As of 1982, about 120 of the contemplated 254 RHUs were reported to be staffed and operating. It was estimated that these units brought primary health care within reach (that is, within four kilometers) of 20 to 30 percent of the rural Kenyan population. A nongovernmental medical observer stated that the staffs in the health centers appeared to be well motivated but that their performance was frequently handicapped by shortages of drugs and other basic medical supplies.

In spite of the MOH's official emphasis on extending primary health care into rural areas, a much greater expenditure is made on services in hospitals. This may be explained in part by historical circumstances—the existence of hospital facilities to which thousands of sick people came for help. Further, both the inpatient and outpatient services of some 80 MOH hospitals are available to everyone at almost no charge. High hospital expenditures also doubtless result from the political strength of the specialists who staff the larger facilities in the provincial capitals and Nairobi. This and other aspects of the MOH will be discussed later, but now I will examine other parts of the organizational structure of the Kenyan health care system.

Other Ministries with Health Functions

Other ministries and nonministerial entities in the government make various contributions to the nation's health care system. Preeminent is the University of Nairobi, which is financed almost wholly by the national government, but which has a semi-autonomous status in the Office of the President. The current president, Daniel Moi, serves as chancellor of the university—a position that, while honorary rather than administrative, symbolizes the university's importance. Since 1967, the university has had a faculty of medicine. In 1974, university programs were established to train pharmacists and dentists, and recently a graduate course for registered nurses, leading to a university diploma, was established.

The Ministry of Water Development has major responsibilities in environmental sanitation. The ministry's work is largely in the cities and small towns, where public water systems are thought to be feasible. (Small-scale rural water supply units and latrines are developed by MOH.) The Ministry of Agriculture operates a modest extension education program, which includes education on family nutrition. The Ministry of Education operates all public elementary schools, in which health education is a small part of the curriculum. (Personal health services for school children have not, however, been developed as yet.) The Ministry of Social Services operates a few facilities for the disabled and the aged, although its objectives are custodial rather than rehabilitative; it also operates ten nutrition centers for women.

Still other health-related functions in government come under the Ministry of Labor. Factory inspectors attempt to visit plants with five or more workers at least once a year, to identify occupational hazards. Safety hazards get the greatest attention, but fumes, dusts, and toxic substances are supposed to be monitored by an industrial hygiene unit. Since in Nairobi alone some 7,000 "factories," or work places, are registered with the Ministry of Labor, the degree of surveillance by that ministry's small staff could scarcely be adequate. Recently, three physicians were trained in occupational medicine and assigned by MOH to the Ministry of Labor, where they examine workers suspected of having acquired an occupational disease. Finally, the Ministry of Labor administers a workmen's compensation program for industrial injuries. Financial compensation is paid to the disabled worker through an insurance fund, but medical services are the responsibility of each industry: if a government facility is used, no payment is necessary, but if the employer wishes to have the injured worker treated in a private hospital, the employer must pay the costs.

Outside the MOH, the Ministry of Local Government bears the greatest official health responsibilities. This ministry oversees and subsidizes Kenya's major cities, which maintain significant health services. These include Nairobi, Mombasa, Nakuru, and Kisumu. The latter three cities operate some 20 health centers, or dispensaries, at their own expense, with some subsidy from the Ministry of Local Government. Standards in these facilities are supposed to be technically supervised by the MOH, but without financial responsibility this seems to have little meaning.

Health services under the Nairobi city council that are not included within the program or budget of the MOH are substantial. There is a maternity hospital with 350 beds that is highly utilized (with 29,000 deliveries in 1981). In addition, there are 11 subsidiary maternity units with 24 beds each. The city operates 24 health centers for preventive and curative services, plus 22 dispensaries for emergencies and other treatment services. To staff this large establishment, there are posts for 120 full-time doctors, although 40 of these posts were not filled in 1982. In addition, the city of Nairobi provides its own environmental sanitation surveillance services, communicable disease control, and health services for school children. A staff of community health nurses and sanitary inspectors does most of this work, under the direction of two medical officers. Not surprisingly, this health program absorbs 60 percent of the Nairobi city council's budget.

Finally, within the governmental sector of the Kenyan health care system, there are two other health activities that are loosely linked to the MOH but that, for all practical purposes, are autonomous. One is the medical research institute, established recently with foreign funding. It is housed in the major health facility of the nation, the Kenyatta National Hospital, and is devoted principally to conducting and coordinating research on tropical diseases in collaboration with the global program of the WHO. The other program is the National Hospital Insurance Fund, a form of social insurance for all or part of the costs of private hospital care. While legally under the MOH, the fund is administered wholly independently, and its financial operations (both revenue and expenditures) are entirely independent. All Kenyans, whether employed by others or self-employed, who earn 1,000 or more Kenyan shillings per month (K.Sh. 10 equal $1 U.S.) are required by law to pay K.Sh. 20 per month into the fund. In 1982, the fund had slightly over 500,000 contributing members; they and their dependents amount to some 2 million covered people. There is no contribution from employers on behalf of their employees, but the employer is obligated to see that qualified workers pay their premiums. A small proportion of the covered persons are individuals earning less than K.Sh. 1,000 per month who enroll voluntarily.

The basic objective of the National Hospital Insurance Fund is different from that of most social insurance programs: its focus is on the more affluent, rather than the poorer, members of society. As stated in a lecture by the fund's director, "It is intended that the scheme should provide for the largest possible number of people in Kenya the opportunity of occupying the hospital beds available in Kenya, for which charges are made, by providing daily allowances to contributors towards meeting those charges." In other words, the fund is oriented toward increasing the use of private hospitals, or private beds in public hospitals, for those whose earnings are high enough to qualify. The benefits payable by the fund have been somewhat less than the usual charges for private hospital care, so the individual must ordinarily pay something extra personally (unless he has supplemental private hospital insurance, which is also available in Kenya). Moreover, there is a limit of 180 days of hospitalization per family per year, although this can be extended by special request from the doctor.

In 1980–81, the National Hospital Insurance Fund collected K.Sh. 71.5 million from its members but paid out only K.Sh. 43.5 million in benefits (including administrative expenses). Since the fund is entirely separate from the MOH budget, these monies are expected to be used for increasing future hospital benefits.

Organized Nongovernmental Programs

There are several organized, nongovernmental programs in the Kenyan health care system, aside from the purely private sector of medical care. Some 15 para-governmental enterprises are engaged in numerous activities related to transportation (railroads, port authority, airline) or agriculture (the tea development authority, the coffee board, and so on). The Ministry of Transport and Communication has certain responsibility for the enterprises in its field, and the Ministry of Agriculture for the others. These semipublic enterprises provide relatively broad health services for their employees and their families. In the sugar industry, some estates and processing plants are para-governmental, while others are purely private.

Private enterprises with 500 or more workers also generally have their own clinics, staffed by nurses and either full-time or part-time doctors. About ten are large enough to have such health services, including the Firestone Tire Co., Kenya Breweries, the British American Tobacco Co., and the Bata Shoe Co. These in-plant health services treat acute illness, whether work-related or not, but, if a chronic illness develops, the case is referred elsewhere for care.

Voluntary, nonprofit agencies are another significant part of the organizational structure of the Kenyan health care system. Most important by far are the religious missions, Roman Catholic and Protestant, which have operated hospitals and clinics since about 1900. Christian missionaries from Europe and the United States learned early that their religious messages were much more effective if they were accompanied by treatment of the physical ailments of the people. Most highly developed are the Catholic missions, which in 1980 operated 27 hospitals (with resident doctors) with 3,565 beds, another 55 health centers with 1,293 beds, and 135 dispensaries and special clinics. Coordinating all these missions is the Kenyan Catholic Secretariat, which has a medical department.

Protestant missions operate 14 general hospitals (with resident doctors) having 1,731 beds, another 29 health centers with 366 beds, and 38 other ambulatory care clinics. These activities are coordinated by the Protestant Churches Medical Association. It is noteworthy that the MOH subsidizes nearly one-fourth of the budgets of the mission medical facilities. The ministry obviously looks upon the missions as providing services complementary to its own and attempts to coordinate the two types of resources geographically. In recent years, the Catholic mission leadership claims that its emphasis is shifting from hospitalization toward primary health care.

Other nonreligious, voluntary health agencies in Kenya include the Red Cross, the Leprosy Society, the Child Welfare Society, and the

Catholic Relief Fund for Malnutrition. These organizations also receive subsidies from the government. The Lion's Club operates a health care program for children.

The Private Health Market

Finally, as in the structure of all health care systems, there is a purely private market for medical care in Kenya—and it constitutes a substantial share of the total health care sector, especially with respect to ambulatory care. Oldest are the traditional healers, who doubtless are the major providers of health care in all of sub-Saharan Africa. These practitioners are of many types, classified by one observer as trance-healers, soothsayers, black magic doctors, herbalists, and bonesetters. They may offer these healing services full-time or part-time, and they charge fees. They practice in both cities and rural areas, although in the latter—where other health services are less available—they play a relatively larger role.

The herbalists, and sometimes the other healers, dispense drugs, which may consist of a combination of traditional and modern remedies (such as penicillin). Drug peddlers, who have acquired stocks of contraceptive pills, vitamins, and sometimes antibiotics, sell them at bus stops and street corners. In addition, nonprescribed drugs may be purchased at almost any general market. (I bought a packet of two 250-milligram tablets of Malaraquin (chloraquine phosphate) from a stall selling candy and toilet articles.) In the cities, pharmacies sell modern drugs both on medical prescription and over the counter.

Most visible in the private market of medical care in Kenya are the private physicians. While estimates differ, it is agreed that at least 70 percent of all doctors in Kenya are in full-time private practice, mainly as general practitioners. In addition, of the 30 percent of doctors working in government posts, the great majority engage also in private practice after official hours. There are relatively few dentists in Kenya, but the great majority of these are also in private practice.

Finally, there are growing numbers of private, proprietary hospitals, over and above the mission hospitals, largely supported by patient fees. There are also private beds in government hospitals. Miscellaneous private vendors, such as opticians and sellers of prosthetic appliances or sickroom equipment, complete the private market for health in Kenya.

PRODUCTION OF HEALTH RESOURCES

The structure of the Kenyan health care system depends on many types of resources, produced both inside and outside the country. Most important is health manpower, but there must also be health facilities, drugs and other commodities, and health-related knowledge.

Health Manpower

In 1981, there were 2,057 physicians recorded in the MOH's official medical registry, but not all of them were in the country and actively engaged in medical work. Adjusting for those away or retired, there were estimated to be 1,685 active physicians, or about 10.5 per 100,000 population. As noted earlier, at least 70 percent of these were in full-time private practice, and most of the remainder practiced privately part of the time. Geographic distribution of doctors is extremely uneven, with about 53 percent of physicians being located in Nairobi, where less than 6 percent of the national population lives. The great majority of the rural population does not have access to a modern physician.

Before independence, all physicians working in Kenya had to be trained elsewhere. In 1967, the University of Nairobi established a medical faculty, which now turns out about 60 medical graduates a year. The course lasts five years, after which a one-year internship is required plus two years of mandatory work in a government hospital. These three years are spent in the relatively large provincial general hospitals or in the Kenyatta National Hospital; the time is not used (as in some countries) to provide medical coverage for rural populations. Of the 1,685 doctors in the country, about 1,200 are Kenyans (trained at home or abroad) and 485 are expatriates.

Dentists numbered 197 in 1981, and trained pharmacists numbered 84. Most drug dispensing is done by the 326 briefly trained pharmaceutical technologists. The most numerous type of qualified health personnel are the enrolled nurses, who have been trained for two years after elementary school. There were 9,190 of these nurses in 1981. Fully trained registered nurses (with three years of training after secondary school) numbered 6,892 or 43 per 100,000 population.

An especially important manpower resource in Kenya are the clinical officers, who head the rural health units. Always male, they have received three years of training in elementary medical diagnosis and treatment after completing secondary school. These essential health workers, particularly for rural areas, are trained in large hospitals, with emphasis on outpatient work. In 1979, there were about 1,000 clinical officers employed in the government.

The number of traditional healers in Kenya, important as they are, is not known. Current law does not call for their registration. Since they are very widely available in rural areas, a rough estimate might suggest one healer per 1,000 people, or about 16,000 in all (considering both full-time and part-time practitioners). Knowledgeable observers report that the magical healers are gradually declining, but not the herbalists or drug peddlers.

As noted earlier, the MOH program for nationwide coverage with RHUs includes a training component. Many of the enrolled nurses have been trained as community health nurses in 12 schools operated by the ministry; this training includes midwifery for home deliveries. The ministry also operates six rural health training centers (in six provinces) with several manpower objectives. They offer basic training for public health technicians, who receive a three-year course in environmental sanitation. They train family welfare field educators, who promote family planning and other preventive health practices. Most important, they offer 13-week courses on managerial concepts and practical problems, designed to help the basic teams of rural health personnel to work together harmoniously in RHUs and subcenters. The standard plan calls for a staff of 15, consisting of one clinical officer (formerly medical assistant), four enrolled community nurses, one public health technician (formerly health assistant), one family welfare field educator, one statistical clerk, three attendants, and four custodial workers.

Current figures on the number of each of the above types of rural health personnel are not available (except for the enrolled nurses of all types, 9,190 in 1981). In 1977, however, there were 1,070 clinical officers, 670 public health technicians, and 580 family welfare field educators; there are doubtless more now. In addition, in 1977 there were other technical personnel engaged principally in urban posts, including 192 laboratory technologists, 196 rehabilitation technologists, 120 radiographers, and 230 nutrition field workers. Voluntary agencies, such as the Kenyan Catholic Secretariat, have also trained primary health care workers, known as public health aides. In 1981 there were 61 of these at 27 posts; they had been trained for five months to provide mainly preventive services for mothers and children.

Health Facilities

As noted earlier, both governmental and nongovernmental bodies sponsor hospitals in Kenya. In 1981 there were 221 hospitals in all, with 28,108 beds, a ratio of 1.77 hospital beds (including bassinets) per 1,000 population.

Statistical breakdown of these hospital resources for the current period is not available, but in 1977 there were 80 government hospitals with 11,941 beds. Reports from the Catholic and Protestant missions

Table 8.1 Distribution of Hospital Beds in Kenya by Sponsorship, 1981

	Hospital Beds	
Sponsorship	(No.)	(Percent)
Government	13,000	46.2
Religious missions	7,000	25.0
Private	8,100	28.8
Total	28,100	100.0

for 1980 indicated a total of 6,955 beds (70 percent in hospitals and 30 percent in health centers). The remainder are in purely private facilities, although some of these are attached to industrial establishments. A report of the National Hospital Insurance Fund categorized 41 hospitals as private in 1982. Making adjustments for the different dates of these figures, and for the expansion of resources in recent years, one may estimate the 1981 distribution of hospital beds by sponsorship in Kenya as shown in table 8.1. Thus, about 46 percent of Kenyan hospital beds are public, including beds for lepers and the mentally ill. The percentage of *general* hospital beds would doubtless be lower. About 54 percent of the beds are in the private sector, with somewhat more than half of them being proprietary.

Other health facilities in Kenya include health centers, subcenters, dispensaries, and health posts—essentially for ambulatory care. In 1981, 262 health centers were reported to be in operation, of which 84 were sponsored by missions and an indeterminate number by enterprises or agricultural estates. The balance of 178, however, were undoubtedly governmental and were staffed by at least a clinical officer, who is capable of treating sickness and injuries. Health subcenters and dispensaries—also mainly, but not exclusively, governmental—numbered 1,130 in 1981. These units are staffed only by auxiliary personnel, who can offer preventive services (including family planning), first aid, and referral to other facilities when necessary.

Health Commodities

Virtually all medical equipment, supplies, appliances, and drugs used in Kenya are imported. For certain drugs, foreign firms have established plants in Nairobi, where tablets or other preparations are made and packaged from imported chemical products. As for traditional herbals, some are imported from Asian countries and some are prepared domestically. Since modern drugs are relatively expensive, requiring scarce foreign currency, there are frequent shortages, especially in governmental hospitals and other health facilities.

Some reflection of the importance of drugs in the entire Kenyan health care system is shown by data on MOH expenditures in 1977–78. In that fiscal year the Ministry had budgeted K.Sh. 72,587,860 for drugs in all its facilities. Actual expenditures, however, proved to be K.Sh. 111,557,120, or 54 percent higher. The total operating expenditures of the ministry that year were K.Sh. 518 million, so drugs absorbed 21.5 percent. (In a developed country, the equivalent expenditure would probably be between 5 and 10 percent.) Furthermore, serious losses of drugs in transit or in facilities are reported.

Health Knowledge

It has been noted that a Medical Research Institute, based in the Kenyatta National Hospital, is doing research on certain tropical diseases. Almost all health-related knowledge in Kenya, however, is acquired from abroad through journals and books. Casual observation suggests that the great bulk of medical literature comes from Great Britain or the United States. Each year, a number of Kenyan medical and public health personnel are sent to Europe and the United States for specialized studies. This is done largely through funding from international health agencies or bilateral aid programs.

The overall picture of health resources in Kenya is one of a meager supply in all categories. Considering the great poverty of the people, one might logically expect most of the resources to be in the public sector. In fact, the great majority of physicians serve a small minority of the population as private patients, and most hospital beds are in facilities requiring private payment for care. The human and physical resources in the public sector for the health care of most of the Kenyan people reflect a lower standard of capabilities. The population is about 85 percent rural, but medical resources are heavily concentrated in Nairobi and three other urban centers.

ECONOMIC SUPPORT

As in all countries, the economic support for the Kenyan health care system comes from many sources. With respect to several of these, only estimates can be made, but it is possible to show the approximate proportions from various sources. The available data may be presented under four headings: MOH, other governmental sources, organized, nonpublic sources, private spending.

Ministry of Health

For the fiscal year 1980–81, the total budget of the MOH was K.Sh. 1.131 billion. About 75 percent of this was for operating expenses and 25 percent for capital expenses (mainly to construct health care facilities). The MOH budget comprised 6.2 percent of the national government budget. Of the ministry's budget, about 11 percent came from foreign aid, multilateral or bilateral.

The breakdown of the MOH budget (table 8.2) shows the basic health policy of the government. The heavy expenditure on hospital services is evident, despite the announced policy of the ministry to put top priority on primary health care for the rural population. Expenditures for district hospitals, private hospital subsidies (essentially to mission hospitals), and funds for central and provincial hospitals together account for 72.9 percent of the total. About half of this, or 36 percent of total ministry expenditures, is devoted to support of the large Kenyatta National Hospital in Nairobi.

Other Governmental Sources

Health expenditures for 1980–81 have been reported for certain governmental agencies, although not for all of them (see table 8.3). Under the University of Nairobi, the support of three professional schools (medicine, dentistry, and pharmacy) is estimated as only K.Sh. 5 million because a substantial share is provided by the Kenyatta National Hospital. Other estimates are low insofar as health activities are only small portions of these ministerial functions. The total estimate for other governmental sources is K.Sh. 154 million.

Organized, Nonpublic Sources

Most important among these sources are the expenditures for the health activities of the religious missions. Data from the Kenya Catholic Secretariat and from the Protestant Churches Medical Association permit calculation of expenditures for 1980–81. The calculation is complicated by the fact that funds spent for operating these health facilities actually come from several sources, and one must avoid counting them twice.

Table 8.2 Ministry of Health Budget in Kenya by Purpose, 1980–81

Purpose	K.Sh. (millions)	Percent
Rural health services		
District hospitals	295.19	26.2
Private hospital subsidies	42.98	3.8
Other health facilities	133.46	11.9
Preventive services	75.78	6.7
Training	72.38	6.4
Supplies and equipment	21.49	1.9
Central and provincial hospitals	486.33	43.1
Total	1,127.61	100.00

Table 8.3 Health Expenditures of Other Kenya Governmental Agencies, 1980–81

Agency	K.Sh.
National Hospital Insurance Fund	43,500,000
Nairobi city council	75,000,000
Other municipal councils (3)*	12,000,000
Ministry of Water Development*	10,000,000
University of Nairobi (health profession schools)*	5,000,000
Ministry of Education (health education)*	2,000,000
Ministry of Agriculture (nutrition education)*	1,500,000
Ministry of Labor*	3,000,000
Ministry of Social Services*	1,000,000
Medical Research Institute*	1,000,000

*Estimates.

The Catholic Secretariat's medical department spent K.Sh. 72 million in 1980–81: about 52 million for hospitals and the balance for other units. Based on the approximate proportions of the two programs, Protestant medical activities must have cost about K.Sh. 25 million, or a total for both of K.Sh. 97 million. The Catholic organization does not provide a breakdown of the sources of its funds, but the Protestant organization publishes such data for each of its hospitals. On the basis of a sample of three of the larger Protestant hospitals, the sources of financing were distributed as shown in table 8.4. Patient and training fees are privately paid and will be considered below. The government grants have already been included in the expenditures of the MOH. These sources account for 84 percent of mission medical expenditures. The other charitable and miscellaneous sources account for 16 percent of total expenditures. Even though this calculation is derived

Table 8.4 Sources of Financing for Three Large Protestant Mission Hospitals, Kenya 1981

Source	Percent
Patient fees (inpatient and outpatient)	59.9
Training fees	0.6
Government (MOH) grants	23.5
Overseas income	2.5
Value of donated services	8.7
Other sources	4.8
Total	100.0

Table 8.5 Estimated Health Care Expenditures of Organized, Nonpublic Entities, Kenya 1981

Source	K.Sh.
Religious mission charity	15,520,000
Para-governmental enterprises (15)	3,000,000
Large business enterprises (10)	1,200,000
Agricultural estates	2,000,000
Voluntary health agencies (for example the Red Cross)	6,000,000
Total	27,720,000

from a sample of Protestant hospitals, it would seem reasonable to apply it to mission health services in general. Accordingly, 16 percent of the K.Sh. 97 million outlay estimated above amounts to K.Sh. 15.52 million.

Regarding other organized, nonpublic sources of health expenditures, crude estimates may be made as follows. For each of the 15 para-governmental enterprises, one may estimate annual health expenditures to average K.Sh. 200,000, or a total of K.Sh. 3 million. For the ten large firms with in-plant medical services, one may estimate annual expenditures of K.Sh. 120,000 each, or a total of K.Sh. 1.2 million. Similarly, other estimates are shown in table 8.5. One might expect the total for voluntary health agencies to be higher, but most of these agencies in Kenya receive government subsidies. Altogether, organized, nonpublic sources contribute about K.Sh. 27.72 million to support health services.

Private Spending

Financial support of the health care system from strictly private sources in Kenya is the most difficult to estimate. On the basis of

studies done in other developing countries, however, it is probably substantial. In Kenya, it was possible to use three methods of estimating.

In 1974, there was a well-organized household survey in Nairobi
that solicited information on recent household expenditures for all purposes. Stratified sampling was done from low-, middle-, and high-income households. Total household expenditures for all purposes were
K.Sh. 14,213 per year, of which K.Sh. 211.44 went for health care. To
arrive at a national average household health expenditure (since the
survey was limited to Nairobi), one could assume the rural household
to spend about two-thirds of the urban amount, or K.Sh. 142. A properly weighted national average comes to K.Sh. 150 per household.
Since the average Kenyan household has about six members, this
amounts to K.Sh. 25 per person per year for 1974.

Since 1974, inflation has occurred at 12 to 20 percent per year in
Kenya. Applying an average of 16 percent per year, the per capita
private health expenditure would have risen to K.Sh. 70.64 by 1981.
For a 1981 population of 16 million, the total health expenditure from
private households would come to K.Sh. 1,130,240,000.

A second method of calculating private health expenditures is to
start from the findings of the 1974 household survey concerning the
percentage of total expenditures allotted to health care. This varied by
household income, as follows: low-income households 0.66 percent,
middle-income households 1.24 percent, and high-income households
2.13 percent. The average health expenditure was 1.49 percent of
household income. For several reasons, however, this percentage should
be higher for 1981. For one thing, the 1974 survey deliberately under-
sampled high-income families (these families spend the highest percentage of their income on health care). Second, general health care
utilization rates in Kenya have been rising in recent years. Third,
overseas support of mission hospitals and clinics has been declining, so
a higher proportion of costs must be met by patient fees. Fourth, an
increasing proportion of physicians and hospital beds in Kenya are
private, and there is abundant evidence that private health care providers generate private demand. For all these reasons, it may be estimated that in 1981, the average Kenyan expenditure on health care
rose from 1.49 to about 1.80 percent of total household expenditures or
of per capita income.

The per capita GNP in Kenya for 1981 was about K.Sh. 4,000; this
is not identical with per capita income, but it is very close to it. Applying the 1.80 percent figure, health care expenditures would amount to
K.Sh. 72. For a population of 16 million, this would yield estimated
health expenditures of K.Sh. 1,152,000,000.

A third method of estimating private expenditures on health care is through a series of estimates of the gross earnings of all types of private health care providers in Kenya. These gross earnings, of course, are derived from the private payments made by patients. Thus, there are approximately 1,180 strictly private medical practitioners, not counting the part-time private practice of government physicians. One may estimate from several sources that full-time private doctors receive in patient fees an average of K.Sh. 30,000 per month. This would indicate gross expenditures of K.Sh. 424.8 million per year. Making equivalent estimates for various types of health care providers in Kenya, one derives the tabulation shown in table 8.6.

Discussions with several knowledgeable persons in Kenya who have been concerned with health services for many years indicate that the estimates in table 8.6 are very conservative. Nevertheless, this method of estimating private household health expenditures yields a figure higher than the other two methods. To be cautious, one may take the average of the three methods of estimating private expenditures (see table 8.7). It is now possible to offer combined estimates of the sources of all health care expenditures in Kenya for around 1981 (table 8.8).

In summary, national health expenditures from all sources in Kenya in 1981 amounted to K.Sh. 2,471,617,000. This money was derived 52 percent from public sources and 48 percent from private sources. The gross domestic product (GDP) (i.e., excluding consideration of imports and exports) of Kenya in 1981 was reported by the World Bank to be K.Sh. 51,608,000,000, a figure lower than the gross *national* product. Overall Kenyan expenditures for health purposes, therefore, were 4.8 percent of the GDP. For a developing African country, this is a relatively high expenditure.

MANAGEMENT OF THE HEALTH CARE SYSTEM

The management component of national health care systems permeates all other aspects—production of resources, organizational structure, and so on. One may briefly consider four main aspects: planning, administration, regulation, and evaluation.

Planning

The major planning for health services is done by a unit within the MOH. Its chief concern currently is the coverage of Kenya's rural

Table 8.6 Estimated Gross Earnings of Private Health Care Providers, Kenya 1981

Providers	Gross Earnings (K.Sh.)
Private medical practitioners (1,180)	424,800,000
Government physicians (505) at 25 percent of private	45,450,000
Private hospitals (about 15,000 beds) at K.Sh. 100 per day and 60 percent occupancy	330,000,000
Drugs purchased in pharmacies, estimated at 25 percent of physician fees	118,000,000
Dentists (150) at K.Sh. 300,000 per year	45,000,000
Traditional healers (16,000) at K.Sh. 1,000 per month	192,000,000
Traditional birth attendants, 80 percent of 800,000 births at K.Sh. 30 each	19,200,000
Other miscellaneous health expenditures	20,000,000
Total	1,194,450,000

Table 8.7 Results of Three Methods of Estimating Health Care Expenditures of Private Households, Kenya 1981

Method	K.Sh.
Household survey of 1974 adjusted to 1981	1,130,240,000
1.8 percent of per capita GNP	1,152,000,000
Gross income of private health care providers	1,194,450,000
Average	1,158,897,000

Table 8.8 Total Health Expenditures by Source, Kenya 1981

Source	K.Sh. (thousands)	Percent
Ministry of Health	1,131,000	
Other governmental agencies	154,000	
Total, public sector	1,285,000	52.0
Organized, nonpublic entities	27,720	
Private households	1,158,897	
Total, private sector	1,186,617	48.0
Grand total	2,471,617	100.00

areas with health centers and health posts, staffed with personnel as reviewed earlier. Although the plans put forward in 1972 were less than half implemented by 1982, efforts are still continuing along the lines of the original blueprint. The planning is done entirely at the central government level, but it is based partly on reports from the provinces and districts. The weakness of the general health information system would seem to be reflected in the fact that the MOH has not issued an annual report since 1968.

Kenya also has a Ministry of Economic Planning and Development (MEPD), which includes a subdivision concerned with health and social services. The scope of this concern, however, is limited essentially to the MOH's program. Neither MEPD's nor MOH's health planning is concerned with the health services of Kenya's private sector, which absorbs 48 percent of total national health expenditures. The Second Development Plan (1970–74) had noted the large private sector, and called on the Ministry of Health to provide closer supervision and integration of services. An evaluation later concluded, however, that "Unfortunately little progress was made in implementing this policy."

Within the MEPD is the central bureau of statistics, which has conducted surveys of household expenditures, including spending for health purposes (as noted above). This bureau also issues such valuable compendiums as the *Economic Survey 1982*, which contains data on the national supply of health facilities, hospital beds, health personnel, and so on.

As noted earlier, in spite of the espoused priority of primary health care for the rural population, some 73 percent of the MOH budget is devoted to the support of hospital services (half of this amount going to the Kenyatta National Hospital in Nairobi). This may reflect a basic disparity between planning or political rhetoric and the realities of the power structure in the Kenyan health care system.

Another discrepancy between planning objectives and reality is seen in the magnitude of the private market in medical care. Of the modest supply of physicians (about one per 10,000 people), 70 percent are in full-time private practice and most of the remainder are in part-time private practice. Fewer than half of the hospital beds are in governmental facilities. As stated in a 1982 MEPD document, *Development Prospects and Policies*, "Since Independence it has been the policy of Government to promote the private sector as a major vehicle for development." It is difficult to reconcile such a policy with the planning objective of achieving universal primary health care, or with the promise of the Kenyan Constitution for free universal medical service. As stated in an evaluative report of a USAID-supported project in 1978: "Uncontrolled growth of a private fee-for-service system of medical care in Kenya will have lasting and negative effects on the cost, quality, and access to basic health services for most of the people most of the time."

Administration

From the account of MOH programs above, it is evident that authority is exercised mainly from the top. This has been particularly so since a change of government policies in 1970. Both provincial and district medical officers are appointed by the central health authorities, and it is their duty to carry out national policies. Drugs and other supplies are distributed from the center to the eight provincial health offices, then to the 41 districts, and from there to the local health units. As noted earlier, under this pyramidal system, shortages are frequent at the local level.

At the provincial and district levels, the administrative responsibility of medical officers theoretically includes both hospital and primary health care services. The district and provincial hospitals, however, come under the technical direction of the central ministry. The hospitals of religious missions are entirely independent, although the subsidies they receive from the MOH imply a certain degree of coordination with the network of public facilities. Poor roads and insufficient vehicles and fuel mean that general supervision is weak throughout the entire structure of the offical MOH system. Appointments of supervisory personnel in the MOH program are theoretically governed by the rules of a civil service or public personnel system, but it is generally recognized that tribal affiliations play a part in such selections.

For some years, public health leadership throughout the world has stressed the importance of involving local people in the management and operation of local health services; with such community participation, it is expected that these services will be more acceptable to the people and more appropriately utilized. Throughout Kenya's 120 operating RHUs, however, such participation is rare. In some externally funded projects, such participation is actively encouraged—as in the Kibwezi Rural Health Scheme of the African Medical and Research Foundation, financed mainly by USAID. Because of the very low educational level of the rural population in Kenya, as in most other African countries, the involvement of people in the management of local health or other social services usually requires strong encouragement from higher authorities. Long colonial domination has typically inculcated a sense of dependency on, and sometimes distrust of, government.

Regulation

Aside from the MOH registration of physicians, dentists, fully trained nurses, pharmacists, and certain other health personnel, the regulation of professional performance is negligible. Likewise, private hospitals are theoretically required to have ministerial permission for their construction, but their operation is not subject to surveillance; the same applies to mission hospitals. Legislation on the sale of drugs has existed in Kenya since colonial times, but resources for its enforcement are very weak. Except for narcotics, almost any drug may be purchased from a pharmacy or an unlicensed drug peddler, with or without a medical prescription. There is no regulation at all of traditional healers or of the remedies they sell.

Probably the most significant regulation in the Kenyan health services takes place within the hierarchical program of the MOH. Since official policy encourages the development of the private medical care market, private providers of care are constrained by a minimum of regulation or surveillance. The weak enforcement of factory regulations on health and safety, due to insufficient inspectors, was noted earlier.

Evaluation

Little is done in Kenya in the way of evaluating health services as a guide to program management. The flow of information on vital health events or the utilization of services is too irregular to permit such evaluation on a regular basis. Occasionally, outside agencies have evaluated selected health needs, such as malnutrition in children or the effectiveness of family planning programs.

DELIVERY OF HEALTH SERVICES

The earlier reference to coverage of 20 to 30 percent of the rural population for MOH primary health care gives a general idea of the inadequacy of health service delivery in Kenya. It is almost certain that the majority of people depend on self-care or on traditional healers for most of their day-to-day health needs. At least 70 percent of deliveries are done by traditional birth attendants. Pure and safe water is inaccessible to the majority of people, and outside the two main cities sanitary disposal of excreta is rare.

The pattern of delivery of personal health service in Kenya varies with the source from which it is sought. A study in one rural district identified some 6,800 complaints occurring in a two-week period. For the largest fraction of these, which were actually minor symptoms, no action was taken; for the next largest fraction, the response was self-medication. The overall distribution of the types of health care received

Table 8.9 Types of Health Care for Illness Complaints by Residents of a Rural District, Kenya 1980

Source of Care	Complaints (Percent)
None sought	37.5
Self-medication	35.2
Governmental health center or hospital	13.8
Church facility	3.5
Private physician	3.5
Traditional healer	4.1
Other or unknown	2.4
Total	100.0

is shown in table 8.9. Many rural people think that it is illegal to consult traditional healers, so these responses are probably underreported. In fact, out of the 35.2 percent of responses categorized as "self-medication," 5.3 percent involved use of traditional herb remedies; added to the percent consulting traditional healers, this would amount to 9.4 percent of the total responses.

Of the various sources of health care, those from governmental and church facilities can be considered organized to some extent. The health teams in MOH health centers have been described. In the church mission units there are also usually nurses, working with or backed up by physicians. The use of mission facilities requires payment of small fees. The principal provider of care in the governmental health centers, it will be recalled, is not a doctor but a clinical officer. Only 20 to 30 percent of the rural population has access to an MOH health center.

Individual, nonorganized care is the normal mode of delivery by a traditional healer, and it is rendered typically in the home of the patient. The private physician, on the other hand, typically sees patients in his office (which is often attached to his home). This same physician may, during official hours, work in a district hospital. Sometimes he owns a "clinic," staffed by a nurse, that he visits periodically. In rural areas, medical fees are very low; otherwise few rural patients could afford care. In Nairobi, on the other hand, where a middle class is developing, the fees charged by private specialists may be very high, such as K.Sh. 200 for a visit to a pediatrician or K.Sh. 250 for an emergency visit to a private hospital.

Medical services in both governmental and mission hospitals are delivered by organized staffs of salaried physicians. Only the private hospitals have open staffs, in which private physicians are paid fees.

The general staffing of public hospitals, however, is very frugal, particularly in nursing and ancillary services. To discourage excessively long stays, patients are required to pay K.Sh. 20 per day. Mission hospitals tend to be better staffed and equipped, but their charges for inpatient care are much higher. Private hospitals are luxurious in comparison with the other types. It was to make private and some mission facilities financially accessible to middle-class families that the National Hospital Insurance Fund was established in 1966.

Before national independence, beds in both public and private hospitals were generally separate, and care was better, for the small population of Europeans and Asians. Special private hospitals were built for Asians in Nairobi and Mombasa. In the large mental hospital in Nairobi, for example, the expenditure per patient-day for the European-Asian wards was five times that for the African wards. Conditions in the latter wards were described in a 1946 government report as resembling a "totally unsuitable prison environment." Such segregation is no longer tolerated on racial or ethnic grounds, but an equivalent separation now occurs on the basis of wealth and social class.

Medical care of the tertiary level is provided mainly at the large Kenyatta National Hospital in Nairobi and at some of the eight provincial general hospitals. Many of the physicians and surgeons on the medical staffs have had specialty training in Europe and the United States and carry on very lucrative practices in their own private clinics after official hours. Even during official hospital hours, 10 percent of their time may be spent seeing private patients; inpatient care for private patients, however, is usually given at a private hospital.

Finally, one may note the organized, general health services available to employees (and sometimes their families) of para-governmental enterprises. Some health care is also provided in large private factories, though only for the worker and for work-related conditions. The Kenyan military services, of course, are also served by an organized program of comprehensive health care.

All in all, health care and general development in Kenya reflect the social policies of a low-income African country recently liberated from colonial rule but committed largely (though not entirely) to a free market economy. Sustaining the private sector are policies that encourage investments by foreign corporations, provide government subsidies to the health facilities of private religious missions, authorize (even encourage) private medical practice by government doctors, and so on. The private health sector is inevitably enhanced by the growing demands of a slowly expanding middle class, by the meager salaries paid to public medical officers, and by the obvious inadequacies of the governmental health services.

On the other hand, public sector health services, both preventive and therapeutic, are sustained by a program of national health planning that aims to make primary health care accessible to the entire population by the hard work and dedication of many public health leaders and by the concern of government for human welfare, if only in the interests of maintaining social stability. With Kenya's one-party political system, free expression is obviously inhibited and discontent among younger military officers and university students can be explosive—as it was in August 1982. Events of this sort, in the long run, are likely to strengthen the public sector, as the government strives to attain health care equity for the general population.

REFERENCES

African Medical and Research Foundation, *AMREF in Action* (Nairobi, 1981).

Family Health Institute, "A Working Paper on Health Services Development in Kenya: Issues, Analyses, and Recommendations" (Washington, D.C.: U.S. Agency for International Development, 1978).

Kenya Catholic Secretariat, Medical Department, "Catholic Health Care, Facilities and Services January–December 1980" (Nairobi, 1981).

Mburu, F. M., "Rhetoric—Implementation Gap in Health Policy and Health Services Delivery for a Rural Population in a Developing Country," *Social Science and Medicine* 13A(1979):577–83.

_____, "Socio-Political Imperatives in the History of Health Development in Kenya," *Social Science and Medicine* 15A(1981):521–27.

Ministry of Economic Planning and Development, *Economic Survey 1982* (Nairobi, 1982), 213–17.

_____, Kenya Development Plan 1979–83 (Nairobi, 1979), 33–34.

Ministry of Finance, Central Bureau of Statistics, *Consumer Price Indices, Nairobi* (Nairobi, 1977).

Nordberg, E. *On the True Disease Pattern in Kibwezi Division* (Nairobi: African Medical and Research Foundation, 1981).

Republic of Kenya, Ministry of Health, *Proposal for the Improvement of Rural Health Services and the Development of Rural Health Training Centres in Kenya* (Nairobi, 1972).

World Health Organization, "Kenya," in *Sixth Report of the World Health Situation 1973–1977* (Geneva, 1980), part 2, 20–22.

9

Progress in Malaysia's
Rural Health Services

In 1953, Malaysia, with some international assistance, launched a Rural Health Services Scheme to improve health care for its large rural population. An evaluation in 1968 showed impressive accomplishments during the first 15 years. By 1982, the program's coverage had been extended to the vast majority of the peninsular population. This chapter describes how this further progress was achieved in Malaysia, a welfare state of developing countries.

In 1953, the British colonial government controlling the Malay Peninsula in Southeast Asia launched a program to improve health services for the rural population. Since the early nineteenth century, the British had dominated Malaya through a complex series of arrangements with various locally ruling sultans. During World War II, the peninsula was occupied by the Japanese; after the war, in 1948, a Communist-inspired guerrilla movement arose in the north. Hostilities continued until the revolutionary movement was finally suppressed in 1953. Then, in order to improve the miserable conditions of rural life (which had contributed to the growth of dissidence), several agricultural, educational, and welfare reforms were started—including the Rural Health Services Scheme (RHSS).

Based on observations made in August 1982, while serving as an external examiner in the Department of Social and Preventive Medicine of the University of Malaya, Kuala Lumpur, Malaysia.

THE RURAL HEALTH SERVICES
SCHEME (1953–68)

The Federation of Malaya achieved independence in 1957, and in 1963 it joined with other former British colonies in north Borneo (Sabah and Sarawak) to become the current nation of Malaysia. The RHSS gradually extended its coverage, which consisted largely of the development of resources (facilities and personnel), to meet the major primary health care needs of defined rural population groups of about 50,000 people. For each such group there would be a main health center staffed by a physician, a public health nurse, a sanitary inspector, and several auxiliary health personnel. Each main health center would have four health subcenters, each serving about 10,000 people and staffed entirely with auxiliary health personnel. Finally, in the villages around each subcenter would be four midwife clinics to handle childbirths for a population of 2,500.

To train the many auxiliary health personnel needed to staff these facilities, special programs were organized by the Ministry of Health (MOH) in two of the main health centers. Assistant nurses, assistant midwives, and health overseers (equivalent to junior sanitary inspectors) were trained in relatively large numbers through short courses emphasizing health promotion and prevention.

The RHSS assigned a hospital assistant to each of the health centers for treatment services. These rural doctor-substitutes were a heritage from the Colonial Medical Service, but now they were receiving more systematic training at large general hospitals. Hospital assistants had to be secondary school graduates and take a course similar in length (but different in scope) to that for registered nurses. They were expected to treat, ordinarily with drugs, all common ailments, referring more complicated cases to the physician at the main health center.

There were 45 district hospitals with between 100 and 200 beds to provide medical backup for the 47 health districts. These hospitals were very modestly staffed, principally with assistant nurses and perhaps two or three doctors, none of them specialists. At the top of the health care pyramid were nine general hospitals, one in each state capital. A fairly wide range of full-time medical and surgical specialists, along with registered nurses, technicians, and other personnel, staffed these tertiary care hospitals.

For administrative backup, each RHSS unit came under the supervision of the medical officer of health responsible for public health work in that district. The public health nurse and sanitary inspector in the district offices served as consultants to equivalent personnel in the rural health centers. The district medical officer, however, had no technical or administrative responsibility for the district hospital. All hospitals, as well as the entire RHSS program, came under the ultimate supervision of the chief medical and health officer of each state. These state officials and all the district health personnel were appointed by the MOH.

All RHSS services were provided free of charge. Costs of the scheme were sustained by the MOH, whose budget was derived from general revenues. While promoting equity, this policy led to one serious problem: the funds available for physician salaries were relatively meager, so the majority of Malaysian doctors chose to engage in private practice. Such practice was invariably in the cities. As a result, virtually all the doctors serving in the health centers of the RHSS were foreign physicians on temporary contracts with the MOH. In 1968, these doctors were mainly from South Korea and the Philippines.

It was in 1968 that I served as a consultant for the World Health Organization to evaluate the accomplishments of the RHSS after its first 15 years.[1] As of December 1967, there had been established 39 main health centers, 139 subcenters, and 703 midwife clinics. The medical staffing of the main centers was entirely by expatriate physicians, and there were frequent vacancies in various other posts. Considering the entire rural population of peninsular Malaysia, the RHSS coverage for primary care was estimated at about 40 percent. In spite of the RHSS's relatively rapid growth, there was much evidence that rural people favored traditional healers in the *kampongs* (villages) over the RHSS resources. For sickness, villagers went most often to the village *bomoh*, and for childbirth to the village *bidan*. If a town was nearby, they might consult a Chinese traditional practitioner or herbalist. The few rural people who could afford it consulted private general medical practitioners.

Enlargement of rural health resources over these 15 years had been substantial. The national infant mortality rate (reflecting mainly the country's 75 percent rural population) declined from 75 per 1,000 live births in 1957 to 48 per 1,000 in 1966. For the Malay ethnic group (about 50 percent of the total population but 90 percent of the rural population), the decline was from 96 to 58 infant deaths per 1,000 live births. Between 1956 and 1965, attendances at facilities of the RHSS rose from 4,492,000 to 6,970,000. There was, nevertheless, clearly room for improvement, both in the quantitative coverage of the RHSS and in certain patterns of its administration. Its weaknesses as of 1968 are highlighted in this summary of the recommendations submitted in my report to the WHO.

1. The nation must be carefully mapped with respect to the ecology of the population, location and coverage of all health facilities, and political lines, in order to identify gaps requiring new construction and to define reasonable districts for combined rural and urban health service administration.

2. At the health district level, the administration of hospitals and all public health services should be integrated, to strengthen the scope and quality of both prevention and treatment.

3. A third echelon of short-stay beds at selected health centers should be added to the current network of district and general hospitals, and relationships among them all should be facilitated.

4. Doctors should be posted at every health subcenter, as well as at main centers in the RHSS, through a system of rural service required as part of medical education prior to licensure.

5. Responsibilities for tuberculosis control and malaria eradication should be delegated, under national standards, to the local health districts so that these and other efforts to control communicable diseases can be integrated into the regular RHSS operations.

6. Consideration should be given to training a combined "assistant nurse-midwife" for a broader range of maternal and child health work and to extending the scope of professional nurse services beyond the field of maternal and child health.

7. The staffing of rural health units with environmental health personnel should be much increased, and their training should be upgraded.

8. Specialists (nonmedical) in health education should be trained and posted throughout the health districts; their work should include educational programs on the hazards of magical healing and unscientific drugs.

9. Training programs, both inside and outside the RHSS, should be strengthened further, and certain personnel policies should be made more flexible to increase staff stability and improve morale.

10. To meet the costs of the above recommendations, consideration should be given to new forms of taxation that would not increase national expenditures, but rather shift the alloca-

tions from the private to the public sector, where health services can be provided more efficiently.

Regarding these recommendations as points of entry to analysis of progress in the RHSS over the subsequent years, one may now consider the Malaysian health scene in 1982.

RURAL HEALTH SERVICE PROGRESS (1968–82)

First of all, the basic trends in the physical foundations of the RHSS should be noted. These are summarized in Table 9.1.

The number of main health centers had more than doubled, and there were substantial increases in the number of other rural health facilities. A new type of facility, the rural health clinic, had appeared by 1982. Further, the staffing of all types of facilities had been much strengthened.

In terms of the 1968 recommendations, overall progress in Malaysia has been impressive. The nation has been relatively prosperous over these years, with a major economic boost coming from the recent discovery of oil. A review of health developments should not, of course, simply attribute these developments to the recommendations. The most that any outside technical consultant in the health field can do is to offer some support for the efforts of certain health leaders in the country.

In the early 1970s, a health planning division was established in the MOH. There had previously been a planning office, which was concerned with architectural blueprints for hospitals and health centers. This function became designated as the microplanning function of the new division, while macroplanning was concerned with achieving geographic health care coverage of the nation. The expansion of rural health facilities increased coverage of the rural population in peninsular Malaysia to 85 percent (from 40 percent in 1968). Special efforts were being made to improve rural health services in East Malaysia (Sabah and Sarawak), which had previously been almost ignored.

Changes in administration at the health district level were not significant. In a few sparsely populated districts, responsibility for the district hospital was integrated with that for the local public health program under the district medical officer. In most of the larger districts where this was attempted, however, it did not prove feasible. Management of the hospital absorbed so much effort that the public health program suffered. Yet, it should be noted that the district medical officer's staff was not strengthened, and the district hospitals were still without any trained hospital administrators. With the growth of

Table 9.1 Trends in the Rural Health Services
Scheme, Malaysia 1960–82

| | Year | | |
Facility	1960	1968	1982
Main health centers	8	39	82
Health subcenters	8	139	249
Midwife clinics	26	703	878
Rural health clinics	—	—	640

population and an administrative framework, the health districts increased from 47 in 1968 to 64 in 1982.

The addition of sick bays with three to five beds was attempted in certain main health centers, but problems developed for provision of 24-hour service to these patients. In a few quite isolated health centers, the pattern was found useful to hold patients until they could be transported to a district hospital. In Sabah and Sarawak, moreover, establishment of a few beds in the main health centers had become standard policy.

The posting of doctors in the health subcenters, recommended in 1968, had emerged as a major policy issue. As a means to this end, legislation was enacted requiring virtually all new medical graduates to devote three years to government service after their medical qualification and one year's housemanship (internship). If the student had received fellowship support for living expenses during medical school years, the obligation for government service increased by ten years to a total of 13 years. So great was the expectation that this would achieve medical staffing of the subcenters, the MOH began to speak of converting the three-tier framework of the RHSS into a two-tier framework. In other words, every health center would serve a population of 15,000 to 20,000 (instead of 50,000) and would be surrounded by several rural community clinics (see below).

This conception was still far from implemented by 1982. The increased number of main health centers (from 39 to 82) since 1968 had been due partly to such upgrading of subcenters and partly to new construction. But there were also 249 health subcenters without medical staffing, although the staffing with nurses, midwives, and sanitation overseers was generally stronger. The young medical graduates putting in their three years of government service were, in fact, posted mostly in district and provincial hospitals. Furthermore, after some years, numerous graduates (about 150 qualifying each year from the University of Malaya) avoided the obligation of government service by getting immediate admission into specialty training programs in Malaysia or other countries. Altogether, some 60 percent of medical graduates were estimated to be fulfilling government service requirements. Many of the 82 main health centers were, as a result, still being staffed by expatriate physicians under contract, as in 1968. The origins of these contract doctors had simply changed from Korea and the Philippines to Indonesia and Bangladesh.

The mandatory government medical service did have a major impact on the staffing of district hospitals that served rural populations. In 1968, a district hospital of 100 to 150 beds might be staffed by two or three general practitioners responsible for all inpatient and outpatient care. In 1982, the norm became five or six doctors in the district hospitals, along with many more nurses and other personnel. The number of hospitals in peninsular Malaysia, furthermore, increased from 54 to 88 (both general provincial and district facilities). Counting only government facilities for short-term care (that is, excluding hospitals for mental illness, tuberculosis, and leprosy), the bed-population ratio remained stationary at 1.59 per 1,000 between 1970 and 1980. The construction of short-term hospital beds only in proportion to population growth over the decade may be regarded as reflecting a high priority for primary health care (in contrast to the all-too-frequent emphasis on hospital bed expansion). At the same time, utilization of the available hospital beds evidently became more efficient. Average length of stay in short-term hospitals decreased from nine to seven days, so more patients could be accommodated in the same number of beds. Put in another way, the average hospital bed served 40.6 patients per year in 1970 and 53.0 patients in 1980.

Regarding the proposed integration of all forms of communicable disease control (especially for tuberculosis and malaria) with other public health activities at the local level, much had been done. With respect to tuberculosis, BCG vaccination of newborns, as well as case finding and ambulatory treatment, have been delegated to the district health officers. Malaria case detection and preventive drug management have also been so delegated. Vector control programs are still conducted by the MOH, and technical guidance is, reasonably enough, provided from the top.

Perhaps the most important program change in the RHSS recommended in 1968 has been the expanded role of the trained rural midwives.[2] My proposal had been to supplement the midwife's training so that she could provide well-baby care and to broaden the training of assistant nurses (in health subcenters) beyond the field of maternal and child health. In fact, the MOH went much further: influenced undoubtedly by the worldwide movement toward strengthening primary health care in rural areas (the WHO-UNICEF Alma Alta Conference was held in 1978), it gave hundreds of midwives six months of additional training in primary health care. As noted earlier, 640 former midwife clinics have been converted into rural health clinics through such supplemental training, along with the provision of certain essential drugs for common ailments and vaccines for immunization. The other 878 midwife clinics, still functioning in 1982, are to be converted into rural health clinics as rapidly as the necessary training can be given.

Progress may also be reported in the environmental sanitation of rural Malaysia. The training of public health inspectors at the Public Health Institute in Kuala Lumpur has been increased from one to three years. Larger numbers of public health overseers have also been trained, and there are nine field training units instead of the two operating in 1968. The overseer's job has also been made more attractive by the establishment of a senior grade. As a result, between 1970 and 1980, the percentage of the rural population of peninsular Malaysia who were provided with safe public water increased from 3.2 to 11.3. Similarly, the percentage of this population provided with sanitary latrines rose from 25 to 45.

The strengthening of health education in the RHSS has been only moderate. Personnel are still trained at the Public Health Institute (operated by the MOH, but without university ties), and their role at the provincial level is being enlarged. The district health offices still do not have health educators, but other personnel—nurses, sanitarians, and so on—have been prepared to carry out health educational activities. For reasons that are doubtless political, however, no attempt has been made to educate people about the possible hazards of traditional healing or traditional medication.

The recommendations on personnel policy in the governmental health services of Malaysia were designed mainly to make public service more attractive to physicians, compared to private practice. Action was taken along these lines by upgrading the rank of doctors doing clinical work so that they would not have to become medical administrators to enjoy higher salaries. It is still often necessary, however, for a physician or surgeon warranting promotion to be transferred to another hospital.

As for health personnel training programs in general, their capacities have been greatly enlarged since 1968. Several of these have been noted above. Regarding medical education, the first medical school at the University of Malaya had yet to graduate its first class in 1968. Since then, some 12 classes of about 150 doctors have been turned out, and two additional medical schools have been started. One is at the National University in Kuala Lumpur, which has graduated a few classes already, and the other has recently been launched in the University of Sciences at Penang. When all three schools are fully operating, about 350 doctors a year will be graduated.

The final recommendation concerned development of new forms of taxation that would, in effect, channel more funds from the private to the public sector in order to strengthen governmental health services. Although new forms of taxation have not been enacted, governmental expenditures for health purposes have increased considerably. A social insurance program for urban wage earners had been contemplated, but it was not carried out. The annual public expenditures for health between 1971 and 1975 were M$183.24 million ($1 Malaysian is equal to $0.40 U.S.), and this rose to M$314.54 million in the 1976–1980 period. For 1981 to 1985, the allocation (usually larger than actual expenditures) will be M$603.54 million per year. These public outlays for health have clearly grown at a faster rate than the population.

These numerous indicators of progress in the health services of Malaysia, particularly for the rural population, reflect the value put on health care activities by the political leaders. Since the vast majority of rural people are ethnically Malays (rather than Chinese or Indian), this coincided with the political interests of the Malayan sultans and public authorities. At the same time, the private sector in health services has expanded. As a result, certain problems persist in the effort to achieve equitable health care. These problems and issues will be discussed, but first the evidence on changes in the population's health status over the last decade or so should be noted.

HEALTH IMPROVEMENTS AND PERSISTENT PROBLEMS

Statistical data on health are reported regularly to the WHO. From these reports it can be seen that, between 1957 and 1975, the life expectancy in Malaysia rose for men from 56 to 65.4 years and for women from 58 to 70.7 years. The infant mortality rate declined from 75.5 per 1,000 live births in 1959 to 30.7 per 1,000 in 1976. For the 1–4 year age groups (highly vulnerable in developing countries), the death-rate declined from 11.0 to 2.6 per 1,000 over the same years. Maternal mortality fell from 2.8 per 1,000 births in 1957 to 0.8 per 1,000 in 1974.[3]

These data apply to the entire national population of Malaysia, but since some 75 percent is rural (populations in places of less than 10,000 people), the improvement undoubtedly reflects rural trends. These facts, of course, do not tell us how much the trends are attributable to the rural or the urban health services, as such, compared with the influence of general standards of living. Housing, education, and other aspects of life have also shown advancement, and these obviously influence health. One can only say that the RHSS probably contributed to improved health status in the population. With the same caveats, it may be noted that the incidence of new cases of pulmonary tuberculosis fell from 90.6 per 100,000 population in 1970 to 73.5 per 100,000 in 1980.

A birth control (family planning) program was operating in Malaysia in 1968 as an autonomous activity outside the MOH (in the Office of the Prime Minister). It was carried out principally through voluntary agencies. This inefficient arrangement obviously reflected certain political considerations. By 1982, the family planning program had become fully integrated with the maternal and child health services of the MOH. Malaysia's crude birthrate in 1957 had been 46.0 per 1,000 population; it fell to 33.7 per 1,000 in 1976. Once again, this progress must surely be attributable to the family planning program, as well as to improvements in the general standard of living. A related trend that could not be quantified, but that was asserted by several health officials, concerned childbirths. In 1968, the deliveries in rural areas were done much more frequently by traditional village midwives than by the trained midwives of the RHSS units; in 1982, this relationship had been reversed.

The increasing output of doctors in Malaysia has been noted; nevertheless, foreign medical graduates were still being recruited for governmental health posts in 1982. As a result, the ratio of doctors to population rose from 18.9 per 100,000 in 1967 to 26.3 per 100,000 in 1980. Over the years, the population of doctors working in the public sector, as distinguished from private practice, rose from 40.5 percent in 1969 to 56.2 percent in 1978; much of this trend was undoubtedly due to the mandatory three-year period of government service. In the last few years, the trend has reversed, and in 1980 publicly employed doctors declined to 51.1 percent. This private sector of medical care explains certain persistent problems in Malaysia. It has the effect of diverting a disproportionate share of health care resources to the minority of the population who can afford to pay for services at the expense of the majority, who cannot.

Another aspect of the private medical sector is specialization. In 1968, virtually all private doctors were general practitioners; care by a specialist was hardly available outside the public hospital system. In recent years, however, mounting proportions of private doctors have become specialists. Although they are usually trained to specialty rank in the governmental system, they have left it to engage in private practice. This trend has been made possible by the rapid growth of private hospitals, where private specialists can treat their patients. In 1968, hospital beds in government facilities or on isolated estates and mines (where hospitals are mandated by law) constituted 95 percent of the total. Scarcely 5 percent of the beds were in private facilities. By 1982, 12 percent of the beds in short-term general hospitals were under private auspices. Only a few of the 100 private hospitals were operated by religious missions (where personal payments are also required). The vast majority were owned by doctors and were operated for profit; they are often called medical centers or specialist centers.

This growth of private specialization in Malaysia has created problems for the provincial general hospitals, which require a wide range of specialists. The prominence of specialization in medicine has also affected the attitudes of the people. Rural and small-town people with conditions that could be perfectly well served at district hospitals bypass these facilities and go directly to the larger provincial hospitals, where specialists are available. As a result, district hospital occupancies have greatly declined (to 40 to 60 percent), while provincial hospitals are overcrowded. The pressures induce the public hospital specialists to leave for private practice—continuing the vicious circle.

Finally, insight on the overall character of the Malaysian health services can be gathered through certain financial data. In 1973, a nationwide survey was conducted on household expenditures for all purposes, including medical or related care and drugs. In peninsular Malaysia, both urban and rural, these health-related expenditures were found to account for 1.7 percent of total household expenditures. This amounted to M$62.64 per household per year. Since the average Malaysian household in 1973 had 5.4 persons, the personal health expenditure was M$11.60 per capita per year. For the peninsular Malaysian population of 9.5 million in 1973, this meant private health expenditures of M$110 million.

Comparable data on *total* governmental expenditures for health purposes are not available for 1973, but MOH expenditures comprise the bulk of governmental health spending. For the period 1971 to 1975, MOH expenditures were M$183.24 million per year. In addition, money is spent on health (mostly for environmental sanitation) by other ministries and by municipalities. It would be reasonable to estimate that those expenditures would bring the total for the public sector to M$200 million in 1973. Accordingly, total health-related spending in that year would have been about M$310 million of which about 65 percent was in the public sector and 35 percent in the private sector. If these proportions are approximately correct, the public sector in Malaysia's national health care system is much stronger than in many other developing countries. Where studies have been made in such countries, private health spending has typically been much greater than public. (In Thailand, for example, the private health sector accounts for 65 percent of the total.) Malaysia, on the contrary, is perhaps a "welfare state" among developing countries.

For 1981–82, the MOH budget was somewhat in excess of one billion Malaysian dollars. The current amount of private spending is not known, but in medical practice and hospitalization the private sector has expanded recently. At the same time, there has been impressive growth in public medical and health services over the years since 1968. In all probability, the progress observed in the RHSS, launched in 1953 after bitter hostilities with a rural guerrilla movement, can be attributed to the substantial allocation of resources by the government to the country's health care system.

NOTES

1. M. I. Roemer, *Rural Health Services Scheme of Malaysia* (Manila: World Health Organization, Regional Office of the Western Pacific, 1969).
2. P. C. Y. Chen, "Providing Maternal and Child Care in Rural Malaysia," *Tropical and Geographical Medicine* 29(1977):441–48.
3. Office of the Prime Minister, "Health and Social Welfare," in *Fourth Malaysia Plan 1981–1985* (Kuala Lumpur, 1981), 369–81.

10

Public and Private Support of Health Activities in Developing Countries

The source of funds to support health care and other health activities reflects, in large measure, the degree of social responsibility assumed in a nation for those activities. Quantitative data on health expenditures have been collected in industrialized countries for several decades, but in developing countries only recently. The relatively small proportions of health care expenditures that come from public sources in most developing countries have serious implications for health care equity and efficiency.

For centuries, a sense of social responsibility for the health of all people has been maturing throughout the world. The pace of this maturation has differed among countries in relation to their economic and political circumstances. In all countries, however, this social maturation has been reflected in increasing public, as opposed to private, assumption of financial responsibility for health services and health-related activities.

Based on a paper presented at the annual conference of the National Council for International Health, Washington, D.C., 16 June 1982.

DEVELOPMENT OF SOCIAL SUPPORT
FOR HEALTH

Economic support for health care in primitive societies was undoubtedly personal, through barter between patient and healer. In the city-states of ancient Greece, however, taxes were used to pay doctors for the treatment of sick freemen (not slaves) who were poor. In Rome, sewers drained wastewater for environmental sanitation at public expense. In the Middle Ages, hospitals were built initially by religious bodies, but in time their maintenance was supported by local governments. After 1600, local governments also paid certain doctors to treat the sick, though "worthy," poor outside a hospital.

With the decline of feudalism and the rise of industry and urbanization, private medical practice arose in the cities. But workers and their families soon found that disabling illness could be devastating, both because of the loss of earnings and because of the costs of medical care. In response, they formed mutual sickness funds, or voluntary health cooperatives. This social responsibility for health care costs was so helpful that after the 1880s it evolved into statutory social insurance. This soon spread to all the industrialized countries and after 1924 to increasing numbers of developing countries, even where industrial workers were only a small fraction of the population.

Throughout the nineteenth and twentieth centuries, the scope of health services, and of other health activities in support of them, broadened tremendously. Organized provision of preventive and health promotive services acquired a definite place in the governments of all countries. Organized programs for supporting medical care of the poor took shape in all industrialized countries. In the developing lands of Asia, Africa, and Latin America—predominantly colonies in the nineteenth century—central authorities built hospitals and introduced some urban sanitation. After liberation, these newly independent countries greatly extended their resources for medical care and public health.

Aside from financing direct health service delivery, public taxes were used for development of resources needed to support health care systems. The training of health personnel was essential, and this was done at universities and other institutions financed mainly by government. Except in the United States, this was true in all the industrialized countries. In the developing countries, education for the health professions and occupations was also overwhelmingly tax-supported. In addition to hospitals, all sorts of health centers and health posts for general ambulatory care were constructed at public expense in most developing countries. Biomedical research was conducted mainly in the industrialized countries, but in all types of countries health-related research depended principally or entirely on public funding.

Side-by-side with the development of these social financing mechanisms for health care systems, purely private financial support has continued. Private spending has been applied mainly to selected components of health care systems. Broadly speaking, the development of public financial responsibility has been more rapid and wider in scope in the industrialized countries. Conversely, private support plays a relatively larger part in the support of health care systems in most developing countries. Exceptions are found in countries like China and Cuba, which have had Socialist revolutions, but what are the facts in countries with free market economies?

MAJOR SOURCES OF HEALTH SYSTEM FINANCING

The development of social responsibility for health in the industrialized countries has obvious implications for the equity of health care distribution. It also is undoubtedly related to the overall share of national wealth devoted to health activities. This is strikingly shown in the United States, where long-term data are available. In 1929, all health-related expenditures constituted 3.5 percent of the GNP; this figure rose slowly to 4.4 percent over the next 25 years. By 1980, moreover, the percentage of GNP devoted to health had risen much more rapidly, to 9.4 percent. During this span of years, the proportion of spending derived from public or other social sources (governmental revenues, voluntary insurance, charity, and so on) rose at a remarkably parallel pace: in 1929 it was 11.6 percent of all expenditures on health care, in 1955 it was 41.9 percent, and in 1980 it was 67.6 percent. This parallelism surely suggests that collectivized financing (most of which is from governmental revenues) results in greater allocations to health than purely private financing.

The same dynamics seen longitudinally in the United States are evident in a comparison of the size and derivation of health expenditures in different countries of the world today. Data on governmental health expenditures are given in table 10.1. The industrialized countries spend 5.0 percent or more of their GNPs on health activities. The developing countries, except for Honduras, spend 4.2 percent or less of their GNPs on health activities. In a word, the industrialized countries spend larger percentages of larger GNPs on health, while the developing countries spend smaller percentages of smaller GNPs. Further, all

Table 10.1 Total Health Expenditures in Selected
Countries, 1970s

	Expenditures	
Country	*Percent of GNP*	*Percent from Public Sources*
Industrialized Countries		
Sweden	7.3	91.8
Netherlands	7.3	69.9
Canada	6.8	75.0
Australia	6.5	76.9
United States	6.3	38.1
Great Britain	5.2	88.5
Belgium	5.0	84.0
Developing Countries		
Honduras	5.1	37.3
Thailand*	4.2	34.5
Ghana	4.0	27.5
Sudan	3.7	59.5
Sri Lanka	3.0	60.0
South Korea[†]	2.7	13.4
India	2.5	16.0
Pakistan	2.4	37.5
Philippines	1.9	21.1
Bangladesh[‡]	—	13.5

Source: principally, World Bank, *Health: Sector Policy Paper*
(Washington, D.C., 1980), 25.

*M.I. Roemer, *The Health Care System of Thailand* (New Delhi:
WHO South-East Asia Regional Office, 1981), 20.

[†]Chong Kee Park, *Financing Health Services in Korea* (Seoul:
Korea Development Institute, 1977).

[‡]World Health Organization, *Financing of Health Services: Report of a WHO Study Group,* technical report series no. 625 (Geneva, 1978), 59–65.

but one (the United States) of the seven industrialized countries derive the great majority of their health funds from government. (Indeed, if voluntary insurance were included in the public sources, this would apply to the United States also.) Among the ten developing countries, on the other hand, all but two (Sudan and Sri Lanka) derive only a small fraction of health funds from government.

The policy implications of these data would seem to be clear: higher relative allocations to the health sector probably require greater governmental expenditures. The implications of such a policy for attaining equity in health care would seem to be equally clear. Moreover, within the health sector there are many components of varying importance for effective operation of the health care system. The proportionate expenditures for these components, derived from public and private sources, have further implications for health policy formulation.

SUPPORT OF HEALTH CARE SYSTEM COMPONENTS

Health care systems may be analyzed in various ways. After studying the structure and functions of these systems in numerous countries, I believe that any national health care system can be described in terms of five components: production of resources, organization of programs, economic support, management, and delivery of services. All five are necessary, but each component may take a multitude of forms.

Under each of these major system components, there are several, more specific elements. The place of public and private economic support will be considered for each of the above categories, with special reference to developing countries.

Production of Resources

The resources required in a health care system are (1) manpower, (2) facilities, (3) commodities, including drugs, and (4) knowledge. As noted in the historical review, the training of health manpower in developing countries has been supported mainly by public funds. When private medical schools exist, as they now do in certain less developed countries (Philippines, Indonesia, Brazil), their number of graduates is small compared with the number from governmental schools. Private financial support for the training of nurses and allied health personnel is rare in developing countries.

Hospitals and other health facilities in developing countries are likewise constructed mainly at government expense. Large cities may have some small private hospitals that serve a handful of rich families. Health centers and health posts for ambulatory care are overwhelmingly governmental in sponsorship. Insofar as religious missions may establish health facilities, their construction is financed from charitable sources that are essentially social rather than personal. The production of knowledge comes from scientific research, which, in developing countries, is dependent almost entirely on government funds.

Only the production of drugs and other commodities is dependent mainly on private economic sources in developing countries. Drugs and other medical supplies and equipment are predominantly imported by these countries from Europe and North America. They are produced almost entirely by private corporations, which may operate plants abroad for local packaging. In some developing countries, a governmental laboratory may prepare various vaccines.

Organization of Programs

Health resources, particularly medical manpower, may engage in a free market for the sale of services to individual patients; the same applies to traditional healers. In all developing countries, however, substantial shares of personnel, facilities, and so on are organized into programs for (1) serving special population groups and (2) caring for or preventing certain disorders.

Programs for certain population groups may focus on children, industrialized or agricultural workers, military personnel, aborigines, or perhaps persons who have contributed to an insurance scheme. Programs for certain disorders may be concerned with the prevention or treatment of tuberculosis or other communicable diseases, the control of cancer, the prevention of accidents and trauma, the promotion of mental health or treatment of mental disorder, the rehabilitation of persons with physical handicaps, and so on. Virtually all of these organized programs are economically supported by socially derived funds. Such funds may come from private charitable sources, although most come from public revenues. The long-term trend, moreover, is for voluntarily supported health efforts to develop eventually into governmental programs.

Economic Support

As noted in the historical review, several mechanisms of financing health activities have evolved over the years: (1) personal, (2) charitable, (3) voluntary insurance, (4) social insurance, and (5) government revenues. Other, less important sources of health funds might be noted, such as commercial enterprises or lotteries.

Broadly speaking, these financial mechanisms fall into two categories: private and all the rest, or social. In developing countries, private support comes mainly from personal or family sources, with some input from charity and virtually none from voluntary insurance. Social support in these countries comes mainly from government revenues, with a lesser but increasing share from social insurance. As observed earlier, the lion's share of total health expenditures in developing countries (in contrast to industrialized countries) comes currently from private sources.

Management

The management of national health care systems encompasses several elements, the chief of which are (1) planning, (2) administration, and (3) regulation. The principal financial support of all of these processes in developing countries comes from public or other social sources.

National health planning is customarily a function of ministries of health or national planning agencies, or both. Health system administration involves the organization of programs, delegation of responsibilities, supervision, information handling, evaluation, and so on. Regulation concerns the surveillance of performance throughout the health care system in relation to standards formulated in various ways. All of these elements of management require personnel and technology that are dependent almost entirely on social financing.

Delivery of Services

The final component in the chain of activities that constitute health care systems is the delivery of services. The ultimate output of the whole system is the health status of a population; but within the boundaries of the system, the final activity is the delivery of health services. These services may be classified in various ways, but to clarify the role played by public and private financing in developing countries, they may be appropriately categorized as (1) health promotion and disease prevention, (2) therapeutic aspects of primary care, (3) secondary care, and (4) tertiary care.

Health promotion and disease prevention encompass many primary care activities, such as communicable disease control, environmental sanitation, maternal and child health services, mass nutrition, health education, accident prevention, and other services. With rare exceptions, these activities are financed wholly by government revenues.

Therapeutic ambulatory care covers a tremendous scope of activities. They involve countless diagnostic and treatment services of doctors, health assistants, or traditional healers in response to the patient with a symptom of illness. The types of sickness, of course, must be counted in the thousands, even though a relatively small number of diagnostic entities may account for most cases. Methods of treatment are highly variable. Drugs play a large part in therapy, and in developing countries they may be at the heart of ambulatory care, in relation to which the diagnostic process is only incidental. In developing countries, physicians in private practice play a substantial part in the delivery of therapeutic ambulatory care (including even some secondary care) in the main cities; in the rural areas of most developing countries, traditional healers, untrained drug sellers, and various health auxiliaries play a larger role.

It is in this health system element, therapeutic ambulatory care, that private financing plays its largest part. The very large private share of total national health expenditures observed in developing countries is doubtless used mainly for this purpose. Among low-income people, who constitute 80 to 95 percent of the population of developing countries, household surveys have found ambulatory medical care and drugs (prescribed or not) to account for nearly all family health spending. Relatively large outlays on personal health by the small fraction of affluent people accounts also for much of these private expenditures— both for ambulatory care and for hospital services at the secondary and tertiary levels. (Exact data on the distribution of these health care expenditures among social classes in developing countries are simply not available.) This is not to say that public funding contributes nothing in the delivery of therapeutic ambulatory care, but the evidence suggests that, in developing countries, private spending is much more important. This includes, of course, private expenditures for out-of-hospital drugs.

The delivery of secondary care is usually interpreted to include the services of medical specialists inside or outside a hospital, plus the full range of services in a front-line or perhaps intermediate hospital. The support of these services is predominantly from public sources. As for tertiary services in highly developed hospitals, these are also financed mainly by government, but a larger input doubtless comes from affluent families who can pay for sophisticated care of even moderate illness.

CONCLUSION AND COMMENT

This review of the distribution of public and private economic support of the five main components of national health care systems in developing countries leads to two principal conclusions:

1. Almost all the activities in the five major components of national health care systems are currently financed mainly from public sources.

2. One element of health care delivery, however—the therapeutic aspects of ambulatory care—is supported mainly by personal

money paid to private health care providers, including the sellers of drugs.

Taken together, these conclusions call for certain comments. The essential infrastructure of health care systems—resource production, program organization, system management, and so on—is financed mainly by expenditures from public sources. The planning and investment necessary to create and maintain this infrastructure are large and costly. They yield no personal profits.

The sole element of health care systems that is predominantly supported by private expenditures, therapeutic ambulatory care, is relatively simple and inexpensive to provide. (Most underlying investment, such as a doctor's education, has been publicly financed.) It is, therefore, widespread in developing countries, among both scientifically trained and traditional health personnel, and it yields significant personal profits to the provider.

Being dispensed in an open market, without programmatic organization or prudent management, these therapeutic ambulatory services are usually inefficient and wasteful. As in the health care systems of industrialized countries, fee incentives inevitably influence the services provided. Surveillance of the quality of practitioner performance is virtually impossible. The lack of health teams established in organized public programs means dysfunctional use of health personnel.

It is sometimes claimed that private sector health services in developing countries reduce the load on overburdened public systems. In fact, the opposite is true. By withdrawing scarce health manpower and other resources from the governmental health services, the private sector heightens pressures within the public system. Private medical practice is so lucrative, relative to the low public salaries paid in developing countries, that few physicians can resist engaging in it.

Therapeutic ambulatory service, with all the negative effects of its strong private support, is nevertheless an important constituent of primary health care. Yet, it is primary health care that the WHO sees as the key to achievement of global health care equity. The WHO concept of primary health care, however, emphasizes health promotion and disease prevention, the integration of preventive and therapeutic services, the delivery of health care by coordinated teams of personnel, the participation of community people in policy decisions, the use of appropriate technology, and much more. None of these attributes of essential primary health care applies to the ambulatory service bought and sold privately in developing countries. This was well summarized in a WHO-UNICEF Health Policy Statement in 1981:

The private medical sector absorbs scarce health personnel trained mainly at public expense. It is predominantly curative in character, and its expensive practices lead not only to inflated total medical expenditure, but to excessive foreign exchange costs for pharmaceuticals and medical equipment. . . . It has a negative influence on medical education. . . . As the economic basis for the medical profession's guild-type associations and their ethos of individualism, private medicine undermines health service attempts to discipline and rationalize diagnostic and therapeutic procedures on a cost-effective basis. . . . In many countries government facilities may come to be in different ways at the disposal of private medicine. For those reasons the private medical sector now has negative effects on primary health care implementation.

From all these implications of the current characteristics of public and private financing of health care systems in developing countries, one major policy decision would seem to follow. If the inspiring goal of "health for all by the year 2000" is to be reached, all countries—especially the developing countries—must do their utmost to minimize private financing and maximize public financing of all the component parts of national health systems. This has been the natural evolution of national health financing in the industrialized countries, and it is the surest path to both equity and efficiency everywhere in the development of comprehensive services based on primary health care.

Part Three

Industrialized Countries

11

The Health Care System
of Norway

Support of health activities in the industrialized countries is greater than in the developing countries, not only in absolute amounts but also in the percentages of GNP. More important, however, is the much higher proportion of health funds typically derived from public, as against private, sources in those countries characterized as "welfare states." A good example of such countries is Norway, whose health care system is described in this chapter. (Since the U.S. health care system is not analyzed in this book, many features of the Norwegian health care system will be contrasted with those of the U.S. system.)

In chapter 3, the diverse national health care systems of the world were classified into nine types. Systems of the affluent and industrialized countries are of three types: (1) permissive, or laissez-faire, (2) cooperative, or welfare, and (3) socialist, or centrally planned. The U.S. health care system is doubtless the prototype of the first category, and the USSR's system clearly represents the third type. Scandinavian countries have often been characterized as epitomizing the "middle way" in socioeconomic affairs, and the Norwegian health care system represents very well that of the cooperative, or welfare, state.

In response to the technical developments of medical science, the rising costs of proper service, and the general spread of democratic

Based on a working paper prepared for the World Health Organization in 1980.

demands for health care as a social right of everyone, many countries have organized their health services much more extensively than has the United States. The economic aspects have usually been organized first, and, under the aegis of government, many other steps have followed (see cell 2/figure 3.3). One now finds that virtually all of the countries of Western Europe, as well as other industrialized nations such as Japan, New Zealand, and Canada, have cooperative health care systems. There are numerous variations in all aspects of these cooperative systems, but space permits only an occasional reference to them. This account is focused on policies and practices in Norway, as a reasonably typical example.

Norway is a relatively small country with a population of about 4 million. Some 57 percent of the population is urban and 43 percent rural, a somewhat larger rural population than in most industrialized nations. Politically, Norway is a constitutional monarchy, although governance is by an elected parliament. Since the end of World War II, the government has been mainly under the control of the Labor party, although on health issues its policies differ very little from those of other, more conservative parties.

The long narrow territory of Norway is divided into 20 *filkes*, or provinces (although the word is sometimes translated as "counties"). Each province is further divided into communes, or municipalities. There are 443 communes, 396 of them rural and 47 urban, including Oslo, the capital. Governmental authority is much more centralized in Norway than it is in the United States or other federated nations such as Canada, Australia, or Switzerland. The provincial health officers, for example, are appointed by the central government's Directorate of Health Services.

The Norwegian health care system may be analyzed according to the five major components described in chapter 3 (see figure 3.2): production of resources, organization of programs, economic support, management, and delivery of services. It will be clearer, however, to start this account with the organization of programs.

ORGANIZATION OF HEALTH PROGRAMS

The basic organizational structure of the Norwegian health services is relatively simple. The most important functions by far come under the authority of the central government's Ministry of Social Affairs. These include the operation of the Directorate of Health Services and the National Insurance Institute. Certain other health functions are performed by other governmental agencies. Voluntary (nongovernmental) agencies contribute also to the national health services, as do many commercial or industrial enterprises. Finally, there is a private market in which personal health services are bought and sold.

The official responsibilities of the Directorate of Health Services are very broad; they are much greater than the purely preventive services often identified with public health. At the national level, for example, there is a division of medical services, which is responsible for the registration of physicians and certain other personnel and for the supervision of a national network of district doctors. Other divisions are responsible for psychiatric services, for dental services, for the control of drugs, for the planning and approval of hospitals, for hygiene (virtually all organized environmental and other preventive services), and so on.

At the provincial level, there is a provincial health office, whose head is appointed by the national directorate. He is essentially the representative of the Directorate of Health Services in the province. His duties include administration of all basic preventive health services; supervision of the work of the district doctors, who serve also as commune health officers; membership on the provincial hospital board; and various other duties. As a member of the hospital board, he is in a position to see that national standards are being met.

At the commune level, health responsibilities are vested in a communal health officer, known more generally as the district doctor. Although he serves as chairman of a locally elected board of health, the communal health officer is appointed by the central Directorate of Health Services. In this capacity, the health officer is responsible for all local preventive services, including the examination of expectant mothers and small children, immunizations, school health services, environmental sanitation, and so on. In the great majority of communes, which have small populations, the communal health officer serves also as a general medical practitioner—hence the term "district doctor." Clinical work takes about half the officer's time, and he is paid for it by the health insurance system. For official public health work, he is paid a salary by the central government. To assist in the public health work there is a community nurse, and in the clinical work there is an office nurse. Sometimes the communal health team includes a sanitarian. In larger cities, of course, there is a larger and more highly diversified public health staff.

The National Insurance Institute, also in the Ministry of Social Affairs, is responsible for various social insurance programs (old-age pensions, unemployment protection, and so forth), including health insurance. Its health insurance functions are carried out through a network of 445 local offices throughout the country. These offices make payments for services to the ambulatory patient (hospital costs are handled separately) and maintain relationships with patients, doctors, and other health care providers.

Among other governmental agencies with health functions is the Ministry of Labour and Local Affairs; this ministry has a factory inspection service that enforces standards for safety and health protection in the work place. It also operates facilities for vocational rehabilitation of workers. The Ministry of Church and Education maintains schools for the blind and deaf and, of course, oversees the provision of health education in the public schools. (Personal health services for school children, however, are provided by the public health authorities.) Health services for the military establishment, under the appropriate ministry, are another part of the structure of Norwegian health services.

Norway has had numerous voluntary health agencies devoted to specific disorders or working in certain local areas. Most such efforts, however, have become consolidated into the large Norwegian Women's Public Health Association (NKS). This organization has 1,300 local branches, and it operates 670 facilities. Its program includes home care of the chronically ill, rehabilitation of the disabled, care of the mentally retarded, operation of nursing homes, nurses' training, and supplemental feeding for children. Little time and effort is spent by NKS members in raising money, since nearly all costs are met from national government grants. It is primarily voluntary labor that is provided by the NKS. With this governmental subsidy, NKS services are well coordinated with those of the public agencies. The same applies to the Norwegian Red Cross and other voluntary bodies.

Industrial enterprises must also be counted as part of the Norwegian health care structure, insofar as on-the-job health services are provided to workers, particularly in large plants. Private health insurance carriers, which play so large a part in the health care systems of the United States, Australia, and South Africa, are virtually nonexistent in Norway.

Finally, a private sector for medical care must be included in the structure of the Norwegian health care system. One might not consider private services as "organized," but the operations of a market with buyers and sellers, prices and competition, constitute a definable program. The private market for health services is relatively small in Norway, compared with that in the United States, because so much health care has been brought under governmental financing and control.

Perhaps the largest part of the strictly private health care structure is dental care for adults. Dental services for children are provided under two nationwide public dental care programs, but the health insurance system does not finance dental services for adults. Thus both the financing and the delivery of adult dental service are in the private health care market. Drugs not included in the official health insurance formulary are in the private market, as is all self-prescribed medication. A few medical specialists are in private practice, although the vast majority is employed full-time in the public hospitals. (The engagement of hospital-based specialists in part-time private practice, previously permitted, is no longer allowed.) The 50 or 60 percent of general practitioners who are not appointed as district doctors are in private medical practice. Both types of doctors, however, are still paid fees for their services by the health insurance program, with some copayment by the patient. A small proportion (about 10 percent) of Norwegian hospital beds is in private hospitals; even their costs are partially covered by the insurance program.

PRODUCTION OF HEALTH RESOURCES

The principal resources on which the operation of the Norwegian health care system depends are health manpower, facilities, commodities, and knowledge. Relative to the developing countries of the world, all four of these resources are abundant in both quantity and quality.

Health Manpower

As are most other countries of the welfare state type, Norway is well supplied with doctors, having a doctor-to-population ratio of about 1 to 590—higher than the United States'. Norway's ratio, furthermore, has been gradually improving. In contrast to U.S. physicians, some 40 percent of Norway's physicians are in community general practice, with correspondingly less specialization. Dentists are also particularly plentiful in Norway, with a ratio to population of about 1 to 1,000, or double that in the United States. (Outside of Scandinavia, however, the supply of dentists in Europe tends to be weaker than the United States.) Fully trained nurses, actively working, are in about the same supply as in the United States, but much less use is made of assistant, or vocational nurses.

Other allied health personnel are generally less plentiful in Norway than in the United States. There are only about half the number of pharmacists per 100,000 in Norway that there are in the United States, probably because of the different patterns of pharmacy practice noted below. Technicians of all sorts are also much less numerous, as are medical social workers and trained health administrators. Only physiotherapists appear to be more numerous in Norway (and in several other European countries) than in the United States, probably because of their frequent employment in schools, spas, and other places outside of hospitals. Considering the great proportion of Norwegian territory that is thinly settled, the geographic distribution of doctors and other personnel is relatively equitable.

Higher education, like elementary education, is state-supported in Norway. The universities that train physicians, dentists, pharmacists, and psychologists are all governmental, under the supervision of the Ministry of Church and Education. This means that no tuition is charged and that qualified students in financial need may receive scholarship support for living expenses. The same applies to nearly all schools for training allied health personnel. The training of nurses is largely hospital-based, although the nursing school administration is ordinarily independent of the hospital.

Health Facilities

Norway, like other Scandinavian countries, is well supplied with hospitals, and they are quite evenly distributed throughout the nation. Considering only short-term general hospitals and other, special ones (such as those for maternity, cancer, or orthopedic conditions) that would come under this statistical rubric in the United States, there are 5.6 beds per 1,000 population, which exceeds the U.S. supply. Most of the hospitals have been built in relatively recent years and are very functionally designed (although this is not as true of hospitals in many other countries of Western Europe).

The ownership and management of Norwegian hospitals are strikingly different from those of U.S. hospitals. In Norway, some 90 percent of the beds, both for short-term and long-term cases, are in governmental facilities and are mainly under local government control. These facilities are not restricted to the poor, but serve the entire population. The average length of patient stay in Norwegian hospitals (about 15 days) is much longer than in the United States; thus, despite the greater supply of beds, the rate of admissions is slightly lower. This pattern characterizes hospital utilization in most other Western European countries as well.

Norway's population, like that of the United States, has a high proportion of aged persons, so there is a substantial need for long-term hospitals, skilled nursing care units, and custodial institutions for the aged and chronically ill. This need is well met by hundreds of relatively small facilities throughout the country, but, unlike the U.S. pattern, these facilities are owned and operated predominantly by local units of government. The cost of care in these facilities is borne mainly by local government rather than by the health insurance system or the individual.

Commodities

Nearly all drugs and supplies used in the Norwegian health care system are produced by private industry, and the bulk of these are imported from abroad. The costs of these commodities used in hospitals or clinics are covered by the health insurance program. Outside these facilities, drugs are sold in pharmacies, both on prescription and over the counter. The Norwegian pharmacy, unlike the U.S. drugstore, limits itself to dispensing drugs.

Knowledge

A great deal of medical research is conducted in Norwegian hospitals, especially in the large institutions connected with medical schools. There are also special research institutes on cancer and certain other diseases. Norway is, however, a small country, and most medical and related knowledge is acquired from other countries and diffused throughout the health care system by journals, conferences, and other forms of communication. Continuing medical education for practicing physicians is emphasized, particularly for general practitioners.

ECONOMIC SUPPORT

As is true of most of the West European welfare states, Norway has had a long history of social action to simplify and equalize economic access to personal health care. In the early nineteenth century, many local mutual aid societies were organized by workers or the residents of rural communities; among other things, these societies paid for doctors' services. In 1911, a law was enacted requiring low-income workers to belong to such a society—a concept initiated by Germany in 1883. For most of the population, health insurance coverage remained voluntary until 1952, when legislation required that every wage earner plus dependents must be insured, thus covering 95 percent of the population. In 1956, health insurance protection in Norway was made universal.

In 1930, the local benefit societies had been converted into branch offices of a National Insurance Institution, a component of the Ministry of Social Affairs. In 1967, the collection of all insurance premiums was centralized, with the money then being allocated to the local branches. In 1971, even this task was unified with general income tax collection.

The national health insurance system supports the great bulk—about 75 percent—of all personal health care costs. For the first two visits to a doctor, however, the patient must copay 33 and 20 percent, respectively, of the officially negotiated fee; after that, and for in-hospital care, the patient pays nothing. Low-income patients (pensioners, widows, and so on) have no copayment obligations, and no one needs to make copayments for diagnostic tests or physiotherapy ordered by the doctor. Drugs for about 35 serious, chronic diseases are paid for entirely by the insurance, but other drugs (accounting for about 50 percent of drug expenditures) must be purchased privately. Visual refractions for children up to age 15 are covered completely by the insurance, but after this age there are various limitations. Seventy-five percent of hospitalization is paid for by the insurance program and 25 percent by the local county government; the patient pays nothing either to the hospital or the doctor. Even travel costs, beyond a certain minimum, are reimbursed by the insurance system. Dental services are not included in Norway's health insurance benefits, although children get publicly financed care from government clinics, as discussed below.

Altogether, Norway spends about 7 percent of its GNP on health services, although the proportion has been rising from about 3 percent in 1950. Around half of the total expenditures is for hospitalization (including the doctor's inpatient services), nearly all of which comes from public sources. About 80 percent of overall Norwegian health expenditures come from public sources, compared with about 40 percent in the United States. Of the approximately 20 percent of total health expenditures coming from private sources, about half is for the dental care of adults.

A few examples of the variability of economic support methods in other countries of this conceptual type may be noted. In Germany, for example, there are no copayment obligations on the patient, although other methods are employed to constrain overutilization. In Sweden, insurance pays only a small portion of hospital costs, the great bulk being borne by local general revenues. Great Britain differs by financing over 80 percent of its entire health care system from national general revenues, with only small fractions coming from social insurance, local revenues, and private payments. The British general practitioner, furthermore, receives fees only for selected services; most of his income is derived from monthly capitation payments made on behalf of each person choosing to be on his panel, regardless of the services provided.

MANAGEMENT

The management component of national health care systems has been described as including planning, administration, regulation, and evaluation. In Norway, health planning is closely linked with day-to-day administration, so these two processes will be discussed together, followed by discussion of various forms of regulation in the health care system.

Administration and Planning

With government playing a much larger role in the management of the health care system in Norway, compared to the United States, administration is much more centralized and uniform. Even though many functions are delegated to the provinces, such as the operation of hospitals, basic policies are laid down centrally. The single, unified health insurance system greatly simplifies the financial aspects of health care both in the hospital and outside. There are no separate programs for the unemployed, the poor, or the aged, all of whom are simply covered by the national health insurance program. In the Norwegian Ministry of Social Affairs, administrative lawyers play a large role, to assure that the administration of health and other policies conforms with the law.

Norway does not lack voluntary health agencies, as noted earlier, but they are fewer in number and larger in size. They spend little effort on fund raising, since most of their costs are met by government subsidies. In Belgium, Holland, New Zealand, and elsewhere, voluntary societies are deliberately delegated to perform certain functions, such as preventive child health or visiting nurse services, for which they receive full government financing.

The planning of various segments of the health care system, such as its economic support, has long been implicitly conducted in Norway and other countries through national health insurance legislation. Systematic and comprehensive planning of resources—hospital construction and health manpower training—has only been undertaken recently at the central level. The most effective planning of the distribution of specialists has essentially been secondary to the pattern of hospital care. As discussed below, the supplies of specialists are determined by the number of beds found to be needed in each specialty. The balance of doctors must ordinarily engage in general practice, and the district doctor system assures rural area coverage.

Norwegian hospital functions are regionalized. The central government's approval is required for the staffing and equipping of all hospital facilities; thus small rural hospitals are not staffed or equipped to handle complex cases that should be sent to appropriate central hospitals. Hospital budget review is done by the Directorate of Health Services, although payments to hospitals are made by the insurance program.

Regulation

The basic concept of professional licensure is quite different in Norway and most other European countries than in the United States. Since all the medical schools are governmental and are supervised by the Ministry of Education, the graduate has only to present proof of his graduation and to meet certain other requirements (such as hospital training and evidence of good character) to be "registered" by the central government. He need not take a second examination, as in the United States. In nursing and certain other fields, the final examinations in the schools contain questions issued by the national ministry (beyond which the school may include its own questions); registration is automatic upon graduation.

Specialty certification in most European countries is supervised by the ministry of health, but Norway entrusts this function to the private Norwegian Medical Association, as is done in the United States. Requirements in the way of hospital training are usually recommended in other countries by nongovernmental committees of specialists, but the final certification is official; some countries require examinations, while others do not.

The major regulation of ambulatory medical care in Norway and countries of this type is through the insurance system. Statistical profiles are usually kept on doctors, so deviant performance is readily identified; physicians suspected of rendering excessive or improper service (presumably for monetary gain) are contacted by consultant, or control, doctors employed by the local insurance offices. If there is no satisfactory explanation of his services, the practitioner is ordinarily given a warning; if the unjustified performance continues, he may be penalized by reduced payments or even suspension from the insurance system for a period of time. Patients may also bring complaints to the insurance agency, which may then investigate them.

Most drugs used in Norway are imported, thus regulation of their manufacture is limited. The number of drugs that can be sold in the country, however, is limited to only about 2,000—a very much smaller number than the tens of thousands (many with identical composition but different trade names) sold in the United States. In some type 2 countries (figure 3.3), the health insurance system encourages the use of the lower-priced generic drugs by their reimbursement policies— that is, by requiring greater cost sharing for brand-name products.

In Norwegian hospitals, regulation is built into day-to-day work by the general structuring of medical staffs. The use of salaries, rather than fees, eliminates any financial incentive for unjustified surgical operations. Even in the nonpublic hospitals of other European countries, where private doctors may serve patients for insurance fees, the highly selective policy of staff appointments and the referral of nearly all patients to specialists by a primary care practitioner seem to reduce the rate of questionable elective surgery. It is small wonder, therefore, that malpractice lawsuits, which have reached crisis proportions in America, are rare in Norway or elsewhere in Europe. Differences in the judicial systems and in the customs of law practice also doubtless play a part, as does the fact that malpractice insurance is typically carried by the medical profession itself (rather than by commercial insurance companies) for small, uniform premiums. Sweden and New Zealand have recently changed their laws governing malpractice, to put it on a no-fault or social insurance basis and thereby remove it from tort law with all its legal complexities for establishing proof of fault or negligence. Proponents of this approach to medical malpractice in the United States will have much to learn from these foreign experiences.

Medical societies in Europe, as in the United States, are expected to monitor the ethical behavior of doctors. The official registration bodies may take action against a doctor found guilty of unethical behavior, but this is done rarely. Separate professional organizations usually handle economic matters, such as negotiation of health insurance fees.

DELIVERY OF HEALTH SERVICES

The methods of delivery of ambulatory care and hospital care differ significantly in Norway from the patterns in the United States. These two aspects of health care delivery will be examined, followed by discussion of the provision of personal preventive services.

Ambulatory Care

General medical practice, as noted earlier, is much stronger in Norway—and in European countries generally—than in the United States. Most general practitioners are in private practice, but about 40 percent of them are district doctors, appointed and employed by the central government and paid a basic salary. For this salary, they supervise or provide basic public health and preventive services, such as well-baby clinics, school health services, communicable disease control, and health education. Half or more of their time is spent giving general medical care to the people of their districts, for which they receive fees from the insurance system. The district doctor posts are located systematically throughout the country so that all rural or low-income populations will have access to them. There are some 600 district doctors for Norway's 4 million people. An equivalent number of U.S. doctors would be more than 32,000; yet there are fewer than 1,000 posts in the U.S. National Health Service Corps, which is intended to serve the needs of rural and disadvantaged populations.

Teamwork among groups of general practitioners and various allied health personnel is encouraged by a policy of central government grants to local communities for construction of health centers. Doctors locating in these facilities are still paid by the insurance program, either by fees or salaries. Under various auspices, health centers for general ambulatory care are being increasingly developed in Great Britain, France, Canada, Australia, and elsewhere to improve the delivery of primary care. This strategy for strengthening primary care seems to be much preferred, in contrast to the U.S. policy of training physician extenders. Nurses and other allied health personnel are members of the health center team, but their functions are essentially procedural; questions of judgment are reserved for the physicians.

Hospital Care

The Norwegian patterns of medical care delivery in hospitals are strikingly different from those in the United States. With very few exceptions, all medical staffs in hospitals—general as well as long-term special facilities—are composed entirely of full-time salaried specialists. Appointments to these hospital posts are made by the provincial hospital boards, but, to assure quality standards, they must be made from a list of three qualified candidates submitted by the national Directorate of Health Services.

Hospital specialists serve both inpatients and outpatients in a framework that puts the most competent and experienced doctors in supervisory positions. Patients are assigned to doctors whose training and experience are appropriate to their particular cases. There is considerable competition for these hospital posts, and the doctors selected (by the county governments that control the hospitals) have great prestige, typically greater than that of private practitioners in general practice. Senior hospital specialists in Norway, as in Great Britain, were formerly free to engage in private practice outside the hospital a few hours each week, although in both Norway and Sweden this has recently been forbidden.

Normal childbirths (about 80 percent of the total) are attended in hospitals by trained midwives; obstetricians serve only in complicated cases. Anesthesia is given mainly by nurse-anesthetists, under the supervision of medical anesthesiologists. Each hospital has a medical director, who usually does some clinical work, and a full-time business manager. Since the funds for hospital operation come almost entirely from two sources (the insurance program and local government), the business tasks are relatively simple and the management staff is small.

Not all Western European countries have so highly structured a hospital system as Norway's, but the pattern is similar in all Scandinavian countries and in Great Britain. In Germany, France, Italy, and other European countries, the Norwegian pattern characterizes the majority of hospitals, but there are also many nongovernmental institutions where private specialists chosen by the patients may serve them and be paid insurance fees. In Belgium, this free choice, fee-for-service pattern predominates. In all European countries, however, only carefully selected specialists may work in each hospital, and general practitioners must refer their patients to one of these specialists if hospitalization is required. Outside of Europe, New Zealand and Australia follow substantially the same practice, but Canada and Japan apply mainly the U.S. open-staff pattern.

Drug dispensing in Norway, as in most West European countries, is done at pharmacies that differ considerably from the U.S. drugstore. The Norwegian pharmacy limits its functions to the distribution and sale of drugs, not a whole range of commodities. (This may explain the much lower supply of pharmacists, noted above, which is quite adequate.) The location of pharmacies, moreover, is not left to free market operations. Every new pharmacy must be licensed, and if an area is already well served by pharmacies, a new one must locate elsewhere; this has largely equalized access to pharmaceutical services throughout Norway.

Personal Preventive Services

The personal preventive services provided through the network of district doctors have already been noted. In the main towns and cities, there are also numerous public health clinics for pregnant women and small children. In contrast to the U.S. model, these clinics are attended by mothers and babies from almost all families, not solely the poor. The insurance system does not pay fees to doctors for routine examinations, so at least 90 percent of all newborns are given periodic preventive services at these public clinics. This is, in fact, the normal pattern for preventive maternal and child health services throughout nearly all type 2 countries (figure 3.3). In France, children's allowances—another social insurance cash benefit—are given to families only when the mother can show that the children have received routine examinations at a public clinic.

Other personal preventive services in Norway include medical examinations of school children and first-aid services by school nurses, public clinics for tuberculosis and venereal disease, health education activities, and immunizations. Case detection for noncommunicable, chronic diseases is not so often promoted by public health agencies in Europe as in the United States, mainly because of less confidence in the value of such screening procedures. On the other hand, public health nursing services are very highly developed, with home visits made for bedside care as well as for preventive services.

Dental service for children, which is really both preventive and therapeutic, is especially strong in Norway. Virtually all children up to 15 years of age are given complete care in dental clinics (staffed by dentists) at government expense. There are actually two networks of clinics—one is in the cities and financed by local governments, and the other is mainly in rural districts and financed by the national government. Similar dental clinics for children are conducted in all Western European countries, although they are not as well staffed as those in Norway because these other countries have fewer dentists. To cope with its lack of dentists, New Zealand pioneered an important innovation in 1920—the training of large numbers of dental nurses. These are young women who receive two years of concentrated training, after high school, in the complete dental care of children. The dental nurses are stationed in all public schools and do almost all the necessary dental work—not only cleaning teeth, but also drilling and restoring carious teeth and extracting teeth (which is rare). Their supervision by dentists is only minimal. New Zealand's dental nurse idea is being gradually taken up in Australia, Great Britain, and Canada, not to mention numerous less developed countries.

All in all, it is clear that the general health care system of Norway is highly organized, both in its financial support and in its patterns of delivery. It is also continually changing in response to changing conditions. In the late 1970s and early 1980s, the rising expenditures for health service, as in most industrialized countries, became a prominent issue in Norway. To reduce the demands on national revenues, actions were being taken or contemplated to shift a greater share of the costs of medical and hospital service to provincial and even local units of government.

12

The British National Health Service and Its Reorganization

Few health care systems have attracted as much worldwide interest as the British national health service. Soon after World War II, and earlier than any other Western European nation, Great Britain boldly reshaped its health care system to make comprehensive services available to every resident. This chapter analyzes that system, along with a major reorganization made in 1974 and more recent trends associated with general political developments.

The British national health service (NHS) has in many ways set a model for the entire world. Although developed in a capitalist democracy—indeed, a parliamentary kingdom—it embodies concepts of equity, of establishment of health service as a social right of everyone, that have influenced health planners in every nation. Its very structure has helped to clarify the anatomy of the health service industry and the dynamic interplay among the ambulatory, the institutional, and the community preventive services.

NATIONAL HEALTH INSURANCE, 1911–48

To understand the NHS and its recent sweeping changes, one must appreciate that it did not arise de novo in 1948. As in all of

Based on a chapter in M.I. Roemer, *Health Care Systems in World Perspective* (Ann Arbor, Mich.: Health Administration Press, 1976), 104–15, with a supplement covering recent events.

Europe, trade unions, fraternal associations, and "friendly societies" had been providing disability and sickness care insurance since the early nineteenth century. Germany and several other Central European countries had made enrollment in such protective bodies compulsory since the 1880s, and that influence was bound to be felt in the more western European countries and the British Isles. In the 1840s, upper-class employers had encouraged and assisted the mutual aid societies as a way of getting lowly paid workers to look after themselves when they were sick; otherwise, they would have been supported by general revenues.

The first National Health Insurance Act was passed by the British Parliament in 1911, under the moderate political leadership of the Liberal party's Lloyd George. Only the doctors opposed the idea, favoring—as in the United States today—continuation of the entirely voluntary health insurance system for the self-supporting, coupled with a strengthened public medical service for the very poor.[1]

The 1911 Act required insurance protection to meet the costs of medical care and wage loss during sickness for all manual workers earning less than £160 (about $780 U.S.) per year. While membership in an approved society was not specifically mandated, all but a small percentage of workers met the law's requirements through such membership. The worker's dependents did not have to be insured but could purchase protection voluntarily through the same mutual aid societies. Payment of insurance contributions was required from both workers and employers, and the government provided funds for the support of administration and the coverage of very low income or indigent persons. The benefits were limited to the services of general practitioners (GPs) and prescribed drugs. Specialization was, in any event, not highly developed at the time. If the GP thought his patient required a specialist, the case could be referred to a hospital outpatient department, where such services were free. Hospitalization was not insured under the law, since open ward service in many public hospitals and some large voluntary ones was provided anyway through local government support or charity. If specialist care in a private office was desired, it had to be obtained privately. Dental or other special services were not covered at all.

Under the original law, GPs were not paid for their services directly by the approved societies, but rather by insurance committees set up by statute in each county or county borough; these committees had to contain a majority of elected representatives of insured workers, with the balance representing the local doctors, local government, and the Ministry of Health. The approved societies were responsible for the enrollment of workers and for the payment of cash disability benefits but not for the basic medical and pharmaceutical benefits; if they accumulated surplus funds, they could finance supplemental benefits such as part of hospitalization costs.

Under the law, the doctors in each insurance committee area could decide how they wished to be paid, whether on the basis of attendances (fee-for-service), capitation (according to the number of persons who chose to be on each doctor's list), or a combination of the two. It is not always understood that it was the British doctors themselves who increasingly chose the straight capitation method; by 1927, this pattern had become universal.[2] Capitation was preferred because it involved less red tape and was least subject to competitive abuse among the insurance doctors in each area. It was only later, with the NHS, that capitation remuneration of GPs became mandatory.

Approved societies could sell insurance for other benefits, such as dental care, or for voluntary medical coverage of persons not coming under the social insurance law, such as dependents or employees with higher incomes. Many approved societies had been set up by commercial insurance companies as nonprofit subsidiaries, and they enrolled several million persons on a voluntary basis; coverage of specialist attendance in hospitals was included. GP services in small private hospitals (nursing homes) were also sometimes covered, especially for maternity cases and relatively simple surgery.

A study in 1923 showed that the average insured person in Great Britain received 3.5 attendances per year. At about the same time (1928–31), the Committee on the Costs of Medical Care showed that persons of equivalent income in the United States, without insurance, were receiving 2.2 physician services per year. Thus, the British doctor was giving 50 percent more service under capitation insurance arrangements than was the U.S. doctor paid fees for each service by noninsured patients.

PRELUDE TO THE NATIONAL HEALTH SERVICE

Over the years, the income threshold for mandatory insurance coverage in Great Britain was gradually elevated so that more workers would be covered. Additional persons and benefits were also insured on a voluntary basis. On the eve of World War II, however, the health insurance protection of the British population was obviously far from complete, both as to persons covered and benefits provided. It was not surprising, therefore, that during the war—among the goals of which was freedom from want—an Inter-Departmental Committee on Social Insurance and Allied Services was set up under the chairmanship of

Sir William Beveridge to "survey the existing national schemes of social insurance and allied services . . . and to make recommendations."
In late 1942, under Winston Churchill's Conservative government, the
famous Beveridge Report was issued.[3]

This classic document explored the deficiencies and need for expansion of all the branches of social insurance, including old-age pensions, unemployment benefits, disability benefits, and so on, as well as
health services. Regarding the latter, in summary the Plan for Social
Security recommended:

> Medical treatment covering all requirements will be provided for all
> citizens by a national health service organized under the health depart-
> ments (of England and Wales, Scotland, and Northern Ireland), and post-
> medical rehabilitation treatment will be provided for all persons capable
> of profiting by it.[4]

In further elaboration of this goal, the Beveridge Report stated that:

> A comprehensive national health service will ensure that for every cit-
> izen there is available whatever medical treatment he requires, in what-
> ever form he requires it, domiciliary or institutional, general, specialist,
> or consultant, and will ensure also the provision of dental, ophthalmic
> and surgical appliances, nursing and midwifery and rehabilitation after
> accidents.[5]

The report explicitly avoided discussion of "the problems of organisation of such a service" as falling outside its scope.

These were the objectives recommended under a wartime Conservative party government in 1942. It remained for a Labour party government, elected after the war, to implement them with the passage of
the National Health Service Act in 1946. Allowing a tooling-up period
of about 18 months, the Act took effect in July 1948.

As in any sweeping social legislation, there was intense debate in
the period between the introduction of draft legislation and enactment
of the final law. The Minister of Health was Aneurin Bevan, a rugged
Welsh former coal miner, who soon found himself at loggerheads with
the British Medical Association. The association, anticipating the postwar mood, had set up its own medical planning commission, which had
recommended achievement of the Beveridge goals through extension of
the existing national health insurance to cover higher income persons,
government grants to voluntary hospitals in order to enable them better to serve the poor, and retention of the private medical market for
higher income persons. Bevan's bill, on the other hand, would not only
cover all residents of the nation for comprehensive services, but would
provide a basic salary for all GPs (to be supplemented by capitation

payments) and a network of health centers from which both preventive services of local health authorities and primary services of GP's would be furnished—as proposed in 1920 in the Dawson Report. All beds in public hospitals, moreover, would be solely for NHS patients; while specialists could continue private practice on a part-time or full-time basis, they would have to hospitalize their patients solely in private institutions.

In the ensuing debate, which involved a threat to strike by the doctors, many compromises were naturally made by both sides. Universal population coverage was retained, but basic salaries—which GPs had opposed for fear that they would gradually be extended to full government employment—were abandoned. Public hospitals were authorized to maintain about 5 percent of their beds for the private patients of consultants. The network of health centers was not to be established, except for a few experimental facilities. On the other hand, financing was to be derived mainly from general revenues, and only a small fraction from social insurance contributions. Top authority was vested in the Ministry of Health. And nearly all hospital beds were put under the control of the national government.

The most important compromises—or perhaps adjustments to the forces at play would be more accurate—in defining the administrative lines of the national health service were in the design of its tripartite structure. Past developments in Britain up to 1948 had given rise in the health services to several principal sets of vested interests: the GPs, the community hospitals with their staffs of specialists, the medical school–affiliated teaching hospitals, and the local public health authorities. To achieve an operational program that would be adapted suitably to these clusters of power required an administrative structure in which substantial sovereignties were retained by each of these groupings. Coordination among the interests, for the sake of good patient care and efficiency, was a secondary consideration, to be tackled deliberately only later.[6]

Ambulatory Services and the Executive Councils

The first interest group, general practitioners, was already represented, and its remuneration handled, by the insurance committees operating since 1911 under the National Health Insurance Act. These committees generally had subcommittees for doctor services and for prescribed drugs. It was a relatively smooth transition, under the NHS, to establish a network of executive councils—138 of them in England and Wales—which would assume the functions of the former insurance committees; in the new program, these functions would be broadened to administer services for the total population and to handle dental care and optical services.

The average executive council administered these ambulatory services for about 350,000 people, although the range was highly variable; one council for part of London covered 3 million people. Most important were the council's responsibilities for capitation payments to and monitoring of the GPs. Each month the GP was paid a fixed amount for every person on his list, irrespective of the person's use or nonuse of services. The person could change to another GP at any time, whereupon his name would be transferred to the other doctor's list. In order to protect quality, the maximum number of persons permitted on a GP's list was 3,500, although in recent years the average has been about 2,200. Furthermore, the rate of capitation payment went according to a slightly descending scale, in order to discourage excessively long lists. In many ways, the GP, or family doctor, as the primary point of entry into the service, underwent many changes in his mode of work, but more will be said of this below.

Also under the responsibility of the executive councils were the dental services. Unlike the GPs, dentists were paid on a fee-for-service basis, but not all procedures were covered by the NHS. For partial dentures, bridgework, crowns, and certain other prostheses the patient had to pay extra fees personally, although complete dentures were fully covered. The supply of dentists in Great Britain, as in nearly all of Europe (and, indeed, most countries), was relatively low in relation to the needs; the demands for care were high; and dentists' incomes in the early years of the NHS were greater than those of the GPs. (Later, adjustments in GP remuneration changed this relationship.) Priority was accorded to children through a free, public dental service furnished by salaried dentists under the local health authorities.

Prescribed drugs obtained at local chemist's shops, or pharmacies, were another benefit administered by the executive councils. At first, these were entirely covered through NHS fees, calculated by a formula (accounting for the wholesale cost, overhead, dispensing service, and so on) paid to the pharmacist. When the Conservatives were returned to power in 1952, they imposed a copayment charge of one shilling ($0.14 U.S.) on each prescription, and later this was raised to two shillings. With the generally rising consumption of drugs and higher costs per item, certain constraints were introduced around 1960. A "recommended list" was issued by the Ministry of Health, and doctors could order products not on it only if they were specifically justified; otherwise, the patient would have to pay the full cost. The deterrent effect of copayments was transitory, and when the Labour party was reelected these changes were dropped. All the while, over-the-counter products remained available to the British people, at their personal expense, and great quantities were indeed purchased. With advertising and old wives' tales, self-medication does not disappear, even under a publically financed health service system.

Finally, the executive councils were responsible for optical services. These included vision examinations by prescribing opticians (the equivalent of optometrists in the United States) and eyeglasses furnished by dispensing opticians. Fees for standard frames were paid by the councils, but the patient was charged extra for unusual or fancy frames. Hearing aids, prosthetic limbs, wigs (when medically ordered), and other special medical devices were further benefits.

Regional Hospital Boards and Specialist Services

The second major pillar of the NHS structure was a network of regional hospital boards (RHBs)—15 of them to cover England and Wales. Just as the executive councils had evolved from the former insurance committees, the RHBs had antecedents, though more recent, in the system of emergency services set up during World War II while Britain was being bombed. The wartime experience obviously educated British hospitals about the feasibility of communications and teamwork among institutions in a region.

For some years before the war, British general hospitals had been confronted with financial difficulties. The public hospitals, depending mainly on local revenue for support, were chronically underfinanced. The voluntary hospitals, despite the long and distinguished traditions of many of them, were likewise hard pressed by the dwindling of charitable contributions and the difficulty private patients had in meeting the ever-rising charges. When, therefore, the Minister of Health took over control of all but a handful (mainly religious) of British hospitals in 1948, there were no significant objections. With nationalization, the government acquired all the property of the hospitals and assumed all their debts and obligations. Overnight, Britain's 2,700 hospitals, with about 480,000 beds (about 80 percent municipal), attained financial stability. The nationalization included all mental, tuberculosis, and other chronic disease facilities, as well as the general hospitals, but it did not include old people's homes or convalescent units.

The hospital regions were mapped out to contain about 2 million to 3 million people and roughly 30,000 hospital beds of all types. The regional hospital boards were appointed by the minister to represent the general population, the medical profession, and the former hospital owners or sponsors. To actually administer the hospitals, the RHB appointed hospital management committees, which were typically responsible for institutions containing a total of between 1,000 and 2,000 beds; this might mean two or three large units or as many as 15 or 20 small ones. The funds for both operation and capital costs of all hospitals in a region were allotted by the central government to the RHB, which in turn distributed them to the management committees. Because of Britain's postwar financial difficulties and competing obligations for housing construction, schools, roads, military purposes, and so on, new hospital construction until quite recent years was not undertaken, and capital expenditures went almost entirely for renovating the old structures. As a result, many U.S. observers have been struck with the antiquated physical features of most British hospitals; the dedication of their staffs and the efficiency of their operations, however, have been equally noteworthy.

British specialists in medicine and surgery, unlike their U.S. counterparts, are attached mainly to the hospitals. Leaving aside the younger doctors in training (registrars, junior registrars, and so on) about 60 percent are on full-time salaries, and 40 percent spend part of their time (typically 20 to 30 percent) in outside private practice. General practitioners, however, who constitute about half of Britain's doctors, seldom have hospital appointments under the NHS, nor did they have such appointments before. In other words, the patient requiring hospitalization (except in emergencies) is referred by his GP to a hospital outpatient department, where the examining specialist decides if he should be admitted. Likewise, he may be referred to the hospital outpatient department simply for a diagnostic workup. In either case—whether admitted to a bed or not—a report is sent back to the referring physician on the specialist's findings.

This separation of general practice from the hospital has been the subject of much criticism in North America, where nearly all doctors, generalist and specialist, have hospital ties. This closed staff pattern is by no means unique to Britain, but prevails in most of the world. While it means that the community GP is deprived of the stimulation of hospital experience and is temporarily separated from his patient, it also assures technically high quality service within the hospital walls. Moreover, under the NHS, the GP was brought closer to the hospital by giving him direct access to the hospital's laboratory and X-ray services for diagnostic tests (without necessarily sending his patient through the outpatient department), by inviting him to participate in the hospital's educational programs, and by sometimes appointing him to work in the outpatient department or other sections of the institution.

Until quite recently, specialist salaries in hospitals were typically higher than the earnings of community doctors in general practice. All specialists and consultants (the highest rank) are appointed by the

RHBs, and there is great competition for these positions. When an opening occurs, it is widely advertised in the medical journals, and the specialist appointed usually acquires permanent tenure. Those not appointed may be frustrated and must face the decision of going into general practice or emigrating. (Quite a few of the ex-British doctors in North America who broadcast the defects of the NHS are those who failed to win a specialist appointment.) Periodically, specialist salaries are raised, with increased tenure or responsibility, and merit awards are granted for outstanding performance. In the light of the conventionally negative attitudes towards salaries in U.S. medicine, it is noteworthy that the most prestigious and coveted positions in Britain's NHS, and indeed in all of Europe, are those offering salaried hospital employment.

The Teaching Hospitals

In tracing the origins of the NHS, the special interests of hospitals linked to medical schools were noted. Usually associated with a long tradition and exceptionally qualified medical staffs, these hospitals in England and Wales objected to coming under the control of regional hospital boards. The 36 of them (26 in London), therefore, each with its board of governors, were made directly responsible to the Minister of Health. The teaching hospitals in Scotland, however, were integrated into their respective RHBs. (In the reorganization of 1974, as we shall see, such integration was finally achieved on a nationwide basis.)

Medical student education, which is invariably associated with a teaching hospital, is simultaneously under the wing of a university. Unlike U.S. medical students, British medical students take a continuous six-year course, rather than a four-year university baccalaureate followed by another four-year medical curriculum. Contrary to some forebodings, after initiation of the NHS the volume of applicants to British medical schools did not decline, but rose. The majority of medical and other health science students are supported by government scholarships.

Local Health Authorities

The final major branch of the British NHS was the network of local health authorities—146 of them in England and Wales. These were responsible for traditional preventive public health services, and for several other activities as well. While the NHS withdrew from local authorities their responsibilities for public hospitals (which, in a sense, weakened their role), it assigned them new functions for ambulance transport, visiting nurse services (bedside care at home, which had been traditionally offered by voluntary agencies), homemaker care for the chronically ill, and the operation of long-term facilities for the aged or chronically ill not needing hospitalization.

Preventive services had long emphasized maternal and child health. The vast majority of pregnant women and infants in Great Britain have been periodically checked by health department clinics. This applies to all social classes, not only to lower income families, as in the United States. One must recall that the GP, being paid on a capitation basis, is happy to have his patients so attended; he loses no fee, it saves him time, and the mother and child are seen by experts in this preventive work. At the child welfare stations, as they are called, infants and small children receive all necessary immunizations, and the mothers are advised on child-rearing practices. Sick children are referred back to their GP. To lighten the load on these health department clinics and to promote integrated care, in recent years GPs have been offered supplementary fees for immunizations and certain other preventive services.

Local health authorities also conducted special clinics for tuberculosis and venereal diseases. Health services for schoolchildren were still financed by the educational authorities, but the local medical officer of health in most jurisdictions was also appointed school health officer. (Under the recently reorganized NHS, these school health services have been brought into the general program.) Environmental sanitation has been another major responsibility of the local health authorities. In the water supply and sewage disposal systems of Britain, which are less modern than those in the United States, close surveillance is necessary. Inspections of housing, for enforcement of minimum standards, were another responsibility of the medical officer and his sanitation staff, and they occupied a good deal of time.

Other Special Services

Separate, large hospitals for the mentally ill and retarded had evolved in Great Britain, as in most of the world, but with the NHS they were brought under the supervision of the regional hospital boards. Commitment to a mental hospital was changed from a judicial to a medical procedure. The vast majority of admissions became voluntary, and in the minority that were mandatory, two doctors (one of whom had to be a psychiatrist) were required for certification, rather than a court of law. After admission, the patient was entitled to a judicial review, but most mandatory admissions were later converted to informal ones. Increasing emphasis was placed on community care for mental illness: in mental health clinics of many types under the local authorities, mental sections in general hospitals, day care centers, and a variety of other special arrangements. The average length of stay in mental hospitals, as well as the total census, greatly declined—as was, indeed, also happening in the United States at that time.

Workmen's compensation for on-the-job injuries was greatly modified under the NHS. The payment of cash benefits for wage loss, financed solely by employers, was continued as before, under the social security system. All medical services, however, were simply integrated with and provided by the NHS system. Since medical care for all illness was fully covered, there was no reason to falsely attribute a worker's symptoms to an employment cause in order to gain financial protection. Great emphasis was put on rehabilitation, and a special center was developed for the treatment of those few workers, often called malingerers, whose disability was mainly psychosomatic.

Medical inspection of factories for safety and occupational disease hazards was one of the few health-related activities not integrated into the NHS; it was retained as a function of the Department of Labour. First aid in the factories, preplacement examination of workers, safety standards, and the like were enforced through periodic visits, and these imposed a responsibility on management. Medical treatment of sick or injured workers, of course, was through the NHS.

Public assistance for the poor, in its financial aspects, was administered by welfare authorities, but medical care was administered through all the normal procedures of the NHS. No special enrollment or identification of the recipients of public aid was necessary. Likewise, any visitor to Great Britain who became ill or was injured was treated by the resources of the NHS, exactly as the police force would be expected to protect a visitor against crime.

FINANCIAL SUPPORT AND VOLUME OF SERVICE

These were, then, the main features of the NHS as it was set up in 1948; they were attainable only through the assumption of substantial financial responsibility by the Exchequer, or general treasury of the nation. Because employer and worker contributions to the old national health insurance had become customary, however, and because the Exchequer was set up to cover many other cash benefits (old-age pensions, unemployment compensation, maternity and disability allowances, and so forth), a share of these funds was assigned to help support the NHS, along with monies from some other sources.

Table 12.1 Sources of Funds for the British National
Health Service, 1970–71

Source	Percentage
Central government	80.0
Insurance contributions	9.0
Local government	6.5
Payments by patients	4.5
Total	100.0

The exact proportions of funds derived from different sources were not identical over the years. In 1970–71, they were as shown in table 12.1.[7]

The central government funds included allotments to local governments to help them carry some of their responsibilities. Payments by patients included charges for prescribed drugs, for prosthetic dental services, for private beds in NHS hospitals, for special spectacles, and for other miscellaneous purposes. Altogether, the NHS cost about £2.38 billion in 1970–71. Expenditures outside the NHS were estimated at about £100 million for self-medication and about £25 million for privately purchased medical care (about 5 percent of the total). For the 55 million people in the United Kingdom, this amounted to an annual per capita outlay for health services of about £45 (about $125). This compares with an expenditure in the United States for all health services in 1970 of about $325 per person per year. (Even if one were to allow an exchange rate of $3 per pound, in recognition of actual purchasing power differentials in the two countries, the British per capita expenditure for health services was less than half the U.S.)

Yet, for this lesser expenditure, British health manpower and facilities provide a volume of personal health services very similar to the levels in the United States. The 4.2 general medical, surgical, and maternity beds per 1,000 population in Britain are about the same as in the United States. Counting all types of hospital beds—including mental and chronic—in 1970, the British supply was 9.5 per 1,000, compared with the U.S. supply of 8.0. In general hospitals, British admission rates are somewhat lower than U.S. rates, but the average stay per case is longer and the occupancy percentages greater, so aggregate days per 1,000 population per year in Britain are slightly more than in the United States.

Patient-physician contacts are somewhat higher in Britain for primary, or GP, care than in the United States and lower for specialist care. Dental services are less frequently received in Britain, especially for adults, because of a lower supply of dentists. Preventive services, on the other hand, especially for children, are undoubtedly more frequent in Britain than in the United States.

A propos of services, it is significant to note that the rate of elective surgery in Great Britain is much lower than in the United States. It has been pointed out that the ratio of surgeons to population in England and Wales is about half that in the United States, and the rate of elective surgery is correspondingly about half.[8] There can be little doubt that this finding relates to the methods of paying surgeons in the two countries: high fees for each operation in the United States and fixed salaries based on merit in Great Britain. The abundance of unnecessary surgery in the United States has been frequently demonstrated, but whether there is, in fact, too little surgery in Britain is arguable. In any case, life expectancy for both men and women is longer in Great Britain than in the United States, in spite of the average per capita incomes (and presumably levels of living) being lower.

SPECIAL FEATURES AND TRENDS

Over the years, the rate of services and volume of expenditures in the NHS have risen, as they have in the health care systems of most other countries, especially the industrialized ones. Yet, the striking fact is how slowly the rise has occurred in Great Britain. Ten years after the NHS started operation, concern for the rise in costs generated a commission of enquiry—yielding the Guillebaud Report in 1960. The surprise was that, while absolute expenditures had risen, the outlay for health as a percentage of the GNP had actually declined, from 3.9 percent in 1947–50 to 3.6 percent in 1958–59. By 1968, this proportion had risen to 4.6 percent of GNP; at the same time, Americans were spending about 6.5 percent of their larger GNP for health services.[9] In 1974, U.S. expenditures on health had risen to about 8.0 percent of the GNP.

Some point to this relatively constrained expenditure for health purposes in Great Britain as a defect, particularly in comparison with the freewheeling escalation of outlays in the United States. The former is attributed to the largely unitary public source of funding in Britain, which is not easily expanded, compared to the pluralistic sources in the United States. But it is not difficult to show that most of the U.S. increase in expenditures is attributable not to a rise in the volume of services, but rather to a climb in the prices of hospitalization, physician and dental care, drugs (prescribed and over-the-counter), and other services—not to mention the large overhead costs of hundreds of private insurance agencies. One must conclude, therefore, that on balance the Briton is getting more for his money under the NHS than the American is getting under his predominantly laissez-faire system.

Trends in the NHS over the years involve many developments besides money. As in all industrialized nations, the relative importance of hospitals has increased, in tandem with the expansion of medical and surgical specialization. As a reflection of this, the expenditures for hospital care in the NHS rose from 55.7 percent of the total in 1951–52 to 62.6 percent in 1970–71. Still, compared with the U.S. scene, this rise in the proportion of resources allotted to the hospital sector was not very great.

More significant are probably the major changes that have been occurring in British community general practice. At the time the NHS was enacted, most GPs held forth in their private one-man surgeries. The Ministry of Health, however, gave financial inducements to medical grouping. The quality of isolated general practice had been criticized in several studies, and group practice, it was believed, could upgrade it; the engagement of office assistants to relieve the doctor of many simple tasks would be more feasible, and a team of doctors would mean convenient opportunities for consultation and general professional stimulation. Government policy was successful, and the grouping of GPs increased steadily. By 1970, over 65 percent were in offices of two or more, most of them in groups of three or more. In such settings, each practitioner would usually develop skills in some special aspect of general practice, such as child care, minor surgery, gynecological problems, emotional difficulties, and the like.

Another government objective was to improve the geographic distribution of doctors. This was done principally through a ban against settlement of new graduates in areas designated as overdoctored (for purposes of payment under the NHS); the result, of course, was to channel physicians to areas where they were needed. As a result, the British population in underdoctored areas was reduced from about 50 percent in 1948 to 20 percent in 1963. Moreover, the sale of medical practices—a traditional custom in Britain, through which a retiring doctor acquired money to live on—was prohibited and replaced with a social insurance pension program for doctors. Accordingly, the high price of buying a practice would no longer inhibit the young doctor from spending money on modern medical equipment.

Improvement in the quality of general practice was also encouraged by supplemental government grants for engagement of allied health personnel, higher capitation payments for aged patients, supplemental fees for various office procedures and for house calls, and other methods. There was a serious pay dispute between GPs and the government in 1965, resulting in a substantial boost in their earnings and making the whole field of general practice more attractive. By 1970, nearly half of GPs' incomes came from the various special fees and grants rather than capitation. A Royal College of General Practitioners made specialist status possible in general practice, and this was associated with an intensified program of continuing education and the establishment of professorial chairs for general practice in the medical schools.

Perhaps the most significant trend affecting general practice, indeed all ambulatory health care, in the NHS has been the movement, starting in about 1965, for establishment of health centers. As noted earlier, such centers figured prominently in the early planning of the system, but they were not implemented, except in a few experimental projects.

In the mid-1960s, first in connection with the development of new towns and later in most large cities, buildings were constructed or redesigned for housing groups of GPs, complemented by public health nurses, social workers, office or practice nurses, sometimes laboratory technicians, psychologists, dieticians, clerks, or other allied health personnel. Usually built by local health authorities, the quarters were rented by GPs who had their regular lists of patients, but most of the ancillary personnel were furnished at local government expense.

By 1971, there were 475 such health centers in operation or under construction, housing about 1,500 GPs with space available for about 1,000 more. In the centers in full operation, there were an average of five or six GPs, and these doctors tended naturally to cooperate with each other, cover the practice of a colleague who was away, consult among themselves, and make much greater use of the allied health workers than would occur when these personnel were stationed in the traditional health department. While some centers used the office or practice nurse as a screening agent more than others (and there was great variation in other features), it appeared in the early 1970s that the health center was in time likely to change the entire image of ambulatory care in the NHS.

ATTITUDES AND OTHER CONSEQUENCES

Almost from the outset, the NHS encountered problems in the remuneration of doctors, both specialists and GPs. A series of enquiries led to continual readjustments, but on the whole the British medical profession became gradually supportive of the essential principles of the service. Among the population as a whole, the NHS was probably the most popular program that had been launched by any political party. A British Gallup opinion poll in 1964 found 89 percent of the population generally satisfied with the NHS. In 1967, a survey by another organization found 95 percent of the people in general approval; of these, 60 percent rated the service as very good or excellent.

Large bureaucratic structures like the NHS are often charged with discouraging local initiative and any incentive for volunteer work to strengthen the program. Yet British voluntary agencies have not declined. Hospital administrators point out that their committees of volunteer workers are as busy as ever. Instead of spending as much time on fund raising as in the past, however, they devote their energies to rendering services in the hospital that help the patients or lighten the task of the staff.

The charge of "deadly uniformity," so often leveled against large governmental systems, does not stand up to scrutiny in the British setting. As one visits different hospitals and health departments in Britain, one is struck with their diversity. While each hospital, for example, is administered by a sort of troika—the hospital secretary (or administrator), the matron (or director of nurses), and the medical chief—whose members must work closely together, the variations in style and emphasis among the different clinical services and departments of an institution are countless. There is plenty of room for innovation, as long as minimum standards are met.

In terms of resources generated by the NHS, the effect has clearly been to yield an increased supply of physicians—from about one per 950 people in 1948 to about one per 830 20 years later and one per 660 in 1977. The availability of about 25,000 midwives for obstetrical services (both inside and outside hospitals) must be noted if one is to compare this ratio with the U.S. ratio of 1 to 595 in 1976. Over this same span of years, in fact, the ratio of doctors to population in the United States remained almost constant (increasing only after about 1967), while the British ratio improved. Medical incomes, meanwhile, for both GPs and specialists, have risen substantially, and doctors' incomes now fall in the upper 2 or 3 percent of the British population.

The general hospital-bed-to-population ratio has not significantly increased in Britain, but since lengths of stay have steadily shortened, rates of admission have risen. They rose from about 67 per 1,000 annually in 1949 to 92 in 1960 and to about 110 in 1970. As noted earlier, this rate is associated with greater use of hospital outpatient departments, admission of more serious cases (clearly in need of hospital care), and a much lower rate of elective surgery in Great Britain than in the United States. Waiting lists for hospital treatment of elective conditions are still a difficulty, but their length has declined. There is no problem about admission of emergency cases.

Perhaps one of the best reflections of the general adequacy of the NHS is the relatively small percentage of the population seeking care through private arrangements outside the official structure. Voluntary health insurance schemes to finance private care have been free to operate, and although they have been intensely promoted by private carriers, their enrollment had grown to only 883,000, or less than 2 percent of the population, by 1969. In fact, between 1965 and 1967, the rate of disenrollments exceeded that of new enrollments. Although less than 5 percent of NHS beds is reserved for private patients, in the last few years this arrangement for "breaking the queue" with affluence has been intensely debated in Labour party circles, and the loophole may eventually be closed. In any event, whether it is left open or not, it would appear that not many patients are displeased with the waiting times or other limitations of the NHS to the point of paying for private medical care.

PROBLEMS OF COORDINATION

Despite this generally favorable picture of achievements, the NHS has not been without problems. There have been controversies about medical remuneration, as mentioned; constraints on the construction of new hospital beds (because of competing demands for government funds) have caused waiting lists for elective conditions; some patients complain about the brevity of their visits to the GP; and costs have risen (although more slowly than in most other countries). The basic concept of the NHS—a strong primary doctor who provides convenient entry to the system and who oversees his patient's use of specialists and hospital services; a preventive program; and the several other parts—is nevertheless a basis for pride by the architects of the structure.[10]

If any feature of the NHS has been continually vexing to the responsible authorities, it has been the maintenance of the segmented administrative structure. A pregnant mother, for example, would get prenatal care from a local health authority clinic, treatment of illness from her GP, and delivery of the baby by a hospital doctor or midwife. Similar fragmentation of patient care applied to the care of children, many chronic disease cases among all age groups, the management of mental disorders, and others. Moreover, economic trends in the NHS showed a gradual escalation of the resources allotted to the hospital sector, while the general practice and other components remained static or declined.

Since its beginnings in 1948, the NHS has had various coordinating committees attempting to achieve integration among the executive councils, regional hospital boards, and local health authorities, as well as among the teaching hospital boards of governors; some overlapping of board or committee memberships was designed for the same purpose. As early as 1962, the Porritt Committee, under the British Medical Association, had advocated unification of all the vertical components at the local community level.[11] Politically, however, in terms of the power centers responsible for the original divided structure, the time did not seem ripe. Not until 1968 did the national government, then under the Labour party, issue its first green paper advocating, for discussion purposes, a merging of the three main sectors of the service at the local level, through 40 to 50 area health authorities.

Responses were quick to come, and the proposal was criticized as vesting responsibility still too remotely from the local areas, while not making adequate provision for larger regional planning. A Conservative government was elected in 1970, and a second green paper was issued in 1971, responding to the criticisms of the first. Then a government white paper, laying out the party's final, official plans, was issued.

THE REORGANIZATION OF 1974

In recognition of demands for greater local controls, 90 area health authorities (AHAs) were contemplated, with a second tier (largely for planning purposes) of 14 regional health (not hospital) authorities. The AHAs would range in size from 250,000 to 1.5 million population and would be congruent with (but independent of) simultaneously reorganized general local government authorities. The regional health authorities would have from 1 to 5 million population; thus each regional authority would contain from one to 11 AHAs, and usually more than three. The larger AHAs would be further subdivided into districts of about 250,000 population—or the catchment area of a district general hospital. The law putting this general plan into effect was passed in 1973, to take effect April 1, 1974.

The reorganization takes account of past realities. While the AHA is responsible for all types of service—ambulatory, hospital, and preventive—within its borders, it will be advised by a family practitioner committee, the successor to the executive council. The AHAs take over the functions of the former hospital management committees (administering the hospitals), and the regional authorities take over the responsibilities of the regional hospital boards (planning the construction of facilities). The teaching hospitals will be absorbed into the system, but they will have especially strong representation on the AHA boards in their areas. The school health services, formerly controlled by educational officials, will also be made a responsibility of the AHAs. Only the industrial health services remain separate.

Nonmedical representation on governing bodies, although the meaning of this point is debated, would be somewhat greater than before. A majority of members of AHA boards will not be health professionals, but, in the interests of improving efficiency, they will be required to have managerial experience. Perhaps of greater importance is the provision for a new type of medical leader—a community medicine specialist—as advisor to each AHA.[12] This individual will replace the medical officer of health. His duties will be not only to administer the preventive services (communicable disease control and environmental hygiene), but also to consult with the AHA and evaluate for it the efficacy and efficiency of all health services in the local hospitals and doctors' offices. He will be expected to provide health education to the people and epidemiological information to the doctors. He will offer planning guidance to other local government authorities, particularly in education and social services, as well as to voluntary bodies.

Consumer representation will be assured through community health councils at the health district level within the AHAs. As well as being a channel for patient complaints, these councils will advise the district management team, composed of the community medicine specialist, a district nurse, a chief administrator, and two clinicians (one a GP and another a specialist) elected by their peers. An ombudsman, called the health services commissioner, will be employed specifically to hear patient complaints.

It is expected that local health centers will continue to be built and, along with extension of group practices, will provide a setting for linkage of the district public health nursing, social work, and other local government personnel with the GPs. Indeed, to some people, the overriding objective of the NHS reorganization is to enhance the importance of the ambulatory and primary care services as a reaction against the enlarging role being assumed by hospitals. The elevated status and strengthened educational support for general practice, with the same objective, have been noted earlier.

To other people, the major purpose of the NHS reorganization is to achieve greater managerial efficiency.[13] A single hierarchy of authorities—from health districts, to area health authorities, to regional health authorities, up to the central Ministry of Health—is deemed more efficient and administratively economical than three or four sep-

arate vertical bureaucracies. Strengthened administrative responsibilities at the local level through AHAs and community medicine
specialists, backed up by various advisory committees of both providers
(family practitioner committees) and consumers (community health
councils), will presumably mean more effective execution of policies
formulated at the national level.

RECENT DEVELOPMENTS

In the late 1970s, a great deal of attention was paid to the uneven
distribution of resources (doctors, hospital beds, and so on) around the
nation, in spite of the entitlement of people everywhere to equal service. In the Ministry of Health and Social Security, therefore, steps
were taken to make allocations to the regional health authorities on
the basis of a formula that would reflect the extent of local needs. The
formula would include not only measurements of existing resources,
but also indicators of health care requirements, such as the percentage
of aged persons in the population or the infant mortality.

Experience with NHS administration through the 90 AHAs
showed that even at this level there was insufficient adjustment to
various local health needs. The viewpoint developed, therefore, that the
principal jurisdictions locally should be the 200 health districts, which
had around 250,000 people each. Such districts already operated
within most AHAs, and they were sensitive to local needs. A major
purpose of the 1974 reorganization had been to attain great managerial efficiency, but the creation of both area and district level authorities had, in effect, introduced a fourth echelon in the NHS. The
health districts achieved greater integration of services than had been
possible previously. The local authorities remain responsible for environmental sanitation and social services, but not for personal health
services (such as child health clinics). At the district level, the management teams bring together for the first time representatives of GPs and
specialists, as well as the community medicine specialist, the district
nursing officer, and the district administrator.[14]

As of 1981, the reorganized NHS faced problems of rising costs
similar to those of other industrialized countries. The Conservative
government of Margaret Thatcher, however, saw the remedy for this as
constraint in the public sector along with enlargement of the private
sector. By holding the line on salaries of specialists, the government
encouraged them to spend greater time in their private practices. At
the same time, more people were growing impatient with the waiting
time for service in the public system and therefore sought medical care

privately. The government encouraged the growth of private health insurance and the construction of small private hospitals. The policy of the previous Labour party government, to reduce the number of private beds in NHS hospitals, was halted and such beds were slightly expanded.

By 1982, the continued constraints on public spending by the Conservative party government created still greater pressures in the NHS and longer waiting lists for hospital care. As was to be expected, this stimulated the further growth of the private sector, particularly through expansion of private health insurance for private medical care. The government deliberately encouraged this by allowing tax concessions to management and labor for private insurance premiums. Coverage was said to have reached 3.5 million people by 1980—about 6.3 percent of the national population—and it is rapidly growing. The private sector was estimated to account for only 5 percent of total British health expenditures in 1982.[15]

To accommodate these privately insured patients, strictly private hospitals were constructed in London and in a few other main cities. Under existing law, no approval by hospital planning authorities was required for any new facility with fewer than 120 beds or for the expansion of any existing facility by less than 20 percent. The previous Labour party government had greatly reduced private pay beds in NHS hospitals, which heightened the demand for such beds in wholly private hospitals. While the approximately 7,500 beds operated in private hospitals by 1982 constituted less than 2 percent of the total supply, their impact was inevitably competitive. By offering higher salaries and more attractive working conditions, private hospitals could draw medical and other health manpower resources from NHS hospitals. Moreover, like proprietary hospitals everywhere, they served mainly low-risk, elective surgical cases, leaving the more difficult chronic and elderly patients to the public hospitals. All these developments were bound to injure the morale of NHS professional personnel.

The Royal Commission on the National Health Service had taken note in 1979 of the growth of a private medical sector, but it concluded that its minor proportions "could have, at most, a marginal and local effect on the NHS . . . it is clear that the private sector is too small to make a significant impact on the NHS except locally and temporarily."[16] A few years later, however, some observers disagreed, and, anticipating the further growth of private medical and hospital care, they called for actions that would deliberately integrate a private sector into the NHS. They advocated including all private hospital construction and technology within the orbit of official health planning, requiring private hospitals to accept all types of patients, establishing uniform salary scales for health personnel in all public and private hospitals, and other measures.

As elsewhere in the world, both in industrialized and developing countries, some people welcomed the growth of a private sector in British health care, on the ground that it brought more health resources (especially hospitals) into the system and lightened the burden carried by the public sector. Others pointed to its aggravation of public sector problems by withdrawing scarce medical and allied personnel for the service of a favored minority. No one could deny that a private sector would increase access to medical care on the basis of personal wealth rather than need for health care. The ultimate question posed by these recent British developments is, How should resources (health personnel, facilities, and so on) in a national health care system be augmented to meet all health needs? One way is by increased private spending, which naturally benefits those who can spend. The other way is by increased public spending, which can benefit everyone. By any criterion of social justice, the answer is manifest; but political decisions in the health sector, as in other sectors, are often based more on other criteria. The future of the NHS, therefore, will inevitably depend on the policies of the political parties elected to power.[17]

Only time will tell to what extent these various objectives of the NHS reorganization are actually achieved. Some persons have viewed the entire metamorphosis skeptically, as a set of new labels for the same old mechanisms. Some of the role definitions of the new entities are not crystal clear, and their final implementation will probably depend on the strengths and weaknesses of diverse groups in each local area. Nevertheless, in my opinion the redesigning of the NHS further confirms a point made earlier in this book: the worldwide trend toward unified and comprehensive health service planning and delivery. Whether through social revolution or incremental changes, the movement seems to be in the same direction.

NOTES

1. G. G. McCleary, *National Health Insurance* (London: Lewis and Co., 1939).
2. I. S. Falk, *Security Against Sickness: A Study of Health Insurance* (New York: Doubleday Doran & Co., 1936), 155–56.
3. W. Beveridge, *Social Insurance and Allied Services*, American ed. (New York: Macmillan Co., 1942).
4. W. Beveridge, 11.
5. W. Beveridge, 158.

6. A. Lindsey, *Socialized Medicine in England and Wales: The National Health Service 1948–1961* (Chapel Hill: University of North Carolina Press, 1962).

7. G. Forsyth, "United Kingdom," in *Health Service Prospects: An International Survey*, I. Douglas-Wilson and G. McLachlan, eds. (London: The Lancet and the Nuffield Provincial Hospitals Trust, 1973), 1–35.

8. J. Bunker, "Surgical Manpower: A Comparison of Operations and Surgeons in the United States and in England and Wales," *New England Journal of Medicine* 282(January 15, 1970):135–44.

9. T. E. Chester, "How Healthy is the National Health Service?" *District Bank Review*, September 1968. Also U.S. Social Security Administration, *National Health Expenditures, Fiscal Years 1929–70 and Calendar Years 1929–69*, research and statistics note no. 25 (Washington, D.C., 1970).

10. G. E. Godber, "The Future Place of the General Physician," the 1969 Michael M. Davis lecture, University of Chicago, Center for Health Administration Studies, 1969.

11. R. M. Battistella and T. E. Chester, "Reorganization of the National Health Service: Background and Issues in England's Quest for a Comprehensive-Integrated Planning and Delivery System," *Health and Society* 51(Fall 1973):489–530.

12. G. A. Silver, "The Community-Medicine Specialist—Britain Mandates Health Service Reorganization," *New England Journal of Medicine* 287(December 21, 1972):1299–1301.

13. K. Barnard and K. Lee, eds., *NHS Reorganization: Issues and Prospects* (Leeds, England: University of Leeds, 1974).

14. S. Jonas and D. Barton, "The 1974 Reorganization of the British National Health Service," *Journal of Community Health* 1(Winter 1975):91–105; K. Barnard and K. Lee, eds., *Conflicts in the National Health Service* (London: Croom Helm, 1977).

15. P. Chubb, S. Haywood, and P. R. Torrens, *Managing the Mixed Economy of Health: Policy Considerations for the National Health Service in Dealing with the Expansion of the Private Sector*, occasional paper no. 42 (Birmingham: Health Services Management Centre, 1982).

16. P. R. Torrens, "Some Potential Hazards of Unplanned Expansion of Private Health Insurance in Britain," *Lancet*, 2 January 1982, 29–31.

17. R. Deitch, "Labour Plans for the NHS," *Lancet*, 8 May 1982, 1080–81.

13

Canadian Health Services
and Manpower Policy

Although bordering on the United States and having a sim-
ilar general structure, Canada has developed a national
health care system very different from the U.S. model. Yet
with its federated structure of ten provinces, each having
great autonomy in the health services, Canadian health care
strategies have special significance for health planning in the
United States. The crucial distinction in the Canadian sys-
tem is its program of national-provincial medical and hospi-
tal care insurance. This chapter traces the evolution of that
program, along with a special focus on policies involving
health manpower.

The Canadian health service experience is replete with possible
lessons for the United States. Very much like the United States, Canada has approached the solving of its health problems incrementally,
with progress in one sector after another. The nature of Canada's incre-
mentalism has been determined in large part by its "constitutional"
definition of health services as provincial responsibilities and by the
relative multiplicity of political parties with markedly different phi-
losophies.

Based principally on a 1975 field study that included eight of the ten Canadian
provinces. A comprehensive report can be found in R. Roemer and M.I. Roemer, *Health
Manpower Policy Under National Health Insurance—The Canadian Experience* (Washington, D.C.: U.S. Department of Health, Education, and Welfare, 1977).

This chapter summarizes the Canadian health service experience and considers its implications for the United States in six main sections: (1) the evolution of the health care system, (2) approaches to the questions of health manpower supply, distribution, and functions, (3) policies on education of health personnel, (4) the regulation of health manpower qualifications and performance, (5) some overall lessons of special salience for current U.S. problems, and (6) major recent developments.

EVOLUTION OF THE HEALTH CARE SYSTEM

From the viewpoint of health manpower and the development of other health resources, the greatest importance must be attached to Canada's federal-provincial health insurance program. This central feature of the Canadian system did not, of course, spring up overnight, and to understand its dynamics (and lessons for the United States) one must understand its evolution. The evolution involved first hospitalization insurance, then insurance for physician care, and finally insurance for and organization of other services. All three of these components of health care financing have had important influences on the patterns of health care management and delivery; all three movements are still in progress.

Hospitalization Insurance

The enactment of the Saskatchewan Hospital Services Plan (SHSP) in 1946 (to take effect in 1947) had its roots in events over at least the previous 30 years.[1] Tax-supported municipal doctor plans had originated in this sparsely settled prairie region in 1916 as a mechanism for attracting and holding physicians in low-income rural areas. The concept of using a cooperative or collective economic process for solving a key health problem in this context made sense, and the idea spread. In the 1920's, funds for hospital construction were raised by the combined efforts of adjacent rural municipalities, which formed union hospital districts. In the larger economic environment, cooperatives of wheat farmers for marketing their produce, purchasing fertilizer, and other purposes were found to be similarly effective.

After the years of economic depression that drove down the world price of wheat in the 1930's, compounded by serious drought in the early 1940's, election to power of the Cooperative Commonwealth Federation (CCF) party could come as no surprise in Saskatchewan. In its campaign for election in 1944, a key slogan was to introduce a program of "socialized health services." With an overwhelming electoral victory, the new government lost no time in converting its promise into reality. Years before, the federal government, following European models, had attempted to enact national health insurance legislation, only to have it nullified by the Canadian high court (British Privy Council) on the ground of federal usurpation of provincial rights; likewise, several other provinces had attempted to implement the idea without success. But the Saskatchewan CCF government was determined to move ahead, and it launched the first social insurance program for health care of the total population of a state or province in North America.

As the trailblazer in this field, Saskatchewan had to solve many problems not faced before on this continent. More hospitals had to be built to provide beds for people wherever they lived. Economy dictated a planned scheme of regionalization, so that common conditions could be treated in a nearby facility, while more complex cases could be referred to a district hospital, and the most difficult cases could be sent to large base hospitals in one of the province's two main cities. Many more nurses, technicians, and other personnel had to be trained to staff the beds. Rates of hospital admission rapidly rose until it was realized that the conventional system of per diem remuneration gave both hospitals and doctors incentives to maximize hospital occupancy at all times—and even to set up additional beds in the corridors whenever feasible.[2]

After a few years, it was recognized that more judicious planning was needed. On the basis of initial experience, the provincial health leadership concluded that 7.5 hospital beds for 1,000 people would be adequate to meet total needs—these beds to be distributed among local, intermediate, and base hospitals. To staff the bed complement in each facility and meet all the other expenses for serving patients at an estimated 90 percent average occupancy, a certain annual budget would be required. The hospital could be paid one-twelfth of this amount each month, regardless of the actual patient load. Thus, there was no incentive to overcrowd. If the budgeted allotment was not fully spent, the hospital could keep the surplus at the end of the year; if there was a deficit because of an epidemic or some other justifiable cause for excessive utilization, the provincial SHSP would make it up.

This whole process required careful review of all hospital program budgets and the stipulation of reasonable standards for the nurses and other staff, laboratory supplies, food, and so on necessary for hospitals of given sizes. Nationally recommended standards (such as 4.2 nursing hours per patient per day) were applied. Salary scales were left up to each hospital to decide; but, with unionization of hospital employees developing rapidly, provincewide collective bargaining for different categories of employees soon followed. Budgets had to be resubmitted and reevaluated each year, as costs of living, wages, and prices of commodities—as well as standards of patient care—changed.

Thus developed the Saskatchewan system of hospital reimbursement, a system that in Canada came to be called global budgeting, and that in the United States is termed prospective budgeting. There are more details to it than given here, and its application requires uniform hospital accounting procedures and a competent staff of consultants at the provincial level. These consultants are not only in the field of general hospital administration and accounting, but also in nursing, laboratory and X-ray technology, dietetics, and the other key functions in hospital operations. This staff carefully reviews hospital budgets; more important, it consults with hospitals on recommended policies. Their advice could as often be to engage additional laboratory technicians, for example, as to hire fewer kitchen helpers—with the advice backed up always by the assurance that necessary costs would be met by the hospital insurance plan.

An important side benefit of the SHSP was a steady flow of information on every patient hospitalized; upon the patient's discharge, the hospital was required to send a one-page summary report to the SHSP. These reports included basic information (name, address, diagnosis, attending doctor, surgical operations if any, condition on discharge, and so on) on *all* patients, even the occasional nonresident served in a Saskatchewan hospital or the occasional resident hospitalized outside the province (for which the external hospital would be paid on an indemnity basis). From these data, analyses could be made to indicate whether the residents of a particular area (rural municipality, town, or city) were being hospitalized at a rate substantially higher or lower than the provincial average. Such information permitted rational decision making on whether additional hospital construction or enlargement was justified in an area or, indeed, whether the number of beds was excessive and should be reduced (or budgeted for a lower occupancy level).

There were virtually no limits on admission or duration of hospital stay, except the doctor's decision, but soon it was found prudent to introduce certain kinds of surveillance. Short stays (one to two days), which might suggest admission only for some diagnostic tests that could properly be done outside the hospital, were scrutinized and, if found excessive for a particular doctor or area, would summon a request for an explanation. Likewise, long stays (over 30 days) required periodic medical reports. If significant amounts of hospital use could not be justified, further abuse was deterred, first with a warning and then, if necessary, a certain reduction in the monthly payment to the hospital. On the other hand, any extra funds raised by the hospital through voluntary donations, extra charges for use of private rooms, and so on could be kept without reduction of the global budget allotments.

Over the years, details in these administrative procedures changed, but basically the strategies worked out in Saskatchewan were adopted by British Columbia when its hospital insurance plan was enacted in 1949. The British Columbia plan imposed a $1 per day copayment charge on the patient (designed to discourage overuse) and modified the reporting procedures in certain ways. When the solvency and qualitative improvements of hospitals in Saskatchewan and British Columbia, as well as the high popularity of the programs with the general population, became evident throughout Canada, interest was naturally kindled at the national level. By 1956, the success of the idea and the political dynamics of the time led the national Parliament, under Liberal party control, to enact the National Hospital and Diagnostic Services Act. Its provision for about 50 percent support of any provincial program meeting certain minimum standards was consistent with the British North America Act, which serves as Canada's constitution. Diagnostic services were included in the Act to pay for outpatient diagnosis that could avert unnecessary hospital admission. By 1957, conditions for the Act to become operative had been met (participation of at least half the provinces with half of the national population), and by 1961 the program had been implemented in all ten provinces. The general administrative and accounting strategies hammered out in Saskatchewan were adopted throughout Canada.[3]

Other provinces learned from Saskatchewan's experiences. Principally, this involved providing for a hospital bed supply lower than 7.5 per 1,000 (the Saskatchewan ratio), since it was found that, under conditions of universal insurance coverage, whatever beds were provided tended to be used. The bed supply ultimately determined the staffing needed (75 percent of hospital operating costs), the supplies consumed, and virtually all the costs. All the provinces found that budget reviews permitted rational planning of hospital functions according to some type of regionalized scheme. Additional training programs for nurses and other personnel were needed. Since heavy hospital costs were being met through a social mechanism, people had more money to enable them to see doctors and pay them, so physicians' incomes rose. With the federal sharing of costs out of general revenues, provincial government expenditures declined, whether these funds were raised by earmarked insurance premiums, a sales tax, general revenues, or through a combination of methods. Each year, the overall costs rose, mostly due to elevated standards (more staffing, shorter workweeks, better supplies, and so on), but the same thing was happening in the United States and elsewhere. Governments and political parties were not greatly concerned, because "free" access to hospital care was extremely popular with the voters.[4]

Within the broad national criteria, there were many variations among the provinces in their hospital insurance programs. Administrative responsibility was assigned to the Department of Health in some provinces and to special commissions in others, though always under the general control of government through the Minister of Health. The provincial funds were raised in different ways. While periodic payment for "readiness to serve" on a global budgeting basis was applied everywhere, details in budget review criteria differed. The optimal bed supply, as suggested above, also differed, as did salaries. In a few provinces, the government bargained directly with professional associations or unions on salary scales. Small extra charges were permitted in some provinces, as long as they did not constitute a barrier to hospital use.

Thus, the Canadian strategy achieved a nationwide program of hospital insurance within a few years, without invading provincial prerogatives. By confining benefits to hospitalization, Canada took a first step toward comprehensive health insurance that was politically acceptable, offered important leverage for health service planning, was agreeable to both hospitals and doctors, and yet met a deeply felt need in the general population. At the same time, the problems in this categorical hospital-linked approach generated further actions to broaden the health benefits and correct inequities.

Insurance for Physician's Care (Medicare)

It was only a few years after Saskatchewan's hospital cost burden was cut in half by the federal matching legislation that the provincial government, still under CCF control (but renamed the New Democratic Party), began to think of extending the scope of "socialized health services." Insurance for doctor's care was the obvious next step to be taken. The rate of hospital utilization was high compared with that in the United States or in other affluent nations, and rigorous controls were not politically feasible. If complete physician's care could be economically supported, hospital abuse might be eliminated, while at the same time early and more prevention-oriented medical attention would be promoted.

As is customary in democratic societies, a study commission was appointed; it recommended a program of action; and in 1962 the Saskatchewan Medical Care Insurance Act was passed.[5] Despite its providing free choice of doctor and fee-for-service remuneration, physicians objected to direct payment by the government and a fixed schedule of fees, even though it would be negotiated. As a result, the Saskatchewan Medical Association called the first strike by doctors, except for care of emergencies, in North American history. The strike settlement, after 23 days in July 1962, retained the basic principles of universal coverage and governmental control, but permitted use of private fiscal intermediaries and allowed doctors to charge patients extra amounts beyond the officially scheduled fees, if the patient chose a doctor who made such extra charges. Initially, the latter mechanisms were used by doctors serving 12 percent of the patients, but the operation of the free market brought this down to barely 2 percent of the patients by 1974.

Once again all of Canada looked to Saskatchewan's experience—doctors, political leaders, and other citizens. The sudden spurt of average Saskatchewan medical incomes from the lowest of the ten provinces to the highest within two years did not escape notice. Despite the bruised relationships left by the strike, the general popularity of the program was clear to both politicians and voters everywhere. A Royal Commission on Health Services that was deliberating at the time decided to call for a national medical care insurance program as its principal recommendation. And this time, instead of a nine- or ten-year gap between provincial pioneering and national legislation, it was only four years.[6] In 1966, the national Medical Care Act was passed—on essentially the same basis of federal-provincial matching, but with a more generous formula for the poorer provinces, as under the Hospital Act of 1956. It took a few years for all provinces to take up the "medicare" offer, but by 1971 it had become a nationwide program.

Variations in the provincial administrative mechanisms were somewhat greater than under the hospital insurance program. Commissions separate from the Health Department were more frequently assigned administrative responsibility, and various forms of fiscal intermediaries were more often used. Despite the trauma of the Saskatchewan battle over the doctors' right to levy extra charges on the patient, some provinces were tougher in restricting this practice than Saskatchewan. They called the practice "opting out" and required that a doctor wishing to employ this indemnification mechanism for any of his patients apply it to all of them. As a result, only a small percentage of doctors in these provinces employed it at all. None of the provinces required copayments from the patient or imposed deductibles. British Columbia was sufficiently confident of the popularity of the program that legally enrollment was voluntary; the "buy" for the consumer was so good (the province covering the indigent) that the minimum federal requirement of 95 percent coverage was readily met.

Utilization and costs under a nationwide medicare program naturally rose, and greater controls by the provincial authorities followed.[7] In some provinces, only one complete medical examination per year would be paid for. Practice profiles, by specialty and diagnosis, were statistically compiled, and deviant physicians were asked for an explanation. Services deemed clearly excessive or unjustified were remunerated at a 50 percent rate or not at all. With insurance of out-of-hospital ambulatory services, hospital admission rates did not decline, but rose—evidently due to an increase in hospital beds available and in the number of cases coming to medical attention, some of them requiring hospitalization. Now that Saskatchewan was no longer alone among the provinces in having medicare, physicians' incomes soared everywhere in Canada, and Saskatchewan's rank among the ten provinces again took a place near the bottom.[8] Doctors and consumers almost everywhere found the program highly agreeable.

Just as hospital insurance generated construction of more hospital beds, the very anticipation of medicare led to a rapid increase in the supply of doctors.[9] Additional medical schools were built, and the established schools increased their enrollments. A rise in immigration of doctors also occurred, not only because immigration restrictions were lowered (medicine was declared a needed occupation), but because the word spread that Canada was a country where medical earnings were high. By 1975, a doctor-population ratio of one to 600 was being approached—well above that in the United States at the time. This ratio was greater than the idealistic recommendation of the Royal Commission on Health Services in 1964. More significant evidence perhaps was the frequent observation that the average number of hours of medical work per week or per year was declining; if a doctor could earn enough to satisfy himself and his family in 40 hours per week, why work 50?

In response to the growing consensus that the supply of physicians was now adequate, steps were taken to limit immigration of foreign medical graduates. Not only was the foreign medical graduate likely to be less well trained than the graduate of a Canadian medical school, but two inequities might be corrected: qualified Canadian applicants for medical school, now rejected, could be accepted; and the brain drain from other nations needing doctors more than Canada would be reduced. It was decided that only if a foreign medical graduate would settle in an area with a shortage of doctors (usually in a northern rural region) for a certain number of years would he be allowed to immigrate to Canada.

Of probably greater importance in the long run was the realization spreading across Canada that the system of delivering medical care should be modified.[10] The essence of the change should be toward developing patterns of teamwork in health service, so that much of the work traditionally done by doctors would be delegated to less expensive, but competent, personnel. This meant training such personnel, but it also meant providing an effective setting in which they could work along with the doctor. Starting with the landmark Castonguay-Nepveu Report of Quebec, published in 1970, province after province issued official statements calling for the establishment of community health centers at which doctors and allied personnel would provide comprehensive (preventive and therapeutic) ambulatory health services. Improved regionalization of both hospital and ambulatory services should accompany this.[11] In 1972, a similar message was broadcast from the national level in the Hastings Report on community health centers, which was commissioned by the national Conference of Health Ministers (representing all of the provinces along with the federal Minister of National Health and Welfare).

In practice, the health center movement proved to be less dynamic than the flavor of the several investigations and reports promoting it. In the main, health centers were organized in areas of medical care shortage. This policy engendered less opposition from the private medical profession, while clearly helping to meet needs where they were greatest. The movement was encouraged by most provincial governments, albeit in varying formats. The combination of the health center pattern with a population enrolled for comprehensive service (as in the U.S. health maintenance organization) was limited to a few locations in Saskatchewan and Ontario, because the free choice of doctor guarantees of the federal medicare law were interpreted as barring such enrollment. As of early 1975, health centers in all Canada numbered fewer than 100, but the number was growing at a steady rate.

Perhaps, as in Great Britain, the rather rapid growth of private group medical practice was achieving purposes similar to those of health centers, though in a different form. By 1970, it was estimated that 31 percent of Canadian doctors were in formal groups—a proportion well above that in the United States at the time. Several provincial governments decided to take advantage of this spontaneous process, seeing it as the natural entry to teamwork service, by assigning public health nurses and other personnel to work with the medical groups.

Other Insurance and Organizations

Both the hospitalization and physician's care insurance programs are administered by the provinces, but they are administered under conditions specified by the federal government. These requirements, on population coverage, services to be provided, public responsibility, and other features, are monitored by the Department of National Health and Welfare as conditions for the substantial federal subsidy.

Other support programs of the federal government have also shaped the health services of Canada's ten provinces. The National Health Grants program, operating from 1948 to 1972, assisted the provinces in construction and renovation of hospitals, in strengthening their basic public health programs, in developing community mental health services, and in preparing for general health insurance. In 1966, in tandem with medicare, a large Health Resources Fund was established to finance over the next 15 years construction of educational facilities that would train the additional health manpower needed across the nation. In every province today one sees impressive educational structures financed from this source that have helped to turn out increasing numbers of doctors, nurses, technicians, and others who have met Canada's escalating demands for personnel. Other federal departments, such as those for veterans' affairs and for manpower and immigration, have contributed significantly to developments in rehabilitation of the disabled. The Canada Assistance Plan, also under the Department of National Health and Welfare, shares with the provinces the costs of health services for the indigent beyond those covered by the social insurance programs.

The most rapidly advancing health programs, however, are those developing within the provinces solely at provincial expense. Just as Saskatchewan initiated the actions that led to national insurance for hospital and physician's care, it and other provinces are continuing to initiate programs for other types of health service. Provision of prescribed drugs seems to be the sector of need most often being tackled by the provinces, although it is restricted to older persons in some provinces, requires some cost sharing by the patient in others, and so on. Nursing home care, also usually with various limitations, is another supplemental provincial insurance benefit. Optometry, hearing aids, podiatry, and even chiropractic service are among the other supplemental benefits. Dental care has been approached very warily because of both the costs and Canada's meager supply of dentists. Saskatchewan has again broken new ground in North America by training school dental nurses to give virtually complete dental care to children, along the lines pioneered in New Zealand in 1920.

Other provincial programs of importance include the operation of mental hospitals, workmen's compensation for industrial injuries or occupational diseases, and the traditional public health services. Regarding the latter, the promotion of regional administrative patterns is especially notable, regions being geographic areas made up of several local governmental jurisdictions. Public health laboratories tend to play a broader role in Canada than in the United States, often doing clinical pathology tests for practicing physicians as well as tests specifically related to public health. Voluntary agencies, often with public subsidies, are active in visiting nurse services, ambulance transport, and emergency care.

Judging from previous developmental patterns in Canada, it seems likely that the insurance initiatives in new sectors of health service, starting now in the provinces, will eventually lead to action at the federal level.[12] If one may hazard a prediction, the national government—eager to place a ceiling on its expenditures for hospital and doctors' care—may strike a bargain, so to speak, with the provinces. Despite provincial objections, it may impose ceilings on the per capita sums it will match for the two basic programs, but at the same time agree to match (probably also with ceilings) the costs of additional benefits for drugs, dental service, nursing home care, and so on.

Thus, the Canadian style of incremental development of organized or socially financed health services may have important lessons for the United States. The initiative of one, then a second, enterprising province demonstrated the soundness of the hospital insurance idea so effectively that after a few years the concept was applied nationwide. Theoretical arguments about hospitalization being the wrong end of the health care spectrum at which to start a national health program were outweighed by pragmatic considerations of political feasibility, popularity with the citizens, and leverage for system planning. The weakness of noncoverage of physician services was soon corrected by the initiative of one province in adding these benefits and—despite a traumatic strike by doctors—demonstrating so well the effectiveness of the idea that it was soon emulated nationally. Now further health benefits are being extended along the same lines. Moreover, abuses in the way of excessive rendering of services by doctors or hospitals generate their own reforms, in the shape of greater quality and cost controls.

The manpower concomitants of Canadian provincial-national health insurance have been conspicuous. The highlights of these developments may now be summarized.

HEALTH MANPOWER SUPPLY, DISTRIBUTION, AND FUNCTIONS

With escalating demands for health services under the medicare program, there could be no political objection to investing more funds to increase the output of health manpower.[13] The Health Resources Fund of 1966 for constructing educational facilities was very helpful, and the provinces took similar actions. Immigration preferences brought thousands of foreign-trained doctors into Canada. A major boost was given to training allied health personnel in technical colleges of many types. By 1975, the prevailing Canadian viewpoint was that, with a ratio of about one doctor to 600 population, an adequate supply had been achieved; there remained problems of geographic and specialty distribution. Beyond this, more ancillary personnel of various types were needed, especially for dental care, as well as more dentists.

With respect to physicians, the greatest concern seems to be the strengthening of family medicine, even though Canada already has more than twice the proportion of general practitioners found in the United States. The College of Family Physicians, with its prescribed training programs, has given a specialty status to the qualified generalist. All 16 Canadian medical schools have organized a department of family medicine or its equivalent as a division of another department. Family practice teaching units are providing ambulatory patient care at every medical school, sometimes at several locations. Continuing education for GPs is steadily increasing. Stronger postgraduate training is provided in the field, and it benefits from the general policy of linking all Canadian internships and residencies to medical schools. Even provincial fee schedules are being adjusted to raise the relative rewards for general medical service, vis à vis the lucrative specialties.

Much attention at the national level is directed to planning for a reasonable distribution of specialists. Utilization data from the medicare program are the basis for studies of requirements by working groups of specialists in each field. It is hoped that eventually residency programs can be adjusted to produce specialists based on population needs rather than on the wishes of departmental chairmen in teaching hospitals. The payment for ambulatory psychiatric care by the medicare program has greatly increased the number of specialists going into this field, as the census of mental hospitals has declined. The pediatrician, being now accessible to people of all incomes, has had to adjust to the demand by becoming more of a consultant, while common ailments of children are handled by the GP.

Improved geographic distribution of doctors has been tackled in a number of provincial actions. Bursaries for living expenses have been offered to medical students, conditional on their future settlement in areas of need, mainly rural. Subsidies or guaranteed annual incomes for rural doctors have been other provincial approaches. Quebec (and more recently British Columbia) has used the British strategy of declaring certain places overdoctored, so new doctors expecting medicare payments must settle in locations of greater need. Small rural hospitals or, more often, health centers are established to attract doctors to isolated areas. In very sparsely settled northern regions, the outpost nurse must still be relied upon.

The exceptionally high supply of registered nurses in Canada is obviously a consequence of the hospital insurance program and the abundant hospital bed resources it has supported. In contrast to the United States, there is not so much need to rely on the less fully trained vocational nurse or certified nursing assistant. Yet nurse wastage, by withdrawal from active work, is still a problem in Canada, as elsewhere; it is being met by higher salaries, part-time jobs, child-care centers in large hospitals, and other adjustments.

The registered psychiatric nurse has long been used for staffing mental hospitals and, more recently, mental health clinics. With much more caution, Canada is approaching the development of nurse-practitioners to extend the arm of the doctor. For outpost stations, the nurse-practitioner is trained in clinical management of common ailments and in providing preventive services. As an office copractitioner with the doctor, despite some impressive demonstrations at McMaster University Medical School and elsewhere, there are divided views on how much the nurse-practitioner should be trained to do without strict medical supervision, how she should be paid, her legal status, and other matters. There is consensus on widening the nurse's role as home visitor and helper to the doctor, but the great importance attached to family physicians in Canada may be responsible for the caution in training nurses for independent clinical functions.

A distinctive Canadian innovation is the school dental nurse, now being trained in two provinces (Saskatchewan and Manitoba) and soon to be in a third (Quebec). The severe shortage of dentists, with little prospect of governmental investment in their increased output, has made this approach politically acceptable. In several ways, Canada has improved on the original New Zealand model—furnishing the dental nurse with better equipment, a dental aide such as the dentist has, and more frequent advice from dentists, all of which increase the productivity and quality of her work.

The combined technician, capable of doing both laboratory and X-ray work in small hospitals, is another Canadian innovation, taking various forms in different western provinces. More recently there has been exploration of the idea of a combined clinical technologist, who would carry out intensive care functions now assumed by separately trained inhalation therapists, renal dialysis technicians, and specialists in heart-lung perfusion equipment. One enterprising medical school is training a Master of Health Sciences, a nonphysician to lead health teams; so far, candidates have come from nursing and rehabilitation therapy.

The Canadian pharmacist, like his U.S. counterpart, is in search of wider functions because the precompounding and packaging of drugs have reduced his traditional responsibilities. Advising the physician on drug interactions, as well as community health education, are the principal new functions being explored.

The community health centers, discussed earlier as a crucial mechanism for modifying the health care delivery system, are providing at the same time a practical setting for new functions of health personnel. The several different patterns being developed correspond with the differing political ideologies and conditions among the provinces. Increasing recognition of the importance of teamwork is the obvious guiding principle in Canada for the most effective use of all kinds of health manpower.[14]

EDUCATION OF HEALTH PERSONNEL

The rapid increase of schools for training all types of health personnel was made possible by the commitment of government, both federal and provincial, to this objective, partly in anticipation and partly in the wake of the two nationwide health insurance programs.

For many years the federal government had been subsidizing various provincial functions under the terms of the tax-rental agreement, which returned to the provinces part of the national income tax revenues. With the Fiscal Arrangements Act of 1967, the substantial federal support of all postsecondary education was made explicit and brought special benefits for the education of health manpower. Approximately 50 percent of the latter operational costs have been met from these federal funds; regarding the balance, nearly all of it has been met by provincial government funds for public institutions and most of the remainder for private ones. Even for the handful of old, private universities in Canada, about 80 percent of the financial support is derived from public revenues, federal and provincial. The operation of various semi-autonomous provincial councils for assigning these funds to the several institutions has served to protect their independence within broad limits.

This public support, it must be emphasized, applies to more than universities. The several types of technical colleges, in which allied health personnel training is so extensive, are similarly supported. In fact, Canada seems to have emphasized these practice-oriented training centers, in contrast perhaps to the mounting tendency in the United States to provide university degrees for more and more types of health occupations. In addition, one must not overlook the training of health workers in hospitals, at the expense of the hospital insurance program, and in public health agencies.

Physicians

Canada, with 16 medical schools, has a greater proportionate number than the United States. Three of them have been established since 1965, and all 16 have expanded their enrollments since the national health insurance programs took effect. To further increase the output of doctors, three schools have concentrated their four-year curriculums into three years by eliminating long summer holidays.

Two of the Canadian medical schools have adopted the organ-system method of teaching instead of the traditional presentation of subjects by departments. All 16 schools, as noted earlier, put relatively strong emphasis on teaching both community and family medicine. Departmental arrangements, of course, differ among the schools, with about half combining these two fields in one department and the others having independent departments of family medicine. In either pattern, the teaching of family medicine is strengthened by the operation of one or more family medicine clinics that are usually separate from the main teaching hospitals. These family units often make use of nurse-practitioners and numerous other support personnel, adding to the general national movement for development of health centers.

One of the most significant Canadian innovations is at the postgraduate level of medical education. Since 1970, all internships and residencies to be approved by the Royal College of Physicians and Surgeons (for specialty certification) must be affiliated with medical schools. This need not mean that all postgraduate training is confined to university hospitals, but rather that all such teaching hospitals must be under medical school supervision with respect to their educational activities.

Contrary to common anxieties previously expressed in Canada and currently expressed in the United States, the advent of universal insurance for hospital and doctor's care did not reduce the availability of teaching material for the medical schools. If anything, the effect has been positive. Every patient in a teaching hospital is a teaching case, and this has evidently caused no problems. The patient knows that, if he enters a teaching hospital, he is likely to receive especially good care—in return for which he may be served by residents under supervision or examined by medical students. Students, moreover, learn to deal with all social classes of patients, rather than solely the indigent. This is important not only in widening the spectrum of diseases observable but also in shaping the attitudes of the maturing student toward patients and his personal relationships to them. (Perhaps the condescending attitudes of many young American doctors towards patients—about which one hears frequent complaints—is due in part to habits formed in teaching hospitals limited essentially to indigent or lower social class patients.)

Nurses and Allied Health Personnel

As noted, the general Canadian tendency has been toward strengthening technical and vocational colleges for allied health personnel, rather than proliferating university degree programs. Being under the supervision of governmental education departments, the standards maintained in these institutions are high. One does not see in Canada the numerous proprietary schools for medical or dental assistants of various sorts found in many U.S. cities, where large tuitions are collected for inferior training programs.

The shift of nursing education from the general hospitals to community colleges might be construed as an exception to the above trends. The transfer, however, has not often been to universities with four years of study, but principally to two-year colleges. As in the United States, which really pioneered the concept, this constitutes a reduction in time from the three-year hospital diploma course, as well as an enrichment of academic content. This is believed to attract into nursing intellectually more serious young persons who are likely to remain active longer. Whatever the two-year college graduate lacks in practical abilities is soon acquired in hospital experience.

The nurse-practitioner training programs, because of Canada's attachment to family medicine, attract less enthusiasm than one sees for them in the United States. At the same time, an explicit national decision of the main professional bodies has rejected any policy for training physicians' assistants—not surprising with Canada's large supply of registered nurses and the absence of any flow of returning military medical corpsmen. Perhaps the most significant U.S. impact on the nurse-practitioner concept has been the decision in several baccalaureate training programs to enrich the teaching of clinical practice as a regular component of the university-based nursing curriculum.

The innovative Canadian training of combined laboratory and X-ray technicians, initially by public health agencies and now by technical colleges, has been noted above. In addition, nearly all the technical colleges have strong two-year courses for conventional, separate laboratory or X-ray technicians. For rehabilitation therapists (physical, occupational, and speech therapy), however, the trends are rather mixed. In a few places they are being trained in nondegree three-year colleges; for the most part, however, the baccalaureate route is being followed. This may well be due to the independent responsibility so often carried by these personnel, in the light of Canada's very small supply of physical medicine specialists. It is also perhaps an outgrowth of the origin of several of these training programs within medical schools, as parts of universities. The influence of U.S. professional societies toward continuously upgrading these fields may also play a part. The earlier Canadian movement for training combined physical and occupational therapists, moreover, has been declining and now continues only at one university; even these graduates later tend to concentrate in one field or the other.

Training in health service administration in Canada has been expanding, although the academic settings have been in ferment. Of six special programs (counting the very youngest one at Dalhousie University), four are lodged in medical schools, usually as parts of departments of community medicine. The recent closing of the School of Hygiene at the University of Toronto and the transfer of its faculty to a major new division of the medical school is being viewed with much interest throughout the continent. While one view may regard this as a downgrading of the status of public health education, another view regards it as an elevation. With the medical school now containing three major divisions—basic sciences, clinical medicine, and community services—the latter may represent a stronger position than that of an isolated school of public health. University authorities in Toronto emphasize that this placement of community services in the medical school does not limit its students to physicians, just as departments of physiology, for example, have long awarded M.A. and Ph.D. degrees to nonmedical candidates.

As for continuing education in medicine and the allied health fields, it is actively promoted throughout Canada on a voluntary basis. Universities, professional societies, hospitals, public health agencies, and other bodies all play a role. In one or two provinces, dentistry and pharmacy have made a minimum amount of continuing education mandatory for relicensure, and this tendency may spread. The Royal College of Physicians and Surgeons is seriously considering such a policy for maintaining specialty status. Nursing is particularly active in this field because of the need to provide refresher courses for older women who return to work after being inactive for some years (such courses are mandatory in some provinces). Likewise, for the diagnostic technologies and for the rehabilitation therapies, continuing education is a high priority.

In medicine, and most actively in Quebec, the detection of deficiencies in a doctor's performance through the health insurance program is the signal to the licensing agency to require him to take instruction to correct his weaknesses in specific fields. The family medicine movement, as noted earlier, encourages GPs to participate in continuing education programs.

REGULATION OF HEALTH MANPOWER

Examination of the system of regulating the qualifications and performance of health personnel reveals several marked trends. First is the drive toward national academic standards for many health occupations, despite provincial autonomy over qualifications and functions of health manpower. Second is enactment, or planned enactment, of strengthened registration and licensing laws, with increased public accountability, expanded scope, and more stringent controls than have prevailed in the past. These reforms are particularly striking in the field of medicine, but they affect other professions as well. Third is use of the health insurance system as a channel for controls over the quality of medical practice, including deliberate linkages to licensing and professional bodies.

National Academic Standards

Although one might assume that substantial federal financing of postsecondary education explains the trend toward national academic standards for health personnel, the government of Canada actually provides this subsidy with no strings attached. Rather, it has been the role of national professional associations in accrediting educational programs and adopting national examinations in many fields that has promoted national academic standards, despite varying provincial requirements for practice.

The Liaison Committee on Medical Education of the Canadian and American associations of medical colleges accredits medical schools in Canada. For postgraduate medical education, the Royal College of Physicians and Surgeons sets standards for specialist training in all fields except family medicine, which is governed by the College of Family Physicians. The Royal College was largely responsible for introducing the important requirement of university affiliation for all residencies, mentioned earlier. For the allied health professions, accreditation of education by the national professional associations, which register or certify individuals, achieves a uniform standard of training that facilitates mobility across provincial lines. (Exceptions to national standards for accreditation of education are in nursing, for which provincial nursing associations accredit educational programs, and in all fields in the Province of Quebec, where the provincial government approves educational programs.)

Probably more important than accreditation of education by professional organizations are the national examinations required in medicine, dentistry, pharmacy, nursing, and other fields. The distinguished Medical Council of Canada gives examinations for a licentiate (LMCC) acceptable to all provinces and has set the pattern for other professions. The LMCC examination, required of all Canadian medical graduates, provides a basis for mobility of doctors across Canada that may be contrasted with the complexities of U.S. arrangements—the reciprocity system (far from complete among the states), the tests of the National Board of Medical Examiners (not mandatory and not recognized by certain states), or the examination of the Federation of State Licensing Boards (FLEX), applied largely for the licensing of foreign graduates. (Admittedly, this mobility may lead to heavy concentrations of doctors in attractive areas, like British Columbia, and shortages in the colder prairie provinces. The same imbalances, however, occur in the United States.) Furthermore, with the new restrictions on immigration of foreign medical graduates, the LMCC will probably be required of non-Canadian as well as Canadian medical graduates, thus applying a national standard across the board. Even though the vast majority of educational institutions in Canada are public, not private, the national examination is regarded as a necessary and effective guarantee of individual competence in medicine as well as in other fields.

Strengthened Licensing Laws

In the sphere of legal regulation of health manpower, the main new initiative was taken by the Province of Quebec, where, under the tradition of French civil law, strong reliance is placed on governance through explicit statutory provisions. The Professional Code of Quebec, enacted in 1973, is a marked departure from typical registration or licensing laws. It accords with the temper of the times in Quebec, where imaginative policies are being directed toward improving life for ordinary people. Moreover, it was the first modernized, reformed licensure law. Ontario has now enacted a Health Disciplines Act, Alberta has a medical licensing law, and other provinces—Manitoba, Saskatchewan, and Nova Scotia—are discussing new proposals.

The Professional Code of Quebec establishes a new system for regulating the qualifications and practice of professionals, both those in the health professions and others. The key mechanism is an independent professional corporation to govern each discipline, with the directors composed of members of the profession and several representatives of consumers. These corporations are endowed with broad regulatory powers and the authority to protect the population with respect to the qualifications of professionals, surveillance of their conduct and practice, and exercise of disciplinary measures. All the professional corporations are coordinated by an interprofessional council, which is monitored by a governmental agency, so that, while self-government of the professions is retained, public accountability is built into the system at the level of each corporation and on an overall, integrated basis.

The Professional Corporation of Physicians, which is the most important of the corporations for the health professions, carries out not only the traditional functions of a licensing agency with respect to validating qualifications, registering physicians, and conducting disciplinary procedures, but also the innovative function of monitoring the quality of medical care. Its professional inspection committee makes periodic visits to hospitals, where it reviews charts, examines services, and confers with the medical staff. The most common sanction for substandard performance imposed by the corporation is a requirement that the physician undertake specified continuing education to improve his skills. The College of Physicians and Surgeons in Manitoba provides somewhat similar surveillance of hospital practice and, in fact, considers this activity its most important one.

The other provinces have not taken the same path as Quebec in creating a radically different type of organization to regulate professional practice, but the directions in Ontario, Manitoba, and Saskatchewan constitute other efforts to increase public accountability in regulation. In several Canadian provinces, the Colleges of Physicians and Surgeons were formerly both the provincial medical associations and the statutory registration bodies. (This double function still applies generally in nursing and several other fields.) Gradually, the professional and licensing functions in medicine were separated, and now in all provinces there are two organizations—the voluntary association, which handles professional matters (including negotiation of the fee schedule under the medicare program), and the statutory body (often elected by members of the medical profession), which is responsible for registration and regulation of the right to practice. This separation of functions was designed to increase protection of the people and to correct the legal defect of delegating a governmental function to a private agency.

The new licensure legislation enacted in Quebec and Ontario and various proposals under discussion in other provinces are designed to carry this objective one step further. The various approaches to achieving increased protection of consumers include: (1) adding citizen representatives to the boards regulating the health professions; (2) expanding the authority of the registration or licensing body to include regulation not only of initial qualifications to practice, but of ongoing performance; (3) broadening the grounds on which disciplinary action may be exercised to include both misconduct and general incompetence (not only egregious acts); (4) encouraging or requiring periodic updating of qualifications so that the right to practice is, in effect, limited in time; (5) providing for limited licensure in accordance with education and experience so that the functions of doctors are restricted in scope (this proposal goes far beyond the current requirement in some provinces for registration of specialist qualifications); and (6) coordinating regulation of the various health professions through a single governmental body.

These are the regulatory mechanisms being developed in various forms and combinations by different provinces. Despite much variation, there is remarkable unanimity on two points—on the need to increase public accountability of the professions and on the need to expand the capacity of the licensing laws to regulate not only initial qualifications of health personnel, but their continuing performance and practice as well. While these innovations in regulation of the health professions are still in an early stage, they already give promise of making professional conduct more responsive to the needs of society, while preserving the tradition of self-government.

Controls Through the Health Insurance System

It is probably no accident that strengthened licensing laws are being enacted simultaneously with implementation of a national health insurance system. If public funds are spent for health care, they must be well spent. For example, specialist fees under the health insurance system are paid only to those who meet the requirements for specialists. The computerized data produced by the health insurance system permit examination not only of the individual physician's performance but also of the patterns of practice in different specialties and in different geographic areas.

This was to be expected. What might not have been expected, however, was the response of the medical profession to development of physician profiles and to analysis of patterns of practice. In all provinces, once the health insurance records reveal poor performance by an individual doctor or improper or unsound patterns of practice (such as excessive numbers of appendectomies or hysterectomies), the insurance authorities turn to the medical profession for remedial action. Either the provincial registration agency or the provincial medical association then is responsible for investigating the problem and for taking appropriate action. Since the health insurance authorities have the power to disallow all or part of the reimbursement to an individual doctor, or to reduce the fee for a particular procedure deemed inadvisable or overused, these agencies are in a position to promote a cooperative attitude on the part of the profession. In fact, as a result of increased experience with this monitoring of quality of care, the profession seems to accept it as beneficial both to patients and to themselves.

This integration of controls by the health insurance system with the functions of the registration agencies and the professional associations is probably the most significant development in regulation of health manpower qualifications and performance in Canada.

In contrast to the experience in the United States, Canada has a very low incidence of malpractice actions, which may be regarded as a method of influencing quality of practice through judicial channels. The reasons are complex and are related, doubtless, not only to the beneficial effects of the national health insurance programs and the more rigorous quality controls on medical performance, but also to the absence of contingency fees in legal practice and other factors. Also in contrast to the United States, the hospital insurance program in Canada has generated relatively strong governmental systems of surveillance of hospital performance; accordingly, less importance attaches to the voluntary accreditation program. In the United States, the growth of such accreditation was largely in response to the weakness of the governmental role in this field. These are two further demonstrations of the wide-ranging impact a nationwide health insurance system can exert on quality control.

GENERAL OBSERVATIONS

In broadest perspective, one may make some general observations about the Canadian health service experience and its impacts on health manpower developments.

The high volume of hospital and medical services being provided in Canada has been noted, despite a somewhat lower percentage of GNP being allocated to health service. The full meaning of this paradox would require elaborate exploration, but surely the constraint on charges levied by doctors and hospitals (that is, prices) under the health insurance programs plays a part.

The costs of the health insurance system are rising. Being quite visible in the public sector, they are of concern to political leaders, who search continually for more rigorous cost controls. It is noteworthy, nevertheless, that the general phenomenon of rising costs is no great popular issue among the Canadian people; one does not hear the talk of a "health care crisis" so common in the United States. So far as the average citizen is concerned, his costs for medical and hospital care are met by the governmental programs, and he is pleased with them. The general taxes he must pay to support these programs do not seem to disturb him greatly. One wonders whether the much lower share of Canada's national budget devoted to military purposes (compared to U.S. military expenditures) contributes to this attitude. Put the other way around, a much larger share of health service costs can come from the public sector without noticeable citizen complaints about high taxes.

The relatively large sums invested in hospitals have increased their stability and quality of performance. In just the first eight years after nationwide hospital insurance, from 1958 to 1966, hospital personnel in Canada nearly doubled, increasing from 135,000 to 256,000 (the majority of these being registered nurses and other professional personnel). Hospital boards of directors and administrators have been able to devote more of their time to program content and less to fund raising.

Yet the strengthening of hospitals did not mean a deterioration in ambulatory care. Outpatient and emergency cases have risen steadily in Canadian hospitals, as they have in the United States. After statutory hospital insurance, and even before similar insurance for doctor's care, voluntary insurance for complete medical care grew. Statutory medical insurance logically followed, with action by Saskatchewan for broad doctor's care coverage in 1962 and national entitlement by 1966. The remaining gaps in comprehensive health service are being filled by social insurance initiatives in the provinces for drugs, dental service, nursing home care, prosthetic appliances, and so on. Federal matching of these expenditures is probably in the offing.

All these expenditures of health care funds on a collective public basis have naturally generated increasing concern for quality controls, as well as expenditures. The provincial medical registration bodies, as well as the medical associations, are exercising more rigorous discipline over physician performance. A constant flow of data from the medicare insurance system provides physician profiles, which greatly simplifies the detection of deviance. One proof of the pudding is the reduction in infant mortality and the rise in life expectancy for both sexes in Canada—now surpassing the United States in both of these health outcome measures.[15] Another reflection perhaps is the very low rate of malpractice actions in Canada, compared with the United States, although many factors in law and custom doubtless also play a part. In any event, patients clearly do not have the angry dissatisfactions that so often generate lawsuits against the U.S. doctor.

Excessive service is being limited by controls over the supply of hospital beds, even reductions in bed-to-population ratios. Since most medical and hospital services are generated by doctors rather than patients, similar constraints are being put on the supply of physicians through immigration restrictions. Though this action has not been motivated by altruistic concern for the brain drain from other countries, its effects are prudent for the welfare of other nations that can ill afford to lose the doctors or other health personnel whom they train.

The many shibboleths that have long marred discussions of health insurance—both governmental and voluntary—in the United States have been dispelled by the Canadian experience. Doctors did not leave the country; greater numbers came in and were trained. Medical school applications did not decline, but rose.[16] Doctors' incomes, already high, grew higher. Doctors were not swamped with work; instead, their numbers rose and their workweek was shortened. The quality of medical care did not deteriorate; by all the evidence, it improved.[17] Free choice of doctor did not disappear, it was enhanced, as all persons of any income could see the doctors of their choice. Copayment was not necessary to control excessive use or abuse; in the limited trial of deterrent fees against ambulatory service in one province, their impact was found to be discriminatory against the poor, and they were soon dropped.

The notion that instituting insurance without changing the delivery system is extravagant can hardly be tested from the Canadian experience without a proper comparison nation or population. It may be noted, however, that all sorts of steps to change the system were soon generated. Health centers, a rapid increase in group practice and other teamwork arrangements, regionalization programs of many types, various measures to improve the geographic distribution of health manpower, all were widely promoted.

Far from causing a deadly uniformity throughout Canada, the national matching of provincial health expenditures has heightened diversity. With basic hospital and doctor services ensured, each province has been free to develop further its own ideas. Even within the nationwide programs, provincial variations in administration are considerable. Provincial government responsibilities for health service have not been weakened, but strengthened. Even when responsibilities have been assigned to agencies other than the health department, the latter agency has acquired new functions, so its role has not been reduced. The trend, moreover, is toward unification of the several health administrative functions at the provincial level.

One might hope that Canadian law will not always be interpreted to bar trial of the concept of health maintenance organizations (HMOs) with their enrolled populations for whose health service the HMO takes comprehensive responsibility. To yield the incentives provided by prudent hospital use in U.S. health maintenance organizations, Canadian HMOs could be paid the *total* per capita provincial health costs for its members; then, when a patient is hospitalized, the organization would reimburse the government, rather than the hospital. Such an arrangement could encourage the growth of programs like the community clinics of Saskatchewan or the prepaid plans of Ontario, which have borne great handicaps, despite their potential for improved services along with economy.

With medical care financing nearly all collectivitized, fresh attention is being directed in Canada toward further strengthening of preventive services.[18] The treatment programs have fostered prevention by making early ambulatory medical care more accessible. But new ways are being sought to promote health actively, to modify human behavior so that disease and accidents will be averted. Political and administrative lines between health promotion and treatment of disease are fading in Canada, as public and social responsibility for the health of the population are enhanced.

RECENT MAJOR DEVELOPMENTS

The escalation of expenditures for health care has been a worldwide phenomenon, but major attention in recent years has been focused on this problem in Canada. To some extent, of course, a rise in expenditures for health purposes is to be expected in any affluent economy; as basic needs for food and shelter are met by lesser shares of national wealth, larger shares become available for services such as health care or education. The greater proportions of aged persons (with chronic disorders), the expansion of medical technology, the rising demands for health service associated with higher educational levels, and

Table 13.1   Health Care Expenditures in the United States and
Canada, 1971–76

	Expenditures on Health ($ billions)		Percent of GNP Spent on Health	
Fiscal Year	United States	Canada	United States	Canada
1971–72	86.39	7.03	7.8	7.2
1972–73	94.24	7.68	7.7	7.0
1973–74	104.24	8.64	7.8	6.7
1974–75	122.20	10.09	8.4	6.6
1975–76	139.30	11.79	8.6	6.9

Source: Canadian Medical Association, report based on data from the Canadian
Department of National Health and Welfare and from the U.S. Department of
Health, Education, and Welfare, Ottawa, 1977.

many other factors contribute to these increased expenditures in the
health sector.

It is worth noting that the rate of mounting health expenditures
in Canada has continued to be less than that in the United States. The
data in table 13.1, comparing recent trends in the two countries, are
instructive.

Thus, in spite of the great rise in the rate of hospital utilization
and the supply of health manpower associated with the national programs of health insurance, the trend toward increased expenditures—
measured as a percent of GNP—has been more moderate in Canada
than in the United States, which has national health insurance coverage only for the aged.

This contrast can probably be explained largely by the whole body
of regulation of the health care system arising from the Canadian
national insurance programs. Restrictions on expanding the number of
hospital beds, the regionalized planning of hospitals with provincial
government budget review and prospective periodic payments, the surveillance of physician services and reimbursement (with negotiated fee
schedules), the incentives for use of generic drugs, the health center
movement—these and other strategies have helped to restrain the
mounting of health care costs. Expenditures for hospitalization and the
services of physicians have indeed risen, but at slower rates than comparable costs in the United States.[19] While the aggregate hospital days
per 1,000 population per year are still higher in Canada than in the
United States, the trend in the last decade, for example, has been
downward in Canada, while in the United States it has been upward.[20]
The cost per patient-day in U.S. hospitals, moreover, is much higher
than in Canadian hospitals.

Another important aspect of health expenditure trends in Canada, clarified only recently, has been their relative impacts on different income groups. Based on detailed studies in Quebec comparing expenditures between 1969–70 and 1971–72 (that is, before and after the introduction of insurance for physicians' care), it has been shown that, although costs rose for all income groups, the relative burden on the higher income group increased, while the burden on the lower income group declined.[21] Thus, in the earlier period, individuals or families (spending units) with annual incomes of less than $5,000 paid 21.3 percent of total national medical care costs, while those earning more than $13,000 paid 17.7 percent. After physician's care insurance, these relative burdens shifted downward to 15.8 percent for the lower income group and upward to 24.6 percent for the higher income group. Contrary to common allegations about social insurance financing, therefore, the relative cost burdens for health care have become more progressive.

A major concern at the national level in Canada has been to slow down the overall rise in health expenditures for all income classes. It will be recalled that, in spite of the various cost-control measures noted above, the federal government was obliged to match (that is, to pay 50 percent or more of the costs) whatever expenditures for hospital and physician's care were made by the provincial programs. In 1977, therefore, the Canadian national government took a major step to induce even greater cost-control strategies within the provinces.[22] The 1977 Federal-Provincial Fiscal Arrangements and Established Programs Financing Act (known commonly as bill C-37) made important changes in the relative fiscal obligations of the two levels of government. Expenditures for hospital and medical care in the provinces were subsidized much less than in the past. The new policy put much greater pressure on the provinces to control the costs of their health care systems.

The details of bill C-37 are relatively complex; to some extent, new benefits are offered to the provinces in compensation for the greater financial burden thrust upon them. The package of provisions of the 1977 law has been well summarized by a Canadian political scientist, R. J. Van Loon.[23] First, the federal contributions to provincial health costs have been reduced from about 50 percent to 25 percent; also, with 1975 set as the base year, subsequent increases in federal support will be limited to the rate of growth of the GNP. Second, recognizing the extension of various health benefits (drugs, dental care, and so forth) in the provinces without previous federal matching, a new annual block grant of $20 per capita will be made to help cover the cost of those new services (with increases also geared to changes in GNP).

Third, the federal taxes on personal and corporate incomes will be lowered so that the provinces may levy proportionately greater taxes on these sources. Fourth, transitional federal adjustment grants will go to the provinces to allay provincial hardship from the changed fiscal arrangements.

One can see in Canada the evolution of health insurance financing that has occurred in many other countries with older systems. First, mandatory health insurance programs are introduced at both provincial and federal levels in response to political pressures for achieving greater equity in health services; at the same time, the patterns of health care delivery are left untouched in the face of conservative opposition to any change.[24] Then, the rise in expenditures and their great visibility generate a whole series of regulatory controls. Among these are deliberate strategies to restrict the growth of health care resources (manpower and facilities), as well as to introduce new patterns of health care delivery (regionalization, health centers, emphasis on prevention, and so on). The 1977 legislation has clearly been designed to intensify the force of this second stage.

A third stage overlaps the second: namely, in response to continued cost-control pressures, more sweeping changes are made in the entire structure of the health care delivery system to achieve greater efficiency and effectiveness within acceptable cost limits. This process has taken place in Great Britain, Sweden, Chile, New Zealand, and in all the Socialist countries.[25] Most recently, it has taken place in Italy, where a complex aggregation of semi-autonomous local health insurance programs is becoming welded into a unified national health service, with salaried personnel being supported by general revenue financing and a quantum leap in organizational structure.[26] Exactly how far Canadian health services will move along this path remains to be seen, but the direction suggested by recent events seems clear.

NOTES

1. M. LeClair, "Historical Perspective: The Canadian Health Care System," in *National Health Insurance: Can We Learn from Canada?* S. Andreopoulos, ed. (New York: Wiley & Sons, 1975), 11–93.
2. F. D. Mott, "Government-Sponsored Care in Saskatchewan," *Hospitals,* 1950, no. 24, 58.
3. G. G. Simms, "Critical Review of Fiscal and Administrative Controls on Costs and Use in Canada from the Point of View of a Provincial Hospital Authority," *Medical Care* (supplement on Canadian-American Conference on Hospital Programs) 7 (November–December 1969):59–74.

4. J. E. F. Hasting, *Monograph on the Organisation of Medical Care within the Framework of Social Security: Canada* (Geneva: International Labour Office, 1968), 73.
5. W. P. Thompson, *Medical Care: Programs and Issues* (Toronto: Clarke Irwin, 1964).
6. F. D. Mott, "Medical Services Insurance: The Next Phase in Canada's National Health Program," *Medical Care Review* 24 (July–August 1967): 521–36, 615–43.
7. S. S. Lee, "Health Insurance in Canada—An Overview and Commentary," *New England Journal of Medicine* 290 (28 March 1974):713–16.
8. S. Wolfe and R. F. Badgley, "How Much is Enough? The Payment of Doctors—Implications for Health Policy in Canada," *International Journal of Health Services* 4 (Spring 1974):245–64.
9. J. R. Evans, "Health Manpower: Issues and Goals in Canada," *Bulletin of the Pan American Health Organization 8 (1974)*:302–10.
10. H. R. Robertson, *Background Study for the Science Council of Canada— Health Care in Canada: A Commentary,* special study no. 29 (Ottawa: Science Council of Canada, 1973).
11. Science Council of Canada, *Science for Health Services* (Ottawa, 1974).
12. A. P. Ruderman, "Canadian Medicare: Can We Use a Plan That Good?" *The Nation* (23 October 1972):369–73.
13. Health and Welfare Canada, *Second National Conference on Health Manpower* (Ottawa, n.d., c. 1972).
14. M. LeClair, "L'Avenir de la Médecine au Canada," *L'Union Medicale du Canada* 101 (November 1972):2329–32.
15. Metropolitan Life Insurance Co., "Progress in Canadian Longevity," *Statistical Bulletin,* October 1975, 5.
16. N. E. Collishaw and R. M. Grainger, "Canadian Medical Student Selection and Some Characteristics of Applicants, 1970–71," *Journal of Medical Education* 47 (April 1972):254–62.
17. M. LeClair, in *National Health Insurance,* 49–52.
18. M. Lalonde, *A New Perspective on the Health of Canadians: A Working Document* (Ottawa: Health and Welfare Canada, 1974).
19. G. H. Hatcher, "Canadian Approaches to Health Policy Decisions—National Health Insurance," *American Journal of Public Health* 68 (September 1978):881–89.
20. National Center for Health Statistics, *Health—United States 1978* (Washington, D.C.: Department of Health, Education, and Welfare, 1978), 308.
21. J. C. Morreale, "The Distribution Effects of National Health Insurance in Quebec," *Journal of Health Politics, Policy, and Law* 2 (Winter 1978):479–507.
22. E. Vayda, R. G. Evans, and W. R. Mindell, "Universal Health Insurance in Canada: History, Problems, Trends," *Journal of Community Health* 4 (Spring 1979):217–31.
23. R. J. Van Loon, "From Shared Cost to Block Funding: The Politics of Health Insurance in Canada," *Journal of Health Politics, Policy, and Law* 2 (Winter 1978):454–78.

24. M. G. Taylor, *Health Insurance and Canadian Public Policy: The Seven Decisions that Created the Canadian Health Insurance System* (Montreal: McGill-Queen's University Press, 1978).

25. M. I. Roemer, "National Health Insurance As an Agent in Containing Health Care Costs," *Bulletin of the New York Academy of Medicine* 54 (January 1978):102–12.

26. F. B. McArdle, "Italy's National Health Service Plan," *Social Security Bulletin* 42, no. 4 (April 1979):38–42.

14

Rural Coverage and Health Personnel Functions in Industrialized Countries

Meeting the needs for health personnel of many types is an essential requirement for the operation of all national health care systems. Adequate numbers of each type of manpower must be prepared and must be (1) located according to an appropriate geographic distribution and (2) assigned functions that they can properly perform. This chapter examines the strategies of five industrialized countries with respect to both of these objectives, focusing for the first on rural health personnel coverage and for the second on innovative personnel functions.

To learn possible options for the United States in health manpower policy, field studies were made in five industrialized countries: Australia, Belgium, Canada, Norway, and Poland.[1,2,3,4,5,6] These five were selected because they illustrate a range of different types of national health care systems, and such systems obviously have an important bearing on health manpower policies. The first four countries have national health insurance that covers all or nearly all the population; the scope of benefits and methods of administration, however, differ in

Based on field studies done for the Department of Health, Education, and Welfare between 1973 and 1976 and partially reported in "Strategies for Increasing Rural Medical Manpower in Five Industrialized Countries," *Public Health Reports* 93 (1978):142–46 and "Innovative Functions of Health Personnel in Other Countries: Lessons for U.S. Health Planners," *Inquiry* 16 (1979):259–63 (adapted and substantially revised).

many respects. The fifth country, Poland, operates a national health service in which financial support is derived almost entirely from general revenues of the economy and all resources (both personnel and facilities) are controlled directly by the government. Perhaps the principal common attribute of the five systems is that most health services in the nation are financed collectively and provided as public benefits.

Four of the countries are parliamentary democracies, of which two (Belgium and Norway) have constitutional monarchies. Two are federations of states or provinces (Australia and Canada), in which there are many differences among jurisdictions regarding health policies. In the constitutional monarchies, there are also provinces or countries, but in the main they carry out policies that are determined by the central government. Poland is a Socialist country, where general control is exercised by the dominant political party.

METHODOLOGY

A literature search was conducted (through the MEDLARS system of the National Library of Medicine) on health manpower articles published in the last ten years in all five countries. Field visits of five to ten weeks were then made to each country during the years 1973–76. Interviews to elicit information regarding health manpower policies, practices, and experience were held with executives of the ministries of health, social security authorities, provincial and local public health agencies, universities and other training institutions, professional associations, consumer organizations, hospitals and other health facilities, regulatory agencies, important voluntary health bodies, individual providers and recipients of health service, and miscellaneous other knowledgeable persons involved in health services. In all interviews, information was sought on health manpower education, functions, and regulation, with special attention to strategies employed to attract physicians to rural areas and to identification of innovative personnel functions. Numerous official reports and unpublished documents were collected wherever possible, particularly to obtain quantitative data on health manpower supplies, distribution, functions, and trends.

A monograph was prepared on each of the five countries from the information gathered. Each monograph presents the findings under six main headings: (1) the national health care system, (2) health manpower resources, (3) innovative functions of health personnel, (4) health manpower education, (5) regulation of health personnel, and (6) salient highlights, issues, and trends. As part of the second general topic—health manpower resources—data were presented on the geographic distribution of physicians, dentists, nurses, and other major categories of health personnel, along with accounts of the efforts being put forth to equalize this distribution in relation to population needs.

This chapter will first examine the findings on geographic distribution of doctors and strategies to attract them to rural areas. It will then consider innovative personnel functions in relation to customary practices in the United States.

ATTRACTING PHYSICIANS TO RURAL AREAS

In all five countries, as in virtually all nations of the world, cities and rural areas had unequal distributions of physicians and other health personnel. The natural flow of people and health services in geographic regions inevitably requires greater technical resources in the cities, but the degree of such urban concentration is usually excessive. To cope with the resultant undersupply of health manpower in rural districts, numerous actions have been taken specifically to strengthen rural resources.

Underlying Influences

Before discussing these specific efforts, one should note several underlying features of national health policy in the five countries that indirectly influence the availability and distribution of all health services, urban and rural.

The impacts on rural areas of many aspects of the national health care systems as a whole should not be overlooked simply because they are not identified as having rural objectives. Most fundamental is the operation in four countries of national systems of health insurance and in Poland of a general tax-supported system covering everyone. These economic support programs mean that the typically lower income levels in rural districts do not directly discourage the settlement of physicians and dentists in rural areas, as is the case in the United States. This basic point should not be exaggerated, since, even with financial protection, rural people do not seek as much medical care as urban people. Under insurance programs paying physicians by the fee-for-service method, therefore, rural practitioners still tend to earn less. Moreover, copayment requirements in Norway, Belgium, and Australia may offer some financial deterrence to low-income families, and these families are commoner in rural areas. Nevertheless, the protection of social financing doubtless reduces one of the barriers to settlement of medical manpower in rural areas.

Second, the general enlargement of the health manpower supply that has occurred in all five countries undoubtedly affects the numbers available for rural service. Whenever there are shortages of physicians or other health personnel, the urban locales that are more attractive for work and life are bound to be occupied first. Even in the freest market economies, however, when urban opportunities for physicians are saturated, rural locations will be sought; thus, a larger overall supply of health personnel is bound to help the rural areas. Obviously, many factors influence the saturation point of a medical market, but the steady expansion of the supply of physicians and nurses in all five countries, as well as the expansion in the numbers of dentists in Norway and Poland, has clearly benefited rural areas.

Third, a national system of health care delivery that is basically organized, as it is in Poland, helps assure personnel for all locations, urban and rural. Where all physicians and dentists must work seven hours per day in the systematized public program, the availability of vacancies on the organization chart is crucial. Although Polish physicians are not ordered to go to one place or another, they will naturally go where positions are available; if ail urban posts are filled, they must take rural posts. This strategy has operated to steadily improve rural health care resources in Poland.

Similar dynamics operate within the hospital services of Norway and, to a lesser extent, Australia. When the medical staffs in hospitals are entirely (Norway) or substantially (Australia) composed of salaried specialists, the physicians trained in various specialties essentially must go where hospital posts are available. The specialist may also engage in private practice outside the hospital, but membership on the closed staff of a hospital is a practical necessity. Thus, the establishment of hospitals in the rural regions of Norway and Australia, as well as in Poland, inevitably attracts health personnel.

Fourth, implementation of the concept of regionalization of health facilities is especially helpful to rural people. To some extent, this policy is being applied in all five countries studied. In Poland, virtually all hospitals, health centers, and health stations are established in accordance with a centrally planned regional scheme. This is also the general strategy for hospital construction in Canada, Norway, and Belgium, which is carried out through the selective awarding of capital grants. To a lesser extent, the strategy is applied to the construction of health centers for ambulatory care in Australia and Canada. The operation of regional public health authorities in Canada and Australia,

moreover, provides a stronger voice for the articulation of rural personnel needs by regional citizen boards.

A fifth broad policy with special rural implications is the movement in all five countries to strengthen general medical practice. The
ways that this is being done will be discussed later, but here it may be
noted that the generalist in medicine has a manifestly greater role to
play in rural than in urban areas. In all five countries, the swing of the
pendulum toward specialization has been slowed down or reversed in
recent years. Specialization is bound to be more concentrated in urban
centers. The principal need of rural people is for general primary care,
after which they may be referred elsewhere for needed specialty services. The newer type of specialist in general medicine has a role par
excellence in rural communities.

Finally, a sixth general policy with special dividends for underserved rural localities is the operation of information systems for physicians and others seeking a place to practice or work. The Norwegian
Medical Association provides such an information service for all new
medical graduates; provincial medical associations in Canada and
state associations in Australia likewise maintain data on communities
needing physicians. In Australia, the national medical association as-
sists small-town physicians in finding locum tenentes so they can take
holidays.

Special Strategies

Numerous other strategies that were more specifically directed at
equalizing the geographic distribution of health personnel were identified in the study countries.

Two years of mandatory service in a rural post, after completing
medical school, were required in Poland from 1948 to 1963. This requirement was ended once Poland had achieved a large enough overall
supply of physicians to rely on voluntary incentives, as is discussed
later. In Norway, a similar period of mandatory rural service was required of new medical graduates but was also abandoned when the
supply of physicians had expanded enough. Of the 18 months of supervised postmedical school training required of all Norwegian graduates,
six months must be spent as assistant to a district doctor (whose role is
discussed later).

In Canada, actions have been taken recently to limit the immigration of foreign physicians. Some provinces grant licenses to immigrant physicians only for practice in underserved rural communities;
this restriction applies until citizenship is gained, which usually requires five years. A sort of reverse compulsion is applied in the Prov-

ince of Quebec; there certain cities are declared overdoctored for purposes of payment under the medical care insurance program. Thus, a physician, in effect, is compelled to settle and practice in a community needing more physicians if he expects to be paid by the insurance system. Smaller towns in rural districts would naturally benefit from this policy.

Much more widely applied in all five study countries are several specific inducements designed to attract physicians to rural locations. In Canada, with its extensive rural stretches, various policies have been implemented. Even before the national medical care insurance program was instituted in 1967, many rural municipalities in the prairie provinces (particularly Saskatchewan) offered public salaries to attract general practitioners; the first of these began in 1914. Provincial governments later gave supplemental grants to these municipal doctor plans. More recently, the Province of Ontario has guaranteed relatively high annual incomes to physicians who settle for a stated period in certain rural localities; the local community assumes responsibility for adequate housing and office facilities. The great majority of physicians entering this program, in fact, have remained in the rural community beyond their initial contract period. Some Australian states have likewise guaranteed physicians minimum incomes for settlement in small towns.

In Poland, as noted, there is no longer any mandatory period of rural service, in spite of the generally structured character of the Socialist health care system. Rural medical and dental posts, however, offer higher salaries than positions with similar responsibilities in a city. Also, more attractive housing is offered than is likely to be available in a city, where, in light of the rapid Polish urbanization, housing is still in short supply. The rural physician also can purchase an automobile on more favorable terms than his urban counterpart. Automobile expenses are paid, of course, for professional travel.

Apropos of traveling expenses, the social insurance systems of all five countries reimburse the physician for these costs incurred in making house calls. In Belgium, the physician making a long drive to a rural patient is reimbursed for travel time, as well as for motor vehicle expenses.

The district doctor system of Norway is one of the most impressive strategies for getting health care protection to rural populations. The national government appoints and pays the physician a basic salary for taking on the public health responsibilities in his area. Half of the physician's time, however, is spent in general clinical service to the local population, for which payment is made by the insurance system. The entire country is covered by some 600 district doctors, each of whom is assisted by one or more public health nurses and sometimes a sanitary inspector. Most districts are thinly settled, and in Norway's Far North, the positions offer longer holidays, subsidized housing, and supplemental credits toward attainment of specialty status later, if that is desired. The Norwegian district doctor soon finds himself a much respected leader in general community affairs; the whole system, with its national status, has a rich tradition that engenders a strong esprit de corps. There are virtually no vacancies in the 600 positions throughout the country. For the U.S. population of more than 200 million, this system would be equivalent to having more than 30,000 primary care physicians (compared to the less than 1,000 in the U.S. National Health Service Corps, which has been developed to help underserved areas).

On a more limited basis, some Australian states have appointed salaried rural physicians, who serve patients without charge during certain hours each day and for fees at other hours. Their salaries are paid partly by the state government and partly by the local community. Since the 1974 social insurance legislation, governmental stipends are simply supplemental to the physician's health insurance earnings.

Both Australia and Canada have long used the device of fellowships for medical or dental schooling in return for equivalent periods of service in rural communities. This approach has been particularly successful in the Province of Ontario. In the other three countries, where almost all professional school students in financial need are supported by national stipends, such a mechanism would have little meaning. Medical schools in Canada and Australia also send students for brief periods of training in certain isolated communities.

Organized transportation is a special strategy for providing medical care to isolated patients in some countries. Australia has its flying doctor service to bring physicians to its vast, thinly settled interior. Several Canadian provinces have special airplane ambulance systems, which bring rural patients to city hospitals any time of the day or night; telegraph or radio communication is part of this process. These programs are all subsidized by government.

Finally, in the very thinly settled regions of Canada's Far North and in the Australian Outback, there are health stations staffed by nurses with extended roles. The substantial responsibility and dramatic overtones of these posts make them attractive to a certain type of woman, and there are few vacancies. These positions are typically financed by government and supervised by a territorial physician, but the nurse does much diagnosis and treatment on her own; she seeks medical help by radio or refers the patient to a distant facility only for difficult conditions. With few exceptions, such broad responsibility is not delegated to nurses in rural villages that are within an hour or two of a city; nor is it found in any of the European countries studied.

Other strategies affecting the geographic distribution of health manpower may be briefly noted. Dental care programs for children in rural areas are well developed in Norway through government support of dental clinics. Some Canadian provinces send dental nurses, trained and authorized to provide virtually complete dental care for children, to work in rural schools. Some states of Australia give priority to serving the dental needs of rural children. Public (governmental) control over the location of private pharmacies in both Norway and Belgium and of the public pharmacies in Poland, has the effect of reducing excessive concentration in the cities and equalizing drug services for the rural population. In Norway, rural pharmacies are even subsidized from a fund raised by a special tax on urban pharmacies.

INNOVATIVE FUNCTIONS OF HEALTH PERSONNEL

If health services are to be efficient and economical, personnel should obviously be trained to have the knowledge and skills reasonable for their functions. Inadequate training endangers the quality of service they can render, and excessive training is economically extravagant. In general, a health care system should have health workers with the *least* elaborate training necessary to prepare them to perform a function *properly*. Clearly, it is wasteful to use the costly services of physicians, dentists, pharmacists, professional nurses, or others to provide services that could be delivered well by personnel whose training is shorter and whose salaries are proportionately lower.

In the five nations studied, several noteworthy features characterize the functions of physicians (general and specialist), nurses, and dental and other classes of personnel; influencing the capacities of all these health personnel is a movement to develop health centers.

Physicians

The most striking feature involving physician functions in the five countries studied, compared with the United States, is not an innovation at all, but rather the retention of an earlier pattern of value that we have almost abandoned. This is the relatively strong place still held by the general medical practitioner. In the United States, the trend to specialization has been so massive that hardly 15 percent of the doctors available for patient care today are generalists; in the five countries studied, the comparable proportion varies from 35 percent in Poland to 55 percent in Belgium.

This basic difference has enormous implications for day-to-day medical care. Virtually every family in these countries has a general physician to whom it can turn for help when needed. He—or in Poland more often she—can handle most of the problems quite adequately, referring the patient to a specialist if necessary. The GP tends to become a friend and adviser, someone to guide the patient through the complexities of the medical care system (which is less puzzling, incidentally, than in the United States). Except for Canada and the United States, where the open pattern of medical staffing in hospitals prevails, referral to a specialist usually means referral to a hospital as an outpatient or inpatient. In either case, on completion of his services—sometimes only diagnostic, sometimes including therapy—the specialist sends a report back to the referring practitioner. There is continuity of care for the patient and surely a great deal more of the understanding that prevails in an ideal doctor-patient relationship, of which we used to hear a great deal in the United States before the deluge of specialization.

As a result, in two of the countries one hears little—and in three of them not a word—about nurse-practitioners or physicians' assistants to take the place of the disappearing GP for provision of primary care. Even with the high proportion of generalists noted, the attitude in all five countries is that still more emphasis is needed on primary care. The solution is not to train shortcut substitutes, but rather to strengthen the arm of the GP; this is done with enriched continuing education, higher fees, merit awards, more office assistants, and the whole teamwork setting of health centers. Extended-role nurses are posted in the Canadian Far North and the Australian Outback, where populations are small and thinly settled. These nurses have continuous radio contact with physicians. In Belgium and Norway, the U.S. physician extender concept is rejected out of hand. In Poland, where the doctor supply was decimated by World War II, *feldshers* were trained and used until 1960; since then, with the supply of physicians expanded greatly, the training of *feldshers* has been terminated. The existing *feldshers* were transferred to special ancillary functions as ambulance attendants, health educators, or sanitarians, with the more competent ones sent on through medical school to become physicians.

Except in Canada, the GP has virtually no connection with hospitals, nor does he covet such connections. He gains his strength from his ties to hundreds of families, not from the right to do an appendectomy in the hospital operating theater. Especially impressive is Norway's network of 600 district doctors, discussed earlier.

Nurses and Midwives

The supply of graduate professional nurses actively working in Australia, Norway, and Poland is roughly the same as in the United States (around 360 per 100,000 population). In Belgium, the ratio is half that, and extensive use is made of a more briefly trained assistant nurse. In Canada, the ratio is twice as large (740 per 100,000). The abundant supply of nurses in Canada is doubtless a result of the nationwide hospital insurance program, which operates in an economy with relatively few other employment opportunities for young women.

Apropos of the relationship of nursing resources to a nation's general employment situation, it is noteworthy that in Poland there are almost no applicants for training as second-level assistant or vocational nurses; the other employment opportunities are so great that virtually every young woman interested in nursing takes the full professional course. This finding serves to remind one how much the large complement of vocational nurses in the United States must depend on a reservoir of unemployed women—largely from ethnic minorities—who are glad to train for these poorly paid jobs.

As for functions, the most striking feature of the nursing scene in all of the five study countries except Canada is the great importance of midwifery. There are, of course, certain differences among the four countries in the training programs. In Australia and Norway, the fully qualified nurse takes extra training to become a nurse-midwife; in Belgium and Poland, there is a basic training curriculum for midwives that is parallel to, but separate from, that for nurses. The functions of both types of childbirth attendant are essentially the same, and in all four countries they handle nearly all normal childbirths, which constitute the great majority.

One wonders why U.S. obstetricians have been so reluctant to accept this well-established manpower policy, applied successfully not only in the countries studied but throughout the world. Obstetricians in Norway and elsewhere still carry the ultimate responsibility for deliveries, but there are no more problems between obstetricians and midwives than one sees between physiotherapists and the physicians who ask them to treat patients. In fact, the relationship between midwives and the obstetrician, or sometimes another specialist in a smaller hospital, is notably strong because they depend on each other so much. Incidentally, the record of maternal and perinatal mortality in these countries using midwives is generally better than that in the United States, and the costs are decidedly lower.

The nurse-anesthetist is by no means unknown in the United States but in most states is resisted by anesthesiologists. In Norway, the nurse-anesthetist handles an estimated 90 percent of all surgical operations under the general supervision of a medical specialist in anesthesia. The results are reported to be excellent, and the idea is being introduced slowly in Poland. Widespread training and use of nurse-anesthetists, under supervision, would seem to be another obvious strategy for conserving medical manpower or channeling more doctors into primary medical care, where the shortages are so serious.

Innovative functions, relative to U.S. practice, also are found for nurses in the field of psychiatry. Postbasic training for psychiatric work is frequently available to the registered nurse in the United States, but in Canada, training for psychiatric nursing can be undertaken from the start. The profession is equivalent in status to that of regular nursing, and the preparation is similar in length but different in content. In Norway, there is an equivalent but separate training program for nurses who wish to work with mentally retarded, and sometimes mentally disturbed, children.

Dental Personnel

In Norway, the supply of dentists is nearly twice as high as in the United States—95 compared with 50 per 100,000 population. Within this abundance are two remarkably well developed public dental programs for Norwegian children. On the other hand, Australia and Canada—with only 33 and 35 dentists per 100,000—have made noteworthy adjustments to their dental shortages, with obvious lessons for the United States.

Since 1920 in New Zealand, dental nurses have been trained, through an intensive two-year course after high school, to give complete dental care to school children. This eminently practical and effective idea has spread to some 20 other countries, including Australia and Canada. In both these latter countries, the pattern has been introduced gradually in selected states or provinces where the shortages were great and the political will of the parties in power was sufficiently strong to overcome the resistance of the private dental profession. In Belgium, where the shortage of dentists is even greater than in the United States, the political will to overcome the resistance of the dental profession has been as lacking as it has been in the United States. Thus, millions of children go with untreated dental disease.

Other Health Personnel

A word may be said about innovative functions performed by other types of health personnel. In Norway and Belgium, the physicians specializing in psychiatry are few, with the gap being filled by psychologists practicing in mental hospitals and clinics. Full doctoral training in psychology in these countries is as lengthy as that in medicine, and the functions authorized are by no means limited to psychometric testing. Indeed, they include the full range of diagnosis and treatment of mental disorders. These psychologists, however, always work in an organized framework and are not reimbursed by the insurance systems for private psychotherapy, as are the handful of psychiatrists so engaged.

In order to staff small rural hospitals on the Canadian prairies, a combined technician has been trained to do simple laboratory procedures and operate X-ray equipment. Some tendency to combine the roles of physical and occupational therapists also may be observed in both Canada and Belgium, but it has not gained momentum.

In countries throughout the world, a great variety of assistants has been trained to extend the capacities of all of the health professions. In Norway, where the supply of pharmacists has been particularly low (33 per 100,000 compared with 71 in the United States), the needs have been met by producing "dispensers," who take a two-and-one-half year course following secondary school. These auxiliaries, composed entirely of women, work under the supervision of pharmacists, who must have a university degree.

Health Centers

In summarizing innovative functions of health personnel found in five industrialized countries, one must note a worldwide trend toward providing a physical setting outside of hospitals for teamwork among many types of health workers. Except for hospital inpatients, Americans have tended to expect the private setting of a physician, dentist, pharmacist, or other health care provider to be the normal place for delivery of service. In a slow but mounting tempo, however, the health center for ambulatory care has been acquiring increasing significance around the world. This is observable in varying forms in all five of the countries studied, and it has the obvious effect of facilitating teamwork among doctors and various other types of health workers.

Staffed by general medical practitioners, the health centers of Australia, Canada, and Norway are typically places for primary health care. In this regard, they differ from the typical U.S. group practice clinic or neighborhood health center with its array of specialists. On the other hand, the Belgian polyclinic and the Polish health center (and polyclinic) are places for the services of specialists—whether in primary care fields, such as internal medicine and pediatrics, or in secondary care disciplines, such as neurology and orthopedics.

Ambulatory care centers of either type mentioned above tend to mobilize the services of public health nurses, social workers, health educators, nutritionists, laboratory technicians, and other personnel much more fully than do separate departments within a public health facility. It seems likely that this health center movement may have greater significance for the United States than any of the other innovative personnel functions that have been reviewed in this chapter. In every instance, the birth and growth of health centers have been influenced by the national systems of economic support for health services.

Even with the U.S.'s fragmented pattern of health insurance and public medical care programs, there is growing evidence that a somewhat similar health center movement—under a variety of public and private auspices—is gaining momentum. With a sound program of national health insurance, one may expect this movement to accelerate and to hasten the day when all categories of health personnel will function in ways that are optimal from the viewpoint of both quality and economy.

SUMMARY AND COMMENT

Several health manpower policies in five industrialized countries (Australia, Belgium, Canada, Norway, and Poland) may be relevant to the solution of problems in the United States—problems with respect to providing medical care to persons in rural areas and problems involving the high costs of medical care.

The many-faceted national programs for economic support of health care in the five countries studied have generated a variety of strategies, direct and indirect, to increase the availability of services to rural populations. These strategies are, in a sense, a political necessity associated with nationally financed health care systems. Since virtually everyone contributes to the support of the health services, everyone has an obvious right to expect them to be available wherever he or she may live. At the same time, the operation of the national health care system offers numerous workable methods for improving the geographic distribution of health manpower.

Limited quantitative data to demonstrate these improvements are available from Norway, Poland, and Canada. In all five countries, however, rural health care handicaps do not now appear to constitute the social issue that they do in the United States, which lacks a national health care system. The precise methods used to overcome maldistribution of health manpower clearly depend on the governmental structure and politcal ideology of each country.

With respect to cost containment, several ways of defining the functions of personnel can yield greater efficiency and economy in health care. Programs for the training and prudent use of some of the types of personnel described above can achieve significant savings in the costs of health services, with no sacrifice in quality of care. Such actions may well call for new legislation at the state level, and the health planner can provide leadership in promoting it. Initiative would be reasonable from planners at both the local level of health systems agencies and the state level of state health planning and development agencies.

Happily, since this comparative international study was carried out, trends in the United States suggest implementation of corrective responses to the problems highlighted by the cross-national comparisons. The 1976 Health Professions Educational Assistance Act contains several incentives for increasing the output of primary care physicians, both in the newly defined specialty of family practice and in *general* internal medicine and *general* pediatrics. Approved residency training programs in family medicine and family practice now exceed 300 and are expanding steadily, with rising interest in them among the current generation of new medical graduates.

Health manpower planning, as a whole, is gaining increased attention from planning agencies at federal and state levels. Training for nurse-midwifery is getting fresh impetus, as is training of nurse-anesthetists. Several states are exploring pilot studies on a wider scope of functions for dental auxiliaries.

The U.S. trend toward training nurse-practitioners and physicians' assistants essentially as substitutes for GPs has been a response to the inadequacies of primary care and has not been seen in other industrialized countries. As the pendulum has swung toward family practice, this movement has lost some of its steam. Moreover, the *role* of the nurse-practitioner is being defined differently—as a true helper and associate of the physician who can extend medical productivity in organized clinic settings, rather than as an isolated substitute for the doctor in rural villages and urban slums. It is noteworthy, incidentally, that even post-Mao China is redefining the functions and upgrading the training of its barefoot doctors.

NOTES

1. R. Roemer and M. I. Roemer, *Health Manpower in the Changing Australian Health Services Scene*, DHEW publication (HRA) 76-58 (Washington, D.C.: Health Resources Administration, 1975).
2. R. Roemer and M. I. Roemer, *Health Manpower Policies in the Belgian Health Care System*, DHEW publication (HRA) 77-38 (Washington, D.C.: Health Resources Administration, 1977).
3. R. Roemer and M. I. Roemer, *Health Manpower Policy under National Health Insurance—the Canadian Experience*, DHEW publication (HRA) 77-37 (Washington, D.C.: Health Resources Administration, 1977).
4. M. I. Roemer and R. Roemer, *Manpower in the Health Care System of Norway*, DHEW publication (HRA) 77-39 (Washington, D.C.: Health Resources Administration, 1977).
5. M. I. Roemer and R. Roemer, *Health Manpower in the Socialist Health Care System of Poland*, DHEW publication (HRA) 77-85 (Washington, D.C.: Health Resources Administration, 1977).
6. M. I. Roemer and R. Roemer, *Health Manpower Policies under Five National Health Care Systems*, DHEW publication (HRA) 78-43 (Washington, D.C.: Health Resources Administration, 1978).

15

Health Policy and Strategies in Europe

Most of the problems in the U.S. health care system have already been faced in the industrialized countries of Europe. A central feature of European strategies to solve them has been the development of nationwide programs for social financing of health care (social insurance and general revenues). From these, there follow numerous policies for the planning and regulation of health manpower, health facilities, and the entire delivery of health services.

It is frequently asserted, in U.S. debates about a national health program, that this country is different from all others and cannot, therefore, learn any lessons from abroad. Yet, when one examines the structure and functions of the U.S. health care system, one finds relatively few features that were not originated on the basis of prior experience in Europe.

The health experience of Europe is relevant for the United States in more ways than simply the obvious one of health insurance legislation. It has meaning for policy formulation on health manpower, hospital organization, medical care delivery patterns, and other features of health care systems. Before examining these in the contemporary scene, a glimpse of history is in order.

This chapter is an adapted and substantially revised version of "The Foreign Experience in Health Service Policy," in *Regulating Health Care—The Struggle for Control*, Arthur Levin, ed. (New York: Academy of Political Science, 1980), 206-23.

EARLY LESSONS FROM EUROPE

When the New World constituted a cluster of European colonies, it was only to be expected that the health care patterns of the mother countries should be transplanted across the the ocean. The 13 English colonies that eventually rebelled and became the United States appointed town doctors to serve the "worthy poor," along the lines of the old Elizabethan Poor Laws. The first hospital, founded in Philadelphia in 1751, was based on the European model, with large wards for the poor and a few doctors appointed to serve them on a charitable basis. When the first outpatient clinic was organized, ten years after the American Revolution and also in Philadelphia, it was a small, free-standing facility for the poor similar to the first dispensary of the Royal College of Physicians founded in London around 1680.

When a U.S. Congress took shape, one of its early enactments for health purposes was the 1798 law establishing special hospitals at the main ports for merchant seamen; costs were to be met by small periodic deductions from the seamen's wages. Alexander Hamilton, who introduced this bill in Congress, based it on a similar program launched in England about a half-century before.

The boards of health established in New York, Boston, and other major cities to cope with epidemics and to institute sanitary waste disposal had European antecedents. As public health agencies matured beyond environmental sanitation to include such programs as maternal and child health services, these advances were also an emulation of trends in France and elsewhere. The tuberculosis sanatorium idea, pioneered in Germany, was adopted in the United States. District nurses to visit the homes of the poor and provide some care for the sick were pioneered in England years before the first visiting nurse association was organized in New York City.

As European industry expanded and caused many serious injuries of workers, the concept of employer liability arose in the law of several countries. Germany in the 1880s enacted the first legislation to mandate employers' insurance for compensation of workers injured on the job. In another 25 years, the same idea was adopted by New York State, and eventually compensation for work-related injuries and sickness—including medical care costs—was enacted into law in every U.S. state.

The concept of insurance for the costs of *general* medical care was, of course, applied in Europe as far back as the artisan guilds of the Middle Ages. With industrialization and urbanization, many forms of cooperative society for coping with sickness—both wage loss and the costs of medical care—took shape in the late eighteenth and early nineteenth centuries. In Germany they were *Krankenkassen*, or sickness chests; in France they were *mutualités*; and in England they were "friendly societies." Largely through the initiative of European immigrants, similar programs to finance medical care were started by fraternal lodges in U.S. cities in the later nineteenth century. Also, when groups of workers were needed at isolated locations, such as coal mines or railroad construction sites, this sickness insurance (or, as we now say, health insurance) idea was implemented to assure the availability of a doctor.

In 1911, Great Britain enacted its first mandatory national health insurance law, requiring that low-income manual workers be enrolled in a local sickness insurance society. Although Germany had passed the first such compulsory insurance law in 1883, the impact on the United States was much greater when its former mother country took similar action. Within four years, similar legislation was proposed in New York State, and between 1915 and 1920 some dozen state legislatures considered the idea. Virtually all these proposals emulated the European model requiring working men to become insured for medical costs through a local organization rather than through a centralized public insurance fund. Although none of these bills passed, the idea did not die. The first *national* health insurance bill, introduced by Senator Robert Wagner in early 1939, proposed grants to the states for helping them to set up health insurance plans. Although aborted by the onset of World War II a few months later, the issue of nationwide social insurance for medical care remained alive for the next 25 years. It was partially implemented in the enactment of the 1965 Medicare amendments to the Social Security Act, which financed services for the aged.

Perhaps 1920 marked a turning point in the tendency of the United States to look to Europe for ideas on the organization of health care, as well as other social issues. After World War I, the United States became a world power; in 1945, after World War II, it became the dominant world power. Instead of the United States' looking to Europe for models of social action, Europe and most nations of the other continents began to look for guidance to the United States. The spread of technology or dissemination of ideas to Asia, Africa, and Latin America, moreover—formerly linked mostly with imperialist domination—became an objective of international "technical assistance." Starting with President Harry Truman's Point Four Program in 1947 and followed by the British Colombo Plan, the planning of socioeconomic development, through technical collaboration, became a major purpose of the United Nations and the central purpose of the World Health Organization and other specialized U.N. agencies.

Because of this realignment of influence among the world's sovereign nations, one can appreciate why the United States now looks so seldom to other countries for guidance in the organization of health services or any other activity. Within the health field, this is perhaps why ideas originating in the United States—such as private group medical practice, or screening tests for early detection of chronic diseases, or health maintenance organizations—are being studied and emulated in other countries.

This current world leadership role should not blind us to the fact that, considering the development of health service systems as a whole, the United States is still a young nation. Regarding most of the components of such systems, other countries, especially those in Europe, have had much greater experience than we. Moreover, in the evolution of the social concepts that underlie most practices in health care organization, many other nations have a heritage of thought and problem solving much richer than ours. We can profitably consider, therefore, the experience of other nations in our current efforts to deal with the pressing problems of health care. Relevant policies of other countries are categorized according to the main features of every health care system.

ECONOMIC SUPPORT MECHANISMS

Most of us would probably agree that the major issue currently confronting the United States with respect to health services is their costs. The most disturbing problem, however, is not so much our aggregate national expenditures for medical care—now amounting to more than 9 percent of our GNP, excluding the costs of medical education and research—but the fact that those costs reduce the access of individuals and families to needed services. (A large fraction of overall resources devoted to health care, as opposed to food and shelter, may be expected in any affluent economy.) Yet this problem of medical costs as a barrier to needed care was largely solved by most European nations long ago. By making insurance for medical and related services obligatory for most of their populations—for all of the population in several countries—financial barriers to care have been eliminated.

When "compulsory" health insurance—as we have come to call it, pejoratively—covers less than 100 percent of the population, it has been the lower paid workers (for whom costs would be most prohibitive) who were first covered, as in Germany. Coverage is gradually extended, but higher paid executives and self-employed persons still typically acquire health insurance protection voluntarily, and unemployed or indigent persons are brought under the same program at government expense. It is noteworthy that Germany, which pioneered this concept of social insurance, has never required any copayment or cost sharing by the patient for physician's care, although other nations, which adopted insurance later, have done so.

We in the United States have applied the social insurance principle only to the costs of work-related injuries and, since 1965, to general medical and hospital care of the aged. Some of the features of our Medicare law suggest that, even within this limited program, we can learn much from Europe. Thus, although doctors and hospitals are paid on a fee-for-service basis, we have no fee schedules; doctors are paid "prevailing and customary" fees, and hospitals are paid "reasonable costs"—whatever these may be. With this essentially blank-check mechanism, it is small wonder that medical and hospital charges rose very rapidly after 1965, much more rapidly than did the consumer price index.

In the European health insurance programs, which pay for each medical service, schedules of official fees are negotiated each year between the national social security authorities and the providers of care. The bargaining power of a national agency to contain prices is obviously greater than that of individual patients. Such price containment would seem to be all the more necessary under an arrangement, as with Medicare, where the doctor may decline to take assignment (that is, to be paid by the program) and can then charge the patient whatever he likes. The patient can thereafter seek reimbursement only up to 80 percent of the prevailing and customary fee, which may turn out to be a fraction of the amount the patient actually paid.

Copayments of 20 percent or thereabouts are imposed in Belgium, Norway, and other countries, but with important differences. First, the fees chargeable are set by a negotiated schedule. Second, they ordinarily apply only to ambulatory service, not to expensive in-hospital medical or surgical care. Third, the share of copayments required usually declines after the first visit or two. Finally, in most countries where cost sharing is required, aged pensioners are exempted from it.

There are probably greater lessons to be learned from Sweden and Norway, where population coverage has been made 100 percent. After many years of trying limited compulsory coverage and extensive voluntary enrollment, protection had reached about 70 percent of the Norwegian population by 1950; through additional mandatory coverage in 1952, the program reached 95 percent. There could be no political opposition, therefore, when in 1956 Norway took action requiring that every resident must be insured. If the person is an employee, he pays the insurance tax through his place of employment, along with a payroll tax paid by the employer. If he is self-employed, he pays through an earmarked part of his income tax. If he is indigent or retired and not a dependent of a taxpayer, then the insurance premium or earmarked tax is paid on his behalf by the government from general revenues.

Universal coverage eliminates the administrative cost of identifying covered persons. It is simpler and less expensive to give care free to the occasional foreign visitor than to mount elaborate administrative procedures to rule out nonresidents. Moreover, obligatory contributions bring everyone into the insurance fund, not only the less prudent individual who might wish to take a chance on not needing medical care, but also persons at low risk of illness to balance those at high risk—the first persons to seek voluntary insurance protection. As the Europeans say, social insurance implements a concept of social solidarity.

Early health insurance programs in Europe were established by local community groups on a geographic or occupational basis. While in Germany and Belgium, for example, these local, nongovernmental "sickness chests" are still viable, they have been subjected more and more to national standards and supervision. A minimum scope of health benefits is required by law, although the more affluent local organizations may offer supplemental benefits. Premium rates—or, more accurately, social insurance contributions—are a specified percentage of earnings, so local chests with higher income employees have more money to spend. When hospitals are paid on a per diem basis (as in France) rather than by prospective monthly budgets (as in Britain), the rates payable to each facility are fixed by the national government.

The analogy to the hundreds of diverse local health insurance plans in the United States—even though they are seldom consumer-sponsored, as in Europe—is obvious. These plans, however, receive only meager supervision from the 50 separate state insurance authorities, and at present there are no nationwide standards. Previous national health insurance proposals in Congress would, in effect, impose uniform minimum standards on these local programs. Greater assurance of standards could be achieved, however, if the United States would adopt the Scandinavian model of essentially absorbing local programs into a national system; then these programs serve as local branches of a central authority. The detailed relationships with patients and providers of medical care can thus still be carried out with the appropriate sensitivity to varying local conditions.

With respect to hospital financing, national health insurance programs in Scandinavia and in Canada have a special lesson to teach. They do not pay for hospital care on a per-item or even a per diem

Table 15.1 Comparative Health Expenditures of Three Countries, 1950–73

| Year | Percent of GNP Spent on Health | | |
	Great Britain	France	United States
1950	4.1	2.9	4.6
1960	3.9	4.0	5.2
1970	4.9	5.5	7.1
1973	5.3	5.8	7.7

basis—a method that furnishes every incentive to keep beds filled, whether the patient really needs hospital care or not. This motivation for maintaining high occupancy levels under U.S. hospitalization insurance has doubtless contributed to the steadily rising proportion of the U.S. health care dollar allocated for inpatient hospital care. In Canada and Scandinavia, by contrast, hospitals are paid a fixed monthly amount to operate, at an assumed occupancy of 80 to 90 percent, regardless of the number of bed-days of care given. There is no financial incentive to admit the patient or to keep him a day longer than medically necessary. This prospective budgeting requires prior review of hospital budgets by a public authority, a process that can eliminate extravagance or waste in staffing or operations. Budget review can also enforce the decisions of planning agencies with respect to the range of technical functions appropriate to hospitals of various sizes and locations. This process is not to be confused with prospective reimbursement of per diem rates, which is much more limited in its possible impact on expenditures for hospital care. Prospective reimbursement simply fixes an average per diem charge allowed, on the basis of a budget review, for a year in advance; it does nothing to influence the number of patient-days of hospital care provided.

Returning to the issue noted earlier about the percentage of GNP devoted to health purposes, the various controls feasible in a national health insurance program evidently result in a smaller piece of the total economic pie's being spent than would otherwise occur. Figures comparing health expenditures in two European countries and the United States are shown in table 15.1.

Thus, even though health expenditures as a share of GNP have risen in both Great Britain and France, with their national financing of health care, expenditures there remain appreciably below those in the United States, without such a program. It may also be noted that the escalation of costs has been more rapid in France, with its insurance financing and fee-for-service remuneration, than in England, with its general revenue financing and more carefully controlled systems of paying hospitals and doctors.

Finally, on the basic issue of financing health care, one may note that all the industrialized countries of the world—including Japan, Australia, and New Zealand, as well as the Western and Eastern European countries—*started* their social programs with the insurance device. First there were voluntary insurance schemes, then obligatory ones. General revenue financing was initially used only for supporting the indigent within a national insurance framework, or for other special purposes. Only after 35 years of national health insurance did Great Britain, for example, move into a national health service supported predominantly by general revenues. It was not until 20 years after the Russian Revolution in 1917 that the national health insurance mechanism was abandoned for urban workers and a unified urban-rural Soviet health care system was established under general revenue financing. Similar evolutions have occurred in the health care systems of other Eastern European Socialist countries; in the German Democratic Republic (East Germany), the social insurance mechanism is still being applied today.

Despite this, some persons in the United States have recently argued that health insurance financing, even if it covers 100 percent of the population, is regressive taxation and that we should avoid it and move immediately to general revenue financing of a national system. (A fixed percentage insurance tax levied on employees with whatever incomes—especially when no tax must be paid on incomes beyond a certain threshold, such as $25,000—is contrasted with progressive income taxes, which impose higher *rates* of taxation as income increases.) These persons seem to overlook the manifest policy, in capitalist parliamentary countries, of using general revenue support at the outset of national medical care programs only for care of the poor or other special purposes. European labor and socialist political parties have clearly been willing to accept this conservative form of taxation in return for the long-term stability and continuity of health insurance programs. Instead of the cutbacks and retrenchments that general revenue health programs encounter at every dip in the business cycle, national health insurance programs have continually expanded the population covered and health benefits offered. In time—as demonstrated in Great Britain and, less dramatically, in Sweden, New Zealand, and other countries—the financial support has shifted more and more to general revenues, and greater shares of health service have come to be delivered through salaried personnel working in governmental health facilities. Most recently (in 1979), Italy took action to convert its complex network of semi-autonomous local health insurance programs—enrollment in which was, however, mandatory—into a unified national health service to be financed by general revenues.

HEALTH MANPOWER POLICY

With respect to the preparation of physicians and other health personnel and the definitions of their functions, there are many other lessons to be learned from abroad. Most, though not all, of the policies and practices stem largely from the systems of social financing of health care just discussed. The more restrained development of specialization elsewhere, largely associated with more structured organization of hospitals, has led to lower ratios of technical and allied health personnel as well. Thus the overall health work force in other nations tends to be relatively smaller than in the United States. Health status outcomes, reflected in life expectancy and infant mortality, however, tend to be better in Western European countries than in the United States, despite its higher general standard of living.

One of the pressing issues in the U.S. medical profession today is its overspecialization. In its laissez-faire setting, the United States has reached the point where scarcely 15 percent of clinically active physicians are GPs. The family doctor, with his great wisdom and warmth (whether real or imagined) has all but disappeared, to be replaced only partially by the internist and pediatrician. The majority of internists and about half the pediatricians have entered subspecialties and seldom play a generalist role except for care of the affluent. Medical leadership has tried to allay anxieties about the critical shortage of general physicians in the United States by counting all the internists, pediatricians, and obstetrician-gynecologists as primary care physicians. But these specialists are not available for the millions of people who seek help in hospital emergency rooms at increasing rates each year.

There have, of course, been responses to the decline of general practice in American medicine. Group practice clinics have multiplied, especially since 1945, although about half of the current number are not combinations of different specialists but single-specialty groups formed more for the convenience of doctors than of patients. In 1969, after long discussion, the specialty of family practice was created, and it has fortunately attracted an increasing share of new medical graduates. Less fortunate, in my view, has been the rise of the physician's assistant and the nurse-practitioner—used all too often not to work with the doctor, but to replace him in the diagnosis and treatment of the poor, particularly persons from racial and ethnic minorities. It is ironic to see the United States embrace the Russian *feldsher* just when the Soviet Union has stopped training these doctor substitutes because its supply of physicians has become adequate.

Some of these developments, such as group practice and specialty status for the generalist (but not the use of doctor substitutes), are seen in Europe also. More significant is the fact that the decline in general practice characterizing the United States has been by no means as great in any other country. While specialization has, of course, increased everywhere, it has been within reasonable limits, so that GPs account for some 40 to 50 percent of clinical physicians in Western Europe, as well as in Canada, Japan, Australia, and New Zealand. The explanation is perhaps not so much a deliberate preservation of the family doctor concept as a limitation of the training of specialists to the numbers necessary to staff hospitals properly.

Whatever the cause, the fact is that Europeans do not have to struggle as Americans do for access to primary care. Virtually everyone in the European welfare states has a general or family doctor to whom he or she may turn in time of need. In the British national health service, this linkage is fortified by a fiscal arrangement in which 98 percent of the population are on the panel of a GP of their own choosing. Similar arrangements prevail in Holland and parts of Denmark. The GP is paid a flat capitation amount each month for every person on his panel, whether that person is seen that month or not. The GP has no financial deterrent to referring his patients for specialist care when necessary. On the other hand, he is bound to treat every condition within his capacity—some 80 percent of cases—if only to keep the confidence of the patient, who is free to leave his panel at any time.

This is not meant to imply that general practice in Britain, or in other countries where fee-for-service payment is customary under national health insurance systems, is without problems. Critics allege mediocrity in much European general practice: they point to the exclusion of most generalists from hospitals, depriving them of the stimulation of colleagues and opportunity to keep up with medical advances. But continuing education is actively promoted for general physicians, and incentives—both professional and economic—are offered for undertaking such studies. Grouping of GPs in clinics is increasing steadily and now involves the majority of those in Britain. The community GP is, of course, welcome to see his patients in the hospital and to make suggestions on their treatment; on the patient's discharge, the GP receives a report from the hospital specialist on what was done.

There may be weaknesses in European general practice, but it is surely superior to a strategy of doctor substitutes, episodic emergency room care, the various phony cults claiming the label "holistic medicine," and other responses to the extreme overspecialization of U.S. medicine. I suspect that we are already learning this lesson as a nation, because the medical pendulum is now swinging back toward rediscovery of the family doctor.

Another lesson to be learned from Europe is in the field of professional education. Virtually all the training of physicians, dentists, nurses, pharmacists, and other health personnel is financed by public funds. In Western Europe, as well as Eastern Europe, only rarely does the student in a professional training school have to pay tuition. For students from poor families, fellowships to cover living expenses are abundant. The basic concept is that, under a national health care system, skilled personnel are an essential resource; their training, therefore, should be financed by society through its government.

By the same token, the content of professional education in Europe is more subject to national standards. Although complete uniformity is by no means required, national ministries of education or special university commissions in government specify *minimum* numbers of hours that must be devoted to various subjects. These standards are usually formulated with the advice of ministries of health and nongovernmental professional groups. Final examinations in nursing and other allied health fields are often prepared by government agencies and must be given in all schools, although the local faculty may pose additional questions. Because of the minimum standards applied to training curriculums in schools, the subsequent licensure of graduates is a very simple matter.

While countries in Europe and other industrialized nations have rejected the doctor substitute for *primary* medical care, there is one field in which nondoctors function extensively to perform services reserved for physicians in the United States—obstetrics. The trained midwife or nurse-midwife in nearly all Western and Eastern European countries handles most maternity care, including prenatal care, childbirth, and postnatal care. In the United States, we are accustomed to regarding midwives as primitive health workers in rural areas doing home deliveries. In Europe, the midwife works mostly in hospitals and local health centers. For normal pregnancies, which are 80 to 90 percent of the total, she handles the delivery herself; an obstetrician is expected to handle only childbirths that are abnormal in some way. Insofar as results reflect performance, it may be noted that maternal and neonatal mortality rates in Britain, the Scandinavian countries, and Holland, where midwives do most of the deliveries, are lower than in the United States.

One could hardly find an easier way to increase the effective supply and use of physicians in the United States than through adoption of European policies on midwifery. Thousands of obstetricians would be released for other types of medical care, and the costs of maternity service would be greatly reduced. Moreover, I suspect that the service would be more satisfactory for most women. The first rule in classical midwifery is patience during the three stages of labor—a policy much more suitable medically and psychologically for most mothers than the all-too-frequent cesarean sections and other methods employed by obstetricians to hasten the birth process.

In summary, one may say that the more collectivized financing and more systematic patterns of delivery of health services abroad have led to more rational and efficient roles for health manpower than we see in the United States.

HOSPITAL FACILITIES: CONSTRUCTION AND OPERATION

For centuries European general hospitals have been sponsored predominantly by local government. These municipal or county hospitals are not solely for the poor, but for everyone. Being under the control of elected bodies, they are naturally sensitive to the problem of costs, and at the same time to the quality of care.

Coming mainly under governmental authorities, although often financed largely by health insurance payments, these institutions are much more amenable to systematic planning than the voluntary hospitals that predominate in the United States. There are also voluntary nonprofit and church-supported facilities throughout Europe, but they tend to be smaller, to be less well developed, and to serve the less complex cases. The contrast with the large public hospitals that serve the poor in most major U.S. cities is obvious—and the implication of the comparison ought to be equally obvious: namely, that public hospitals should serve everyone in the community and should be supported largely by national health insurance payments. There is probably no other practical way to solve the widely recognized crisis in public hospitals in the United States, which has led to the deterioration and closure of so many of them over the last 20 years. Local taxation and even Medicaid funds are unable to sustain a proper level of patient care in hospitals limited essentially to serving the poor.

Inspection and licensure of hospitals in Europe are typically responsibilities of ministries of health in the central government. Since the hospitals are predominantly entities of local government—constructed and managed, in the first place, according to national standards—the process of periodic approval is relatively simple. It is usually delegated to local public health officials. There is more deliberate surveillance over the policies and practices of the smaller private hospitals, whether charitable or proprietary.

Regionalization of hospital service is another policy widely preached in the United States but far more widely practiced in Europe. Under our Hill-Burton hospital construction program, new hospitals are built according to regionalization concepts, but little has been achieved in the way of hospital *functioning* along regionalized lines. Under national health insurance systems of financing, however, where hospital budgets are reviewed by a public agency, payments can be made to cover costs that are appropriate for each facility's role in a regionalized network. It would be impossible, for example, to have the senseless multiplication of CAT scanners in several hospitals of one region of France or Norway that one sees among competing hospitals in a U.S. city—Los Angeles, for instance. Thus, the payments for services made to each hospital by the health insurance program, whether through prospective monthly allotments or through per diem payments, are based on budgets approved by the ministry of health. Such approval for the costs of operations (including depreciation) of a CAT scanner would be given only in hospitals where such sophisticated equipment is considered reasonable and appropriate.

Not that local hospital initiative is completely suppressed in Europe. Local pride and inventiveness are still strong, but there are limits to what will be paid for in a 50-bed rural hospital, compared to an 800-bed urban medical center. In Western Europe, the regionalization concept has been carried farthest under the British national health service, where all the hospitals in a region come under the coordinated control of a single regional health authority. To achieve this, in 1948 almost all the hospitals had to be nationalized. Although this is not likely to happen in the United States in the foreseeable future, the more permissive type of regionalization implemented in Sweden should be quite feasible, with appropriate leverage from national health insurance legislation.

With respect to the internal organization of hospitals, the predominant pattern throughout the world (except in the United States, Canada, and Belgium) is for the medical staffs to consist of a relatively small group of carefully selected and salaried specialists. Such closed staff hospitals are not universal; every non-Socialist country has some open staff hospitals, but the pattern of tightly organized, full-time medical staffs is more predominant. The sometimes negative impact of this pattern on community GPs has been mentioned earlier, although it was also noted that the policy results in larger numbers of such generalists. The influence of closed medical staffs on general hospital operation and performance is probably more important.

When hospital appointments are limited to the best qualified specialists in an area, rather than being open to almost all doctors, the quality of medical care given to inpatients is likely to be better. The whole range of hospital personnel can work together more efficiently as a team when there is a relatively small group of physicians in the facility throughout the day. The magnitude of nurse's notes in the typical U.S. general hospital, compared to their European counterparts, reflects the contrast. The U.S. nurse must record copious observations to inform the doctor of his patient's progress during the many hours each day when he is not present. The European nurse has only to speak to the in-hospital doctor if she observes anything unusual about a patient. The European specialist is clearly a member of the hospital team, which yields greater efficiency in the functioning of all hospital personnel.

Closed staff hospitals are not unknown in the United States. Aside from federal hospital systems such as the Veterans Administration, there are many notable closed staff institutions associated with group medical clinics or health maintenance organizations. Perhaps more significant is the general growth of contractual physicians in almost all hospitals, starting with pathologists and radiologists, and extending to full-time chiefs of clinical departments, postgraduate education directors, emergency physicians, rehabilitation specialists, and others. Many medical school teaching hospitals, with an academic staff and large numbers of interns and residents, approach the European model. Trends suggest that, if only in the interests of efficiency and economy, not to mention the quality of inpatient care, an increasing proportion of U.S. general hospitals will adopt medical staff patterns that now characterize most hospitals in Europe and elsewhere.

DELIVERY OF AMBULATORY CARE

The organized arrangements that are taken for granted in hospitals may also be applied to the delivery of ambulatory medical care. This has occurred most extensively in the Socialist countries, where private medical practice has dwindled to trivial proportions, but it is also seen to an increasing extent in many other nations.

Health centers or polyclinics that provide organized ambulatory services to a surrounding population are perhaps the hallmark of Socialist health care systems. Teams of salaried doctors and allied health personnel in these units furnish both treatment and preventive services. The standard medical staff of a facility for primary care in Eastern Europe consists of an internist (or GP), a pediatrician, an obstetrician-gynecologist, and a dentist. More elaborate polyclinics in cities may offer the services of many more specialists, while rural units may have only a GP. Nurses and other allied personnel are always on the team.

In a sense, the multispecialty private group practice clinic has been the U.S. response to the need for coordination of various specialists in a free enterprise setting. The neighborhood or community health centers established in slum sections of many U.S. cities may represent the concept more accurately, with their teams of salaried personnel offering both treatment and preventive services. One could hardly expect the latter model to be applied in every neighborhood of the United States today, as it is in the USSR or Poland. The British, Swedish, New Zealand, and Canadian versions of health centers, however, should not be difficult to emulate. In these models, physicians (usually GPs) continue their private practices alongside nurses, technicians, and others employed by a local public authority. The doctor derives most of his income from the national health insurance or health service system and pays rent for his quarters; rentals are relatively low, to encourage this pattern of ambulatory care. Although many of these units were initially established in newly settled areas where doctors were lacking, they have by no means been limited to serving the poor. National policy in the above nations, and in nearly all the developing countries, favors using health centers for delivery of primary care as rapidly as they can be constructed.

The various European strategies for getting balanced geographic distribution of doctors in a country have a great deal of relevance for the United States. The economic support offered by national health programs is basic, but beyond this are such policies as the British one of classifying all localities as underdoctored or overdoctored. New graduates are, in effect, channeled to underdoctored areas, since they would not be permitted to receive payments from the NHS in overdoctored areas; purely private practice would be permitted anywhere, but not many physicians could expect to earn a living this way. Many developing countries (and all the Socialist ones) require almost every new medical graduate to work for a period of one to three years in a rural area; this requirement is generally associated with publicly supported medical training, for which graduates are expected to pay back their debt to society by service in rural areas.

One of the most effective strategies for assuring rural populations access to primary medical care has been the district doctor system of Norway. The nation is divided into some 400 districts, in which there are positions for about 600 GPs, who receive modest basic salaries from the central government. Theoretically, the salaries pay for the provision of local preventive health services—immunizations, examinations of schoolchildren, and so on—but most of the district doctors' earnings come from medical care remunerated by the national health insurance program on a fee basis. The local community provides a low-rent home and office combined, and the salaries of one or two nurses are shared between the community and the national government. At one time, all new medical graduates were obligated to serve as district doctors for a year or two; after Norway's overall supply of doctors increased to an adequate level (about one doctor per 540 people in 1977), voluntary applicants for these posts filled all the vacancies.

The much stronger place of the general practitioner in European and in most other countries—indeed, the very fact that he is usually separated from the hospital as a *community* doctor—establishes a strategy for coordination and continuity in health care. When patients are discharged from the hospital, reports on the findings and treatment of each case are ordinarily sent to the primary physician. Thus, the GP can serve as the overall manager of his patient's care, making sure that follow-up measures are carried out, that referrals are made, that any necessary social counseling is received, and the like. The simple availability of GPs, in other words, helps to assure appropriate use of the diverse resources of any modern health care system.

REGULATION AND PLANNING: OTHER FEATURES

With respect to overall regulation of the health care system, certain other policies in Europe and elsewhere are relevant for the United States. As indicated earlier, universities and other schools training health personnel in Europe come under much more governmental surveillance than do those in the United States. As a result, graduates of a recognized institution are accepted as being properly qualified, and licensure calls for no further examining process. Registration with a ministry of health or sometimes a province is merely pro forma. There are no constraints against a doctor's moving from one province to another, as there are for interstate movements in the United States. (Although the National Board of Medical Examiners in the United States has done much to facilitate interstate mobility, barriers are still significant in certain states, such as Florida and California.)

The closed staff pattern of medical work in hospitals, discussed earlier, means that physicians observe each other's performance daily. There need be no elaborate mechanisms for peer review in order to monitor post hoc the work of the independent private practitioner. Not only are there no Professional Standards Review Organizations, one

seldom finds tissue committees, record committees, infection committees, or the many other surveillance mechanisms that U.S. hospitals
have been compelled to establish in response to the freewheeling autonomy and independence of their attending staff physicians. Self-dis-
cipline is built into day-to-day medical work.

For out-of-hospital medical care, the national health insurance
payment process permits review of each doctor's work in relation to
various standards. There are often statistical mechanisms for detect-
ing deviance from a norm, but these are typically followed up with
more detailed investigation by a medical consultant. If some improper
performance is clearly identified, the physician may receive a warning
or a reduction in the fee paid; additional episodes of poor performance
may result in suspension from the health insurance program temporarily or permanently.

The extremely low rate at which malpractice suits occur in other
countries, compared with the United States, is noteworthy. The explanation cannot be simple, because medical, legal, and juridical differences all play a part. National health insurance protection against
disturbingly high costs for the patient and the counseling role of a
family doctor are probably relevant. The usual absence of contingency
legal fees, in addition to trial by a judge, not a jury, in noncriminal
cases, are likewise surely involved. Even so, it is instructive to note the
conversion of medical malpractice to a risk covered by social insurance
compensation in Sweden and New Zealand. The astronomical premiums for malpractice insurance paid by U.S. physicians—and passed
on to their patients—would surely justify careful analysis of the reasons for the wholly different experience in Europe and elsewhere.

In Europe, the regulation of drug production and distribution has
probably been less highly developed than in the United States, where
numerous abuses by pharmaceutical companies have generated since
1906 increasingly rigorous legislation. Little, however, has been done
in the United States to restrain the enormous multiplication and sale
of products whose differential values no physician could be expected to
fully understand. Thus, the many thousands of drugs marketed in the
United States may be compared to the approved list of 2,000 products
issued by Norway's Directorate of Health Services. Such discriminating
regulation, which is still quite permissive compared with the WHO list
of 200 essential drugs, promotes both quality and economy in medical
care.

A systematic approach to health planning in the United States
dates only from 1966, although less comprehensive actions (for example, on certain types of hospital construction or preventive child health
services) were taken long before. The 1966 Comprehensive Health

Planning Act financed a nationwide network of state and local (or area-wide) agencies, whose major responsibilities concerned the construction or modification of *all* hospitals, not just facilities subsidized with federal grants. The National Health Planning and Resources Development Act of 1974 provided broader mandates and greater funding for a nationwide network of planning agencies, although, in spite of its sweeping title, the Act's functions have largely centered on the traditional issue of hospital bed supply and distribution.

Health planning legislation in the United States puts decision making mainly at the local level. Central standards are limited essentially to guidelines, and even authority on the state level consists principally of confirming or rejecting local decisions. The vast bulk of local health planning under current legislation, moreover, is vested in nongovernmental bodies. The weaknesses and inadequacies of this approach are becoming more evident every day.

Health planning in virtually all European countries is not only a role of government (and it is hard to think of any aspect of the health system that is more properly so placed), but mainly of government at the national level. The allocation of a nation's resources for health or any other objective would seem by definition to require central study and decision. Certain tasks may be delegated to local bodies, but the necessity for centralizing the basic health planning process seems to be taken for granted in every other nation.

Perhaps it is the operation of nationwide systems of health care financing throughout Europe that makes this so obvious. The much greater public control of hospitals, around which so much health planning occurs, would also appear relevant. Even such commonplace features as closed medical staffs in hospitals greatly simplify health manpower planning; the demands for medical, surgical, obstetrical, and other specialized types of beds readily indicate the needs for specialists in each field. Thus, the complement of surgical beds found to be needed in a province or nation, for example, dictates the number of specialists required to serve surgical cases, and thus the number of surgeons to be trained. A surgeon not holding a position on a hospital staff could scarcely expect to make a living. A similar method is employed for estimating the need for ambulatory care personnel in Socialist countries, where the empirical rates of utilization of health centers determine the numbers of doctors, nurses, and others to be trained.

One should not infer that all European countries employ exclusively centralized strategies for planning health resources and services. Much of the policy described above is carried out in a relatively flexible and pragmatic manner, without clear-cut blueprints or regulations. There is a great deal of give-and-take between central and local authorities, and political considerations naturally play a large part in final decisions almost everywhere.

It is principally in the USSR and other Socialist countries that the allocation of virtually all resources is made on the central level. In Poland, for example, if more pediatricians are needed in a certain region, the budget for the staffing of health centers and hospitals in that region will be approved for more pediatric posts; hence, newly qualified pediatricians are inevitably attracted to those places where vacancies exist. The same sort of central decision making applies to overall national funding for health services in the Socialist countries. National ceilings on all health expenditures are not as rigid in the non-Socialist, free market countries, with the exception of Great Britain; there, the NHS allotment of Exchequer funds, equivalent in 1977 to about 5.6 percent of the GNP, effectively sets limits on expenditures for about 95 percent of the total outlay for British health care.

TRANSFERABILITY OF EXPERIENCE

How transferable to the United States are these health experiences from Europe? One might speculate that, in the highly decentralized, free enterprise setting of the United States, very little could be transferred.

The same might have been said about a centralized social insurance system for old-age pensions before the Social Security Act was made law in 1935. Had one listened mainly to the testimony of Alfred Sloan, president of General Motors Corporation in 1934, the proposed legislation was going to spell the end of free enterprise in the United States. The fact is that this and many other major innovations, which eloquent voices of conservatism branded as alien and inappropriate, have been introduced in the United States. The bitter opposition to statutory medical care insurance for the aged on the part of nearly all physicians in private practice between 1957 and 1965 will not soon be forgotten.

Health care organization, in contrast to many other social issues, such as foreign policy or land ownership, does not lie close to the heart of a capitalist economy. Changes in it—even sweeping changes—pose no serious threat to the nation's power structure. Various modifications may be made in the financing and delivery of health services without jeopardizing the basic dynamics of the nation. Indeed, social insurance for general medical care, the most hotly contended issue of all, was introduced in most European countries under conservative governments. The working-class benefits provided by such legislation were regarded as a small price to pay for maintaining peace and stability in the socioeconomic structure.

Indeed, as we have seen, most of the regulatory concepts in health care financing, manpower, facilities, delivery patterns, licensure, and planning in Europe have already taken root in the United States to some extent. The lessons from abroad discussed here concern mainly the *degree* to which these ideas might be promoted. In almost every facet of health care systems, we are moving in the same direction of greater organization and regulation as Europe. The transmission of ideas is always done with some adaptation to a new environment, as is seen all too clearly in the structure of our hospitals or the procedural details of our Medicare law. But perhaps half a lesson is better than none. Problems have a way of rising to the surface and then generating their own reforms. Rising costs in the United States (and the resultant inequities in access to medical care) are the foremost problem facing us in health service today: efforts to control these costs will doubtless move us forward along many paths toward a more efficient and more equitable health care system.

16

Mortality in Developed Countries with Differing Health Care Systems and Social Policies

---

The merits of various systems of health care, as measured by national health status, are frequently debated. Yet so many social and environmental factors influence a population's health that it is difficult to determine the impact of the health care system itself. Data on health for countries that are similar in most respects, except for their health care systems and social policies, may permit some causal inferences. Using mortality rates and life expectancies as the indexes of health, this chapter compares selected pairs of developed countries.

In its simplest form, the question posed in this chapter is, "How have social policies and health care systems in developed countries affected the mortality and morbidity of populations"? To answer this question, one may compare data from selected countries with different social policies, different health care systems, or both.

SOME DEFINITIONS

First, some definitions are in order. By "social policies" I mean those policies in a nation that affect the standards of living, whether

Based on a paper presented at the third meeting of the International Union for the Scientific Study of Population, Paris, France, February 28 to March 4, 1983.

the policies are explicit under law or implicit. Thus social policies include all public and private actions influencing income, occupation and employment, housing, nutrition, education and literacy, opportunity for culture and recreation, transportation, and so on. All of these factors may be influenced by deliberate policy decisions of governments as well as by the extent and character of free market operations and the level of economic development. Even among developed countries there are substantial differences in economic levels.

By "health care systems," I refer to all activities whose primary purpose is the prevention of disease, as well as the diagnosis and treatment of it. A health care system includes the many activities necessary to support the delivery of health services, for example the production of resources (health manpower, facilities, and so on), mechanisms of economic support (insurance, revenues, private payment, and so on), methods of management (health planning, administration, regulation, and so on) and the organization of programs for particular population groups or disorders.[1]

Social policies inevitably influence the structure and function of health care systems. Both affect the health status of populations, but their relative strength has varied over the centuries. It is generally agreed that, until about a century ago, social policies in currently developed countries had a much greater influence on health than did health care systems. In recent decades, however, the relative impact of preventive and curative health services has doubtless increased enormously, although the exact proportion is subject to debate.[2] My task in this chapter is made much easier by examining the *combined* influence of these two sets of forces.

GENERAL TRENDS IN MORTALITY AND MORBIDITY

The general trends in mortality in developed countries over the last century or so are well known. Crude deathrates have declined steadily, except for the relatively brief upsurge around 1918 due to the influenza pandemic.[3] The major reason for these lower rates has been the precipitous decline in the deaths of infants and small children. At the same time, there has been a steady, though less regular, decline in birthrates, resulting in an increasing proportion of middle-aged and elderly persons. In most developed countries, the proportion of persons age 65 and over exceeds 10 percent, reaching 14 percent in France (1977) and 16 percent in Sweden (1979). The implications of these changes for morbidity are very great, as are their impact on the types of problems faced by health care systems.[4]

In all developed countries, these demographic changes have been associated with great improvements in general standards of living, nutrition, and conditions of work, but they have also resulted from numerous interventions of the health care system. The most important of these have been developments in environmental sanitation, particularly in sewage disposal and the provision of clean water supplies in cities. After about 1900, immunization against several communicable diseases saved the lives of millions of children who would otherwise have died.[5] The earlier detection of tuberculosis in young adults, with isolation and treatment of cases in sanatoriums, greatly reduced the mortality from this major cause of death during the first half of the twentieth century; after 1950, streptomycin and other drugs converted tuberculosis to a very minor problem in developed countries. Antibiotic drug therapy has almost eliminated disability resulting from gonorrhea and syphilis, in spite of the frequency with which these venereal infections still occur. The incidence of infectious diseases of children and young adults declined so rapidly in developed countries that by about 1950 the major cause of death for the age group 1 to 35 was accidents.[6]

This extended survival resulted in a great paradox: reduced mortality in the young led to a greater volume of noninfectious disease and disability in the survivors.[7] This does not mean a higher *rate* of disability in the aged (although this may apply to certain types of cancer and other diseases in some countries), but a larger overall amount of disability, simply because there are proportionately more elderly men and women (particularly women, because they live longer) in the population. Thus the social consequences of preventing disease are unlike those of preventing other hazards, such as fire or crime. If fires are prevented, communities need less fire-fighting equipment, and a reduction in crime lessens the need for prisons. The prevention of disease, however, creates the need for *more* hospitals and other resources to cope with the problems of the survivors, who become sick and disabled.

Since about 1960 or 1965, a new type of prevention has become prominent in the health care systems of many developed countries. It is the encouragement of living habits, or life-styles, that can reduce the chances of acquiring chronic noncommunicable disorders, particularly cardiovascular disease and cancer.[8] A prudent diet (one low in saturated fats and not excessive in total calories), adequate sleep and exercise, elimination of tobacco smoking, and moderation in alcohol consumption can extend life. (We have yet to determine how to prevent the psychophysiological stress that may lead to unhealthful life-styles.)

The detection in early stages of certain chronic diseases, particularly selected types of cancer, may increase the prospects of a cure.[9] All of these strategies, of course, cannot eliminate the current medical paradox of demography. Extending lives beyond ages 75 or 85 increases the demands upon the health care system and the society as a whole.

CROSS-NATIONAL COMPARISONS OF LIFE EXPECTANCY

There are substantial differences in per capita wealth among developed countries and one must be cautious when comparing national mortality rates and drawing inferences from them. I try, therefore, to compare countries that are reasonably similar in gross national product per capita. If the *distribution* of income in two countries with a given per capita GNP differs, this does not invalidate the comparison, since such differences may be reasonably attributed to different social policies.

The general social policies of most modern, developed, industrialized countries with free market economies have evolved along remarkably similar lines.[10] Social insurance for old-age pensions, public assistance for the poor, unemployment compensation, factory surveillance for occupational safety, special nutritional programs for children, and so on have been established in virtually all of these countries. Their health care systems are perhaps more diverse than their social policies, but even these systems have been moving in the same general direction—namely, toward assuming major responsibility for personal health services, both preventive and therapeutic.

One of the few industrialized, highly developed nations in the world that has not yet established national insurance or other social financing of general health care is the United States. Canada, a country of similar demographic and cultural characteristics and with a roughly equivalent degree of urbanization, has had since 1962 a provincial-federal program of medical and hospital insurance covering virtually its entire population.[11] Canada has a less temperate climate than the United States and a somewhat lower GNP per capita. In 1979, the GNP for the United States was $10,630, and in Canada it was $9,640.[12] One would ordinarily expect life expectancy to be lower in countries with lower GNPs per capita, insofar as this economic index reflects average standards of living. In spite of this, for 1977 (the last year with data from both countries), the life expectancy at birth in Canada for both sexes was 74.35 years, compared with 73.35 years in the United States.[13] Another country with almost universal insurance protection for health care and a GNP similar to Canada's is France ($9,950 per capita in 1979); its life expectancy at birth in 1977 was almost identical with Canada's, at 74.45 years.

One could cite other examples along these lines (Japan and the Netherlands), but any such cross-national comparisons with the United States call for comment. It is often said that comparisons of this sort are "unfair," insofar as the United States has a heterogeneous population with many ethnic minorities from Africa, Asia, and Latin America—more than are found in most European or other indus- trialized countries. These minority groups are said to account for the lower U.S. life expectancy. There is no evidence, however, that persons with these ethnic backgrounds have less biological capacity for good health than white persons of European background, *given the same social conditions and health services*. The considerably poorer health record of nonwhite, compared with white, populations in the United States (and, indeed, in several other industrialized countries) is associ- ated almost entirely with their lower socioeconomic status.[14] Insofar as nonwhite populations reduce the overall health record of the U.S. popu- lation, this must be attributed to social policies and health services.

Lest there be doubts about this interpretation, one may examine mortality data in the United States for the white population alone, compared with the total population of other, somewhat similar coun- tries. A recent study calculated the mortality rates (number of deaths per 1,000 persons per year) of white and nonwhite men in the United states for 1976–77, along with overall mortality rates for men in sev- eral other countries—all adjusted for age (the United States in 1940).[15] In 1976–77 the age-adjusted overall mortality rate for U.S. men was 8.2; for nonwhite men it was 10.6, and for white men alone it was 7.9. The overall mortality rate of Canadian men (including the Metis and other minorities) was 7.7; in the Netherlands it was 7.2; in Switzerland it was 7.0, and in Sweden it was 6.8—all appreciably lower than the rate of 7.9 for white men in the United States. For white women in the United States, compared with the overall population of women in other countries, the differentials were approximately the same.

For one age group in the United States—persons 65 years old and over—a nationwide program of social insurance for medical care (Med- icare) was enacted in 1965. It would be enlightening, therefore, to compare the mortality of this age group in the United States with that of the same age group in the other countries considered both before and after the Medicare program. In 1966–67, when the Medicare program was just getting started, the mortality rate for women age 65 and over in the United States was 45.8, while in Canada it was 43.3, in the Netherlands 44.7 and in Sweden 45.5; in Switzerland the rate was 47.2.

After a decade of Medicare, these mortality rates were completely reversed. By 1976–77, the deathrate for U.S. women age 65 and over had declined to 36.0, including both white and nonwhite population. The rate declined also in Canada and in the other three countries, but not as much. The mortality rate for elderly Canadian women in 1976–77 was 37.5, in the Netherlands 38.4, in Sweden 38.6, and in Switzerland 37.7. The apparent influence of the Medicare program on elderly American men was not quite as dramatic, but it was significant. Before Medicare, U.S. men age 65 and over died at a rate of 69.2 per 1,000, compared with 64.2 for Canadian men; after a decade of Medicare, these deathrates became virtually equal, at 61.3 in the United States and 61.2 in Canada.

Other cross-national comparisons can be useful if one takes into account differences in national wealth, as well as in social policies and health care systems. Two countries that are geographically and economically comparable (with similar degrees of urbanization, although different religious compositions) are Belgium and the Netherlands. As of 1979, the per capita GNP in Belgium ($10,920) was slightly higher than that in the Netherlands ($10,230). Both countries have national health care systems that include social insurance for medical care, but the Belgian system has many laissez-faire and entrepreneurial features. Belgian physicians, for example, are paid on a fee-for-service basis for both ambulatory and in-hospital care, and significant copayment requirements put a special burden on the poor.[16] The benefits of the Netherlands' health insurance program are more comprehensive: primary care physicians (GPs) are paid on a capitation basis, and almost everyone has access to them without any copayment. Preventive services have traditionally been emphasized, and almost all specialists are salaried members of the medical staffs of the hospitals.[17] Despite a per capita GNP that is 7 percent lower than Belgium's, people in the Netherlands have a life expectancy of 74.85 years, compared with 72.20 years in Belgium. These relationships are probably more than accidental.

Another interesting comparison may be made between Austria and England and Wales. Austria's GNP per capita in 1979 was $8,630, 37 percent higher than England and Wales' $6,320. In 1948, Britain had introduced its National Health Service, which entitled every resident to health services, both curative and preventive, of much greater scope than those offered by the long-established social insurance program of Austria.[18] As of 1976, life expectancy at birth in England and Wales was 72.75 years, compared with 71.65 years in Austria.

Still another comparison of probable significance may be drawn between Australia and New Zealand. Both countries are in the South

Pacific, and both were settled mainly by the British in the late eighteenth and early nineteenth centuries. Australia, however, has become much more industrialized; its per capita GNP in 1979 was $9,120, 54 percent higher than New Zealand's $5,930. One would expect such a large difference in per capita wealth to be reflected in a substantial difference in standard of living, which, in turn, would affect life expectancy. In 1978, however, Australia's life expectancy at birth was 73.85 years—only slightly greater than New Zealand's 73.05 years. Perhaps the life expectancy in New Zealand is, partially at least, a result of its national health insurance program, introduced in 1939 and covering 100 percent of the population for comprehensive medical, pharmaceutical, and hospital services.[19] Australia has had a national pharmaceutical benefits program since 1952, but beyond this the population's medical care costs have been covered mainly by voluntary insurance, with major gaps in health care benefits and population coverage. A broader health insurance program was enacted in 1974 but was rescinded shortly thereafter.[20]

A particularly interesting cross-national comparison can be made between the Federal Republic of Germany (FRG) in the West and the German Democratic Republic (GDR) in the East. The division of Germany into two parts after World War II resulted, of course, in two very different socioeconomic orders, including sharply contrasting health care systems. The FRG essentially continued the national health insurance program dating back to the 1880s; most health practitioners are in private practice and are paid fees for their services by hundreds of semi-autonomous "sickness insurance funds".[21] Health care benefits vary with the insurance fund. In the GDR, a totally different health care system was developed by the postwar socialist government.[22] Virtually all medical and related health personnel became civil servants, working in organized teams for both ambulatory and hospital care; prevention was strongly emphasized, and comprehensive health services became available to the entire population without charge (except for small payments for drugs). The per capita GNP of the FRG, however, is 82 percent higher than that of the GDR: $11,730 compared to $6,430. In spite of this enormous difference in per capita wealth, the life expectancies of the populations in the two Germanies are almost identical: 71.95 years in the FRG and 71.70 years in the GDR.

The large differences in per capita wealth between the two Germanies—or, indeed, between the socialist countries of Eastern Europe and the free enterprise countries of Western Europe generally—are beyond my competence to explain. It is generally acknowledged, however, that in the socialist countries personal incomes, while by no means equalized, are more nearly so than in the capitalist countries;

yet the productivity per worker in the socialist countries is reported to be decidedly less, and numerous other factors doubtless contribute to the generally lower material standards of living in those countries. It must also be realized that Western Europe as a whole has a much longer history of industrialization and parliamentary development than does Eastern Europe. These comments are offered by way of introduction to the discussion of infant mortality rates in the next section.

CROSS-NATIONAL COMPARISONS OF INFANT MORTALITY

The infant mortality rate—that is, the number of infants who die during their first year per 1,000 babies born alive—has long been regarded as a sensitive indicator of the general standard of living of a population. At the extremes of the range of infant mortality rates, this concept is obviously valid. For example, in 1975 the infant mortality rate of Nigeria (GNP per capita $420) was 163, compared with 11 in Norway (GNP per capita $8,550).[23] This vast differential (15 to 1) is clearly due much more to the many hazards of the physical and social environment of Nigeria than to differences between the two countries' health services.

Environmental deficiencies and general standards of living probably have the greater impact on infant mortality rates of about 20 or more; if the rate is lower and if most infant deaths occur within the first 28 days of life, then the adequacy of the medical care provided to pregnant women and newborn babies is probably the greater influence. This interpretation applies mainly in recent years and, of course, should not be applied rigidly. It may, however, help to clarify the meaning of recent comparisons of infant mortality rates among and between developed countries. Examining the same five sets of industrialized countries for which life expectancies have just been reviewed, what do the data on infant mortality show?

In 1978, the infant mortality rate in the United States was 13.8; in Canada it was 12.0, and in France (with a very similar GNP per capita) it was 10.7. Since average standards of living in the United States, as reflected by the GNP per capita, are doubtless somewhat higher than in the other two countries, these differentials probably reflect mainly the impact of health care systems. Insofar as personal income in the United States may be less evenly distributed than in Canada or France, the disparities in infant mortality rates would also reflect the influence of social policies.

Life expectancy at birth was greater in the Netherlands than in Belgium, despite Belgium's slightly higher GNP per capita. The comparison of infant mortality rates in 1978 was even more striking, being 13.8 in Belgium and 9.6 in the Netherlands.

Life expectancy was greater in England and Wales than in Austria, despite their substantially lower GNP per capita. The infant mortality rate in England and Wales in 1978 was 13.2, compared to Austria's 14.7. The comparison between Australia's and New Zealand's rates is also roughly parallel to their relative life expectancies.

With respect to the two Germanies, the comparison of infant mortality rates is particularly interesting. The FRG and GDR life expectancies were almost identical, although that of the FRG was slightly greater, and the FRG's GNP per capita was substantially larger. For infant mortality, however, the GDR rate in 1978 was significantly lower, being 13.1 compared to 14.7 in the FRG. It is very likely that this differential reflects the special emphasis on preventive and therapeutic maternal and child health services in the health care system of the German Democratic Republic.

Any discussion of infant mortality rates in developed countries today should take account of certain surprising trends recently reported in the Soviet Union. In 1980, the U.S. Bureau of the Census issued a report bearing the somewhat sensational title: *Rising Infant Mortality in the USSR in the 1970s.*[24] It is rare for U.S. government reports to be reviewed in general publications, but this report was regarded as having major political implications and was extensively reviewed and debated.

According to Soviet sources, the infant mortality rate in the USSR reached a low of 22.9 in 1971, after a steady and impressive decline following the 1917 Revolution. The trend then reversed: the rate rose quickly to 27.9 in 1974 and has remained at around 28 since 1978.[25] Various explanations have been suggested. Hostile critics have referred to a "health crisis in the USSR," interpreting the rise as evidence of a deterioration of the Soviet health care system, as well as of Soviet society as a whole.[26] Others have suggested influences such as: (1) improved housing, so that young married couples need not live with their parents, but thereby forfeit grandmother's care of the baby while the mother is working; (2) increased employment of Soviet women, requiring the placement of more infants in public créches, with the attendant hazards of cross-infection; (3) several influenza epidemics in the 1970s, which affect infants and the elderly more than other age groups; (4) the presence of relatively high infant mortality rates in the Asiatic republics of the USSR, even though these rates are substantially lower than those in ethnically similar South Asian countries such as Afghanistan, India, or Pakistan; (5) a high and rising rate of abortion as a method of limiting family size, a method that heightens the risks of subsequent childbirths; and (6) the exceptionally large Soviet expenditures on defense, which reduce funds available for achieving better standards of living.[27]

Whatever the reason, one wonders why that rate of about 28 since 1978 should be so much higher than the rates of other countries with roughly equivalent per capita GNPs. In socialist Hungary, for example, the 1979 infant mortality rate was 24.2, and its per capita GNP ($3,850) was only slightly below the Soviet Union's. In Greece, with a GNP per capita of $3,960 and with undoubtedly less equally distributed income than either Hungary or the USSR, the rate in 1979 was 18.7. The health care system of Greece, furthermore, has been dominated by the private sector (54 percent of its hospital beds, for example, are private), which ordinarily means very uneven access to health service.[28] Are these differences in deathrate real, or are they artifacts of reporting or calculation? If they are real, can one identify causative factors in the health care systems, the social policies, the family life, or other aspects of life in these countries?

CIVILIZATION AND MORTALITY

There is no question that there have been long-term downward trends in mortality throughout the world and that these have been associated with general advances in civilization. Based on World Health Organization data for 1950 to 1975, this trend has been observed in both developed and developing countries: life expectancy at birth increased from 64.3 to 70.3 years in developed countries and from 42.5 to 53.2 years in developing countries.[29] Civilization has meant urbanization, greater production of food and other essential goods, education, and countless other developments contributing to good health, as well as medical care and disease prevention programs. We noted earlier the paradox of contemporary demography—more disability resulting from reduced mortality—and it may be appropriate to end this discussion with some further comments on this paradox.

In the United States, where mortality statistics have been reasonably complete for some years, there has been a striking extension of life expectancy associated with socioeconomic and scientific developments. Life expectancy at birth increased from 47.3 years in 1900 to 72.8 years in 1976. As noted earlier for developed countries as a whole, most of this gain was due to fewer deaths of infants and small children from communicable diseases. It is perhaps more remarkable that, even at age 65, after which classical public health measures have relatively little influence, life expectancy increased between 1900 and 1976 from 11.9 to 16.0 years, a gain of 34 percent.[30] This advance has doubtless been due partly to the provision of effective medical care, but also partly to prevention in the form of modification of behavior and late twentieth century life-styles.

Evidence for this interpretation is found in the U.S. data on deathrates from cardiovascular disease, the disorder most clearly affected by life-style. From 1900 to 1950, death rates from cardiovascular disease rose in every age group. Then, *adjusted for age*, these rates began to decline, from 308 per 100,000 population in 1950 to 262 in 1970, a reduction of 14 percent. Adjusting the figures for age is a statistical manipulation that does not nullify the paradoxically higher burden of chronic diseases in U.S. society, since the crude (unadjusted) deathrate from cardiovascular disease rose over the same two decades from 357 to 366 per 100,000. Analysis of mortality by age groups, however, does suggest the benefits in cardiac health achieved in the United States between 1950 and 1970 by reduced cigarette smoking among adults, reduced consumption of saturated fats, increased exercise by sedentary workers, widespread detection and drug therapy of hypertension, and general improvements in the provision of medical care. (It is noteworthy that deaths in the United States from cancer did not decline on either an overall or an age-adjusted basis during that same period.)

A probable confirmation of this interpretation is found in reports on death from heart disease during the same general period in the Soviet Union. While the exact definitions and time intervals differ somewhat, between 1964 and 1975 there was an 18 percent increase in age-adjusted Soviet mortality caused mainly by cardiovascular disease.[31] Careful investigation has shown that, between 1965 and 1977, the population's diet changed, with a decline in consumption of potatoes and grain products and a large rise in the consumption of meat, eggs, milk products, and other lipid-containing foods. Between 1960 and 1977, Soviet tobacco consumption rose by 60 percent (while that in the United States declined by 15 percent). Studies during 1975–77 showed that the incidence of hypertension among Soviet men age 40–59 was twice as high as it was among men in the United States. Alcohol consumption between about 1958 and 1974 rose by 5.50 percent per year in the USSR, compared with 2.25 percent in the United States. In summary, the Soviet population seems to be suffering from the same mortality trends, as reflected by death from cardiovascular disease, as the U.S. population did a generation earlier. That is, the USSR is paying the price for its advancement in standards of living, as reflected in the pattern of consumption of food, tobacco, and other products. Somewhat analogous is the explanation for a rising Soviet infant mortality in a period of improved housing and greater employment of women.

Conditions in the United States and certain other developed countries suggest that another stage has been reached, or at least has been started, one in which new health strategies are being devised to fight back against the "diseases of civilization".[32] The general sequence is similar to that observed in the urban centers of many developing countries, where part of the price of "progress" is having heart disease and cancer replace diarrhea and enteritis as the leading causes of death. In those countries, as in the USSR and elsewhere, the diseases of civilization are stimulating new social and medical responses. Old-fashioned killers such as influenza and pneumonia must still be fought, as reflected in a recent decline in life expectancy in the United States due to a 14 percent increase in those disorders.[33] There is every reason to believe that, in due course, social policies and the strategies of health care systems will evolve to meet the changing challenges of morbidity and mortality in all countries.

NOTES

1. M. I. Roemer, *Comparative National Policies on Health Care* (New York: Marcel Dekker, 1977).
2. T. McKeown, *The Role of Medicine: Dream, Mirage, or Nemesis?* (London: Nuffield Provincial Hospitals Trust, 1976).
3. P. F. Basch, *International Health* (New York: Oxford University Press, 1978).
4. E. Shanas *et al.*, *Old People in Three Industrial Societies* (London: Routledge and Kegan Paul, 1968).
5. G. Rosen, *A History of Public Health* (New York: MD Publications, 1958).
6. *World Health Statistics Annual: Vital Statistics and Causes of Death* (Geneva: World Health Organization, 1981).
7. K. Hazell, *Social and Medical Problems of the Elderly* (London: Hutchinson Medical Publications, 1973).
8. M. LaLonde, "Beyond a New Perspective," *American Journal of Public Health* 67 (April 1977): 357–60.
9. American College of Preventive Medicine, *Preventive Medicine USA* (New York: Prodist, 1976).
10 D. Fulcher, *Medical Care Systems: Public and Private Health Coverage in Selected Industrialized Countries* (Geneva: International Labour Office, 1974).
11. M. I. Roemer and R. Roemer, *Health Care Systems and Comparative Manpower Policies* (New York: Marcel Dekker, 1981).
12. *World Development Report* (Washington, D.C.: World Bank, 1981). All monetary figures hereafter are expressed in United States dollars ($).

13. World Health Organization, *World Health Statistics*. Unless otherwise indicated, all data on life expectancy and infant mortality rates are from this source.
14. U.S. Department of Health, Education, and Welfare, *Health Status of Minorities and Low Income Groups*, DHEW pub. no. HRA 79–625 (Washington, D.C.: Government Printing Office, 1979).
15. Metropolitan Life Insurance Company, *Statistical Bulletin* 62, no. 4 (October–December 1981): 10–13.
16. Roemer and Roemer, *Health Care Systems*.
17. Regional Office for Europe, *Health Services in Europe*, 3rd ed. (Copenhagen: World Health Organization, 1981), 133–39.
18. R. Levitt, *The Reorganized National Health Service* (London: Croom Helm, 1976).
19. G. M. Emery, "New Zealand Medical Care," *Medical Care* 4 (1966): 159.
20. Roemer and Roemer, *Health Care Systems*.
21. D. A. Stone, *The Limits of Professional Power: National Health Care in the Federal Republic of Germany* (Chicago: University of Chicago Press, 1981).
22. K. Winter, "Health Services in the German Democratic Republic, Compared to the Federal Republic of Germany," *Inquiry* 12, no. 2, suppl. (1975): 63–68.
23. World Bank, *Health Sector Policy Paper* (Washington, D.C.: World Bank, February 1980).
24. C. Davis and M. Feshbach, *Rising Infant Mortality in the USSR in the 1970s*, ser. P-95, no. 74 (Washington, D.C.: U.S. Bureau of the Census, 1980).
25. S. Schmemann, "Soviet Affirms Rise in Infant Mortality," *New York Times*, 21 June 1981.
26. N. Eberstadt, "The Health Crisis in the USSR," *The New York Review of Books*, 19 February 1981, 23–31.
27. A. Szymanski, "The Health Crisis in the USSR: An Exchange," *The New York Review of Books*, 5 November 1981, 57–58.
28. A. Ritsataki, "The Changing Health Care System in Greece," in C. O. Pannenborg, A. van der Werff, G. B. Hirsch, and K. Barnard, eds., *Reorienting Health Services* (New York: Plenum Press, 1982), 347–56.
29. T. Fülöp, and M. I. Roemer, *International Development of Health Manpower Policy* (Geneva: World Health Organization, 1981), p. 145.
30. M. I. Roemer, "Health-Disease Trends To Shape Hospital's Role," *Hospitals*, 1980, no. 1, 86–88.
31. R. Cooper and A. Schatzkin, "Recent Trends in Coronary Risk Factors in the USSR," *American Journal of Public Health* 72 (May 1982): 431–40.
32. U.S. Public Health Service, *Healthy People: The Surgeon General's Report on Health Promotion and Disease Prevention* (Washington, D.C.: U.S. Department of Health, Education, and Welfare, 1979).
33. "Life Expectancy Dip Is Linked to Outbreaks of Flu, Center Reports," *American Medical News*, 23 October 1981.

Part Four

Socialist Countries

17

Health Services in the
Soviet Union—Contrasting Views

The first national health care system developed in a fully Socialist country was in the Soviet Union, following the Russian Revolution of 1917. Over the years this system has evolved in many ways, but it has seldom been free of controversy. Many foreign observers give highly favorable accounts of Soviet health achievements, as does the Ministry of Health in Moscow. Other foreign observers are highly critical. This chapter offers a brief overview of the Soviet health care system, followed by book reviews of two reports with sharply contrasting viewpoints about the operations of that system.

Following the Russian Revolution of 1917, the Union of Soviet Socialist Republics developed the world's first system of health services designed and implemented according to Socialist principles. Whether or not one considers these principles desirable, they have come to be embodied in the health care systems of numerous other countries that have adopted Socialist political structures, particularly since World War II. Non-Socialist countries, both developing and industrialized, have also adapted many Socialist principles in their health care systems. If the spectrum of health care systems of the world is to be understood, one must have a clear picture of the main features of health services in the USSR.

The two-part book review in this chapter was published in *World Health Forum* 1 (1980): 187–89.

HIGHLIGHTS OF SOVIET HEALTH SERVICES

The central principle of Soviet Union's health services is that they are basically a public, or governmental, responsibility. Access to health services has been established as a right of citizenship, similar to access to the public highways, to police protection, or to basic education. Implementation of this social right has required abandonment of a free market in health care and its replacement with a systematically and largely centrally planned system for producing and using resources that provide health care.[1]

In completely free markets, health services are produced for profit and sold to those who wish to and can afford to buy them—just like shoes or potatoes. Many persons with great sickness needs, however, cannot afford to buy the medical services that could cure them. Medical services are quite complex, furthermore, and the average buyer may not realize what kind or how much of a certain service he should purchase for his own welfare. Even the most entrepreneurial societies have come to recognize the inequities and tragedies resulting from these characteristics of disease and medical care in populations, and they have set up numerous government-financed programs of health service for the poor, for prevention of contagious diseases, for regulation of dangerous drugs, and for other interventions in a free medical marketplace.

The Soviet Union has extended the principle of deliberate national planning much further. In order to assure health services to everyone on the basis of need rather than purchasing power, it established a central Ministry of Health (MOH) as well as branches in each of the 15 constituent republics. The MOH is responsible for both production and use of health resources—manpower (doctors, nurses, technicians, and so on), facilities (hospitals, ambulatory care units, and so forth), and physical items (drugs, supplies, equipment, and so on). In prerevolutionary Czarist days, those resources were utterly inadequate to meet the needs of the country's vast population; they were barely adequate to meet the demands of the tiny fraction of rich people in the main cities.

An enormous program of education, construction, and manufacture was necessary to create appropriate resources. This took time, of course, and required allocation of manpower and supplies from other important sectors of society, such as housing, education, food production, and military defense. During World War II (1939 to 1945), a great part of health care and other resources that had been created in the previous 20 years were destroyed, and these had to be built up again.

Since health services were to be assured to everyone, rather than being a market commodity, the government had to control and allocate them according to the location and needs of the population. This meant, of course, that doctors and other health personnel became employees of the government (similar to public school teachers in the United States), and all facilities were similarly made governmental. Money for support of these resources (salaries, rent, and so on) was derived from the earnings of all productive industry, which was also governmental rather than private.

In order to make the most efficient use of all resources, they would have to be deployed in ways that U.S. business would call cost-effective. Thus, doctors and hospitals would be used only for functions that required the relatively expensive skills of these personnel and facilities; it would obviously be wasteful to use a physician for giving a simple injection that could be done perfectly well by a nurse. Extension of this principle of efficiency meant that nearly all primary and other ambulatory health care would be given by teams of health personnel— doctors, nurses, and others—in health centers or polyclinics that were gradually constructed to be within easy reach of practically everyone. Likewise, hospitals would be available in regionalized networks. For simple conditions (such as childbirth, minor accidents, and common infections), a local hospital was made available; for progressively more complex conditions (such as heart disease, cancer, serious trauma, and rare or multiple disorders in the same patient), hospitals with more elaborate resources (specialists, advanced equipment, and so on) would be available at the district or next higher level.

Because prevention of disease is obviously preferable to treatment (and is usually less costly), preventive strategies were incorporated throughout the system. Thus, instead of separate public health agencies for prevention, with private doctors for treatment (familiar in the United States and elsewhere), all services were united. Immunizations, health education, early case detection, and other preventive measures were offered at all primary care centers and hospitals, along with treatment of the sick. Other preventive services, such as environmental protection or surveillance of working conditions in factories, were carried out by "sanitary-epidemiological stations." All facilities in a geographic district, however, were under unified direction, just as the whole system nationally came under the MOH.

The unification of responsibility for all health services in the Soviet Union is sometimes difficult for persons from free enterprise countries to understand. The MOH and its peripheral branches plan and supervise not only the delivery of preventive and treatment services, but all other components of the system. Thus the MOH controls the medical schools and other training institutions. (This integration was not achieved overnight. Medical schools were traditionally part of semi-autonomous universities, as elsewhere, for 20 years after the revolution, but in 1937 they were transferred to MOH control in order to assure that the numbers and types of doctors trained coincided properly with the health needs of the population). The MOH also determines the drugs to be manufactured (by the chemical industry) and controls the pharmacies that dispense drugs. Medical research is also a MOH function and is carried out through hundreds of special research institutes. In order to assure that doctors and others are informed about advances in medical science, continuing education is mandatory every year or two.[2]

The USSR has huge rural areas, where life is typically less attractive than in the large cities; but the rural people must receive health services. To cope with this problem, the government requires medical graduates to spend three years in a rural post; after this, they are free to leave, but they are offered higher salaries (than for equivalent urban posts) and other benefits as inducements to remain. In addition, the USSR has continued the training of medical assistants, or *feldshers*, principally for service in isolated rural areas—a practice started in Czarist times. As more physicians have been educated, however, the output of *feldshers* has been reduced.

Many Western visitors are surprised to discover that the majority of Soviet doctors—not to mention nurses and *feldshers*—are women. This has come about for several reasons, of which the most important is probably equality of opportunity for medical education. It has also been due to the scale of social values in Soviet society; with its great need for industrialization, the highest salaries were offered to engineers, managers, and skilled workers. Hence, talented men entered mainly these fields rather than medicine or law. Another influence has been a policy of occupational mobility; thus many medical students come from the ranks of nurses or *feldshers* (who are mainly women). Still another influence has been the shorter workday (six hours) for physicians, since it is regarded as a stressful occupation, and this coincides with the greater family responsibilities of women. The killing of thousands of male doctors in World War II was another factor. Finally, the Soviet health care system puts heavy stress on the training of pediatricians to take care of all children, and this type of health service has been considered particularly appropriate for women, for obvious reasons.

The use of pediatricians rather than GPs for providing health services to children follows from a general priority assigned to children in the Soviet health care system. Another priority group is industrial workers. There are clinics staffed with physicians at almost all work places—not solely for prevention and treatment of occupational diseases and injuries, as in other countries, but for comprehensive health care. Several small factories may be jointly served by one industrial clinic, while large plants will have their own. The worker is free to use the industrial facility or the health center near his home, whichever he prefers. Medical records are interchanged.

To facilitate the proper staffing and equipping of all ambulatory and hospital facilities, the MOH promulgates norms—for example, one doctor for 330 people (more than in the United States), with this number divided among general adult physicians (often called therapeutists), pediatricians, obstetrician-gynecologists, and many other specialties. Establishment of these norms is based on a complex planning process, in which empirical studies are made of the health needs of the people, the working time of doctors and others to meet those needs, and the judgment of medical experts on needs that may lie below the surface and not be expressed empirically (such as latent chronic disease or the requirements of preventive medicine). Estimates of needs for personnel and facilities are also submitted to the MOH by local public health authorities, based on their field observations. From all these inputs, desirable standards are formulated, but the resources can seldom be produced immediately. There are competing needs in other socioeconomic sectors, and there are constraints of medical teachers, building materials, and so on. This whole process of estimating health needs, creating resources to meet them within the nation's capacity, and formulating how to deploy the resources is carried out periodically; perception of needs and the capacity to respond to them obviously change over time. Since 1926, this process has been carried out every five years, yielding the well-known Soviet five-year plans in health care, as in all other sectors.[3]

This account of the world's first Socialist system of health services is far from comprehensive, but it may be enough to demonstrate the great differences between it and the health care system in the United States and other free market countries. It may also show how various features of other health systems (such as those in Canada, Norway, or Great Britain) are similar to the Soviet system—for example, the use of governmental financing, the regionalized organization of hospitals, and the coordination of health personnel in teams. Yet everyone knows what vast ideological and philosophical differences underlie the political economies of the Socialist and capitalist countries, even when the latter have intervened in the operations of the free market in medical care, as well as other goods and services.

These ideological differences have led to very different types of descriptions of the Soviet health care system and its consequences. A rather dramatic illustration of these contrasting accounts is found in two books on the organization of health services in the USSR, both published in 1978. The first was written by I.P. Lidor and colleagues, who are officials of the MOH in Moscow.[4] The second was written by a British scholar with a manifestly negative attitude toward Socialist ideas.[5] The following review of the two books may demonstrate how differently the same national health care system may be described by observers with diametrically opposite points of view.

AN OFFICIAL ACCOUNT
OF THE SOVIET SYSTEM

The book by three Soviet health authorities presents a concise, comprehensive account of the health service system of the USSR—its underlying principles, its historical development, and its current detailed characteristics. Like similar accounts of national systems emanating from Washington, London, Paris, Peking, or other national capitals, it describes the structure and function of its health services in a positive and proud spirit. Yet, by reviewing developments and changes in policies and practices since the 1917 Revolution, the writers indicate clearly certain deficiencies and even mistakes in policy made along the way and later corrected.

The book begins with consideration of the significance of various health care systems in the larger social setting of nations. Three basic types of systems are distinguished, associated with (1) developed capitalist nations, (2) developing countries of Asia, Africa, and Latin America, and (3) Socialist countries. Perhaps this is an oversimplification in the interests of brevity, because two or three major subtypes can be readily distinguished under each of these main categories.

Five fundamental principles underlying the Soviet health care system are then explained: (1) its state (governmental) character, (2) free health protection for everyone, (3) emphasis on prevention, (4) the unity of science and practice, and (5) participation by the people. Implementation of these principles has been made possible by an enormous expansion of all resources—both health personnel and facilities—through government action. This, in turn, has depended on growth of the whole Soviet economy and continuing allocation of substantial investments to meet the health needs of the population.

The chapter tracing step-by-step developments since 1913, before the revolution, is especially enlightening. The miserable conditions of life in Czarist Russia, particularly in the vast rural areas are explained: the infant mortality rate, for example, was 269 per 1,000 live births per year. We learn how, from 1925 on, increasing attention was given to establishing health facilities in rural regions—first simple posts staffed only by *feldshers*, then gradually health centers staffed by doctors and polyclinics staffed by teams of specialists. At the same time, special medical units were set up in major industrial plants. The sanitary-epidemiological stations took shape by 1930, for control of environmental health hazards and prevention of infectious diseases. A new conception of medical education—oriented toward meeting objective health needs, such as the emphasis on training pediatricians for the large population of children—was launched. Medical research was systematized and promoted through the All-Union Institute of Experimental Medicine in 1932. Not only hospitals and ambulatory care facilities, but also sanatoriums and spas were increased many times over by 1940.

The USSR suffered massive destruction in World War II—losing 20 million of its people and 30 percent of its national wealth. Some 40,000 hospitals and health units were destroyed. In the postwar reconstruction, administrative policies evolved toward greater coordination of hospitals and ambulatory care clinics. All health services were more systematically organized in regional networks of facilities staffed by personnel ranging from generalists at the periphery, up to highly trained specialists at regional medical centers. Between 1940 and 1976, the supply of physicians expanded fourfold, from 79 to 335 per 100,000 population; the increase in nurses and other middle-level personnel was even greater.

The final chapter gives abundant details on the current Soviet health care system. The production of drugs, supplies, and medical equipment has been improved by the organization of a Ministry of Medical Industry. Medical education has been extended to six years, plus a year of internship. Continuing education has been strengthened for both physicians and allied personnel. Hospitals have expanded to nearly 12 beds per 1,000 population—more than in most other industrialized nations. Emergency care systems have become highly developed in the main cities. While very thinly settled rural areas are still served by *feldshers*, these auxiliary personnel are closely supervised and are being gradually replaced by physicians. The USSR now has one doctor for about 300 people and three allied health workers for every doctor, but its plans call for even greater numbers to achieve its intended standards in both urban and rural areas. Although rural populations are still less well served than urban, the imbalances are being steadily reduced. As the USSR continues to industrialize, increasing attention is being directed to the protection of workers against toxic chemicals, as well as control of water and air pollution. Medical research is expanding steadily in the 400 special research institutes. In virtually every aspect of a health care system, the Soviet experience demonstrates the enormous achievements possible within the framework of a Socialist society.

This valuable summary of the main features of the Soviet health care system concludes with a series of useful statistical tables on demographic, socioeconomic, and health service features in the USSR.

A HOSTILE ACCOUNT OF THE SOVIET SYSTEM

The second book is part of a British series of studies on social policy, but one can only regret how far it descends from the usually high standards of British scholarship. While purporting to be objective, it presents an incredibly distorted view of the Soviet health care system. The author's bias is evident on page one, where we learn that the focus is on developments "from 1950 onwards"—thereby ignoring the enormous Soviet achievements after the 1917 Revolution and the vast reconstruction programs needed after the devastation of two world wars.

The book starts with a description of the political jurisdictions of the USSR—its republics, provinces (*oblasts*), districts, and towns. Great importance is attached to the existence of certain separate departmental programs of health care—such as those of the Ministry of Transport or the military services—in addition to the main system (which operates for example 96 percent of the hospital beds). This attempt to belittle the Soviet claims about its integrated system ignores such massive achievements as the adjustment of medical education, drug production, and health science research to the needs of the health services under a single, unified Ministry of Health.

Expenditures for health are traced from 1958 to 1974, and Ryan finds fault with the discovery that they have remained relatively stable at about 4 percent of "net material product" (the Soviet equivalent of GNP). He overlooks the crucial fact that this constant percentage applies to a rapidly enlarging national income, so that it has meant an increase in health expenditures from 128 to 394 billion rubles per year—a growth of over 300 percent, or an average of 18 percent each year (1 ruble = $1.10 U.S.). He likewise gloats over the differential spending in the republics, ranging from 15.4 to 25.3 rubles per capita; one might only wish that this small a range (about 1.65 to 1) characterized the differentials in health funds among regions of other large countries, such as the United States or India. Ryan's distorted interpretation of statistics is illustrated by his claim that, between 1960 and

1970, interrepublic expenditure differences "widened"; in fact, health expenditures in the poor republics rose by greater percentages than they did in the more prosperous ones.

Ryan also finds evil connotations in the existence of an estimated 130 polyclinics (out of some 35,000 outpatient units in the USSR), where patients pay for services. Knowledgeable observers usually commend the flexibility that this feature demonstrates in the Soviet system—similar to that in Great Britain and other Western nations. The patient who wishes to spend the money may get the reassurance of a second diagnostic opinion, although Ryan admits that such patients typically return to the public system for treatment. The fees for these private services, moreover, are admittedly "low," and they are paid not to the doctor, but to the clinic, which is an open and officially managed facility.

Ryan attempts to belittle the enormous growth of Soviet medical manpower by stressing the differentials among republics. Once again, however, he overlooks the crucial fact that between 1950 and 1974 the doctor-population ratio in the republic best supplied with doctors (Georgia) rose by 40 percent, whereas in the republic with the poorest supply of doctors (Tadzhik) it increased by 133 percent.

Being concerned only with negative interpretations, Ryan states that, after the three years of rural service required of all Soviet medical graduates, the great majority return to a city. The more remarkable fact is that this socially oriented policy provides great numbers of young doctors for the rural areas during three-year periods (no such policy exists in India, for example, or the United States); moreover, about 12 percent of them remain. The high population of women in the Soviet medical profession is viewed by Ryan not as evidence of equal opportunity, but simply as an effect of low medical salaries. One wonders if he finds merit in the overwhelmingly male-dominated medical professions of most countries, where the fee-for-service pattern of remuneration leads to huge medical incomes at the expense of patients.

Increasing specialization is another feature of Soviet medicine that Ryan condemns. The fact is, of course, that this trend in worldwide and is much more moderate in the USSR than elsewhere, such as the United States. Much more important is the fact that Soviet specialists work together in teams (both in hospitals and polyclinics), so their special knowledge and skills are properly coordinated. The largest specialty, moreover, is pediatrics, which in the Soviet setting is really not a specialty at all, but a general health service for children. If one takes proper account of the data in Ryan's statistical table on this question (adding "general physicians," "pediatricians," and "residual groups"), one finds that 47.4 percent of Soviet doctors are truly generalists—a reasonable balance with the 52.6 percent who are specialists. In discussing "paramedical" personnel, Ryan deprecates the occupational mobility that has allowed some 15 percent of physicians to have risen from the ranks of *feldshers* or nurses. In most countries, such mobility is prohibited by rigid rules of academic credentialism. Rather than "creaming off" the best allied health personnel, as he alleges, this policy, with its opportunities for advancement, doubtless inspires Soviet health personnel to be diligent in the performance of their jobs. Another bizarre distortion is Ryan's negative interpretation of the fact that a large proportion (33 percent) of the high rate of ambulatory services in the USSR (about nine per person per year in 1974—greater in cities and lower in rural areas) is for preventive purposes. The extremely low level of preventive medical contacts in most countries is an object of concern in the public health world. The overall Soviet rate of nine ambulatory services per person per year, moreover, was about double this rate in the United States.

The linkage of Soviet polyclinics and other ambulatory care units with hospitals after 1947 has been regarded by most observers as a strategy for coordination that many other countries would like to emulate. The alternation of a doctor's duties between the ambulatory care clinic and the hospital, moreover, is generally regarded as promoting quality in both places. To Ryan, however, these sound policies are condemned as "fragmenting" medical care. He also deprecates the continuation of house calls in Soviet medical practice—apparently oblivious to the widespread regret that this patient-oriented service has almost disappeared in most Western countries.

In spite of the amazing expansion of the Soviet hospital bed supply between 1950 and 1974, from 5.6 to 11.6 beds per 1,000 population—an achievement unmatched in any capitalist nation—Ryan manages to find examples of delays in construction projects. Considering the enormous task of postwar reconstruction of housing, schools, factories, and all, one can only marvel at Soviet achievements in building so many ambulatory and inpatient health facilities. Once again, Ryan stresses the uneven supply of hospital beds among the republics, ignoring the greater *rates* of hospital bed expansion (between 1950 and 1974) in the poorest republics. The rate of hospital admissions among rural people, which is usually lower than the rate among urban people, had actually surpassed the urban rate by 1973.

A final assault in the Ryan vendetta against Soviet health services is his account of the practice of having special facilities for high public officials. This practice can be found in virtually every nation in the world and is justified by the recognized social value of a nation's leaders. In the Soviet health care system, such priority services are based on a person's functional importance in the society, not on personal wealth or inherited status. As for the special services provided for railroad workers, Ryan seems to be unaware of identical policies basically for logistical reasons, followed in scores of other countries.

Only the more glaring distortions in Ryan's account of Soviet health services are noted in this review. His vulgarization of the Soviet emphasis on physical therapy as "white magic" deserves no comment. His criticism of the increasing average patient stay in Soviet hospitals, without reference to the changing age composition of the population, discloses his basic lack of knowledge about health needs. Perhaps nothing reveals the combination of ignorance and bias in this book as well as the author's comparison of infant mortality trends in the USSR and Great Britain. Presenting absolute rates—which are of course lower in Britain today than in the Soviet Union—he ignores the all-important fact that, between 1949 and 1974, the British rate declined by 50 percent while the Soviet rate declined by 65 percent. With these trends, one may reasonably expect the Soviet infant mortality rate to decline to lower levels than the British in the future.

The book by Lidor and colleagues may present an utterly rosy picture of the Soviet health care system, with its weaknesses recognized mainly through reports of their correction, but it is accurate and historically valid. The Ryan book is, above all, a demonstration of how much an author's hostile attitude and biased presentation can distort the reality of a great and internationally recognized achievement in health care organization.

NOTES

1. An early and classic account of the health services in the USSR is given in H. E. Sigerist, *Socialized Medicine in the Soviet Union* (New York: Norton & Co., 1937).
2. A more recent and somewhat critical account of Soviet health service is M. G. Field, *Soviet Socialized Medicine: An Introduction* (New York: The Free Press, 1967).
3. The methods of Soviet health planning are described in G. A. Popov, *Principles of Health Planning in the USSR*, public health paper no. 43 (Geneva: World Health Organization, 1971).
4. I. P. Lidor, A. M. Stochik, and G. F. Tserkorny, *Soviet Public Health and the Organization of Primary Health Care for the Population of the USSR* (Moscow: Mir Publishers, 1978).
5. M. Ryan, *The Organization of Soviet Medical Care* (Oxford: Blackwell, 1978; London: Robertson, 1978).

18

National Health Policy Formulation in Socialist Poland

After World War II, Poland and several other Eastern European countries adopted Socialist forms of government. They came under considerable influence from the Soviet Union in most sectors of society, including the health services. In each country, nevertheless, the application of Socialist principles was inevitably shaped to some degree by the national heritage. The methods of health planning and policy formulation in Socialist Poland are presented in this chapter.

In the United States, it is conventional to decry the "interference" of politics in decision making on matters of health and medicine; only scientific and humane considerations, we are told, should determine health policy. By contrast, in Socialist countries, the preeminent importance of politics in policy formulation in the health care system and in virtually all other aspects of life is openly and repeatedly emphasized. The priority of political considerations is itself a major principle in Socialist thinking. The reality in the United States, in fact, may not be so very different, but it is customary to deny it.

DEVELOPMENT OF THE SYSTEM

After World War II, when most of Poland had been occupied by the Nazis, a new government was formed by the United Workers party,

This chapter is an adapted and substantially revised version of "National Health Policy Formulation in Socialist Poland," *Journal of Health Politics, Policy and Law* 3(1979):155–62, that was based on a 1976 field study in Poland supported by the U.S. Department of Health, Education, and Welfare.

which unified the prewar Communists and left-wing Socialists. Their first task was to rebuild the country which had been devastated by the Fascists, and their highest priority went to housing and industrialization. The next order of business was to redesign and expand the nationwide systems of education and of health services as public benefits. Private medical practice was never banned; it is still found today. The policy of the governing party, however, was to strengthen the public medical service as rapidly as possible, so that private health care would decline through gradual loss of its market. This policy has been largely successful.

Another basic principle of the United Workers party was to develop a unified health care system, with major policy decisions made — after partywide discussion — at the national center. The implementation of policy would be at the level of the provinces, which originally numbered 17 but were recently redesigned into 49 smaller units. The unification of the system, with the objectives of efficiency and effectiveness, meant that all health services would come under the direction of a single Ministry of Health and Social Welfare (MHSW). Thus, unlike Western European countries, Poland's social insurance program, which financed most medical costs, was not under a different ministry and the hospitals did not remain under the control of local government. All health service resources, whether fiscal or professional, preventive or curative, institutional or ambulatory, were placed under a central ministry. Each province would have a department of public health, with equivalent broad responsibilities, reporting to the MHSW.

Unified administration applied not only to the delivery of all personal and environmental health services, but also to the distribution of drugs through public pharmacies. It included the training of doctors and all "middle medical," or allied health, personnel. Not everything was achieved at once, but in 1952 (seven years after the War), the faculties of medicine, pharmacy, and dentistry were withdrawn from the universities (under the Ministry of Higher Education) and put in separate medical academies (under the control of the MHSW). Thus, health manpower development would be, as closely as possible, consonant with the health service needs of the population; moreover, the surveillance of quality in the health services could be best conducted by the medical faculties if they were fully integrated into the health care system. The training of nurses and other middle medical personnel was similarly woven into the MHSW fabric. Likewise, research was to be directed primarily toward health problems of greatest importance in the population—rather than of greatest personal interest to the scientist—and was developed principally in 14 national research institutes under the MHSW.

The principal physical resources for health care delivery in Poland are nationwide networks of ambulatory care centers and hospitals, staffed entirely by salaried medical and allied personnel. Entry of any patient into the system, for either treatment or preventive service, is through the primary care center in his neighborhood. These units are staffed normally by teams of a general physician (sometimes an internist), a pediatrician, an obstetrician-gynecologist, and a dentist, plus nurses, technicians, clerks, and other middle medical workers. (In isolated rural areas, the core staff may simply be a generalist and nurse.) Referrals, when necessary, are made to a polyclinic with more specialized personnel or to a hospital at the local district or central provincial level, depending on the severity of the case. In recent years, closer links have been forged between primary care centers, polyclinics, and district hospitals in local "integrated health service areas" (ZOZs), which vary from about three to ten per province. For historical reasons, the purely environmental, epidemiological, and health educational services are operated by a parallel local network of *Sanepid* stations, which are integrated with the personal health care system only at the provincial and national level.

In this unified health care system, all health workers are public employees; but, as noted earlier, private medical and dental practices have never been prohibited. In the mid-1950s, however, when the supply of health manpower was rapidly increasing, the MHSW required that all medical and dental graduates devote seven hours a day to the public system; after this, they could engage in private practice, although not in the public facilities. Private practice now takes two forms: individual practice and medical cooperatives (which we might call group practice clinics). The latter are rather tightly regulated by the provincial departments of health as to fees charged, conditions of work (a maximum of two hours per day per doctor), and so on. It is estimated that 10 to 20 percent of ambulatory services in Poland is currently obtained at personal expense through these private arrangements, so the national goal has not yet been reached. Hospitalization, however, is exclusively public.

In accordance with Polish Socialist principles, modeled largely after those of the Soviet Union, special priority is given to children—there is a notably high proportion of doctors engaged in pediatrics—and to industrial workers. In addition to the community health facilities described above, large factories also have comprehensive health care programs (curative, emergency, and preventive) for workers, who are free to use these as well as their neighborhood units. Peasants, who still predominantly own their own land, have received lower priority, and it was only in 1972 that they became entitled to the same range of health services, without any personal charges, as urban workers.

THE NATIONAL HEALTH PLANNING PROCESS

This comprehensive and essentially unified system of public services for health protection in Poland was not achieved overnight. Immediately after World War II, Poland's health care resources, human and physical, were drastically depleted. Physicians numbered only 37 per 100,000 and nurses only 27 per 100,000; there were 3.5 general hospital beds per 1,000 theoretically available, but staffing was woefully inadequate. By what process were the numbers and distribution of resources increased to the current level, which is essentially equivalent to that of the United States and in several respects better than that of many other, wealthier countries? To reverse the usual question, how did they get from there to here?

As in most Socialist countries, especially those substantially influenced by the Soviet Union, Poland's current health care system has been developed through centralized planning. The basic policy decisions, made by the governing party, were clear enough: (1) health service should, as rapidly as possible, become a public benefit available to everyone without charge; (2) all health administration should be unified under a single ministry, including medical research and the education of personnel; (3) while centrally planned and directed, implementation of health policy should be delegated to the provinces; (4) preventive and treatment services should be integrated in delivery, with priority for children and industrial workers; (5) a private sector should not be banned, but it should be discouraged by rapid strengthening of the public services; (6) quality should be promoted by the closest possible links between the educational institutions and the health services, including widespread provision for continuing education.

One rather pervasive policy affecting health care should be mentioned. Polish socialism is sometimes described as socialism of a flexible type. Incentives, rather than commands, are used to encourage certain social ends. To attain more equitable distribution of doctors in rural areas, for example, attractions such as higher salaries and other perquisites are offered. Likewise, continuing education is not mandatory, but participation in it gives a basis for more rapid advancement.

Implementation of these health policies is never as simple as one might expect, even with the high degree of centralized authority found in a Socialist country. The method is well illustrated by the process of planning to meet the nation's needs for health manpower, in appropriate numbers and types.

The heart of health manpower planning is the formulation of long-term goals and then short-term norms to guide both the preparation and use of health personnel. The long-term goals are formulated by the MHSW, which has an office for planning that draws upon the resources and views of all branches of the ministry. Formulation of the short-term norms, however, must take into consideration the capacities and potential outputs of many sectors of the economy. It is a complex process, involving a National Commission for Planning, and it must be repeated periodically because of changing economic and social conditions. This is done typically at five-year intervals—hence, the well-known five-year plans of the Socialist countries.

Thus the formulation of goals and of norms requires input from many sources. It constitutes, in a sense, a blend of technical, economic, and political considerations. The technical aspect calls for estimates of the human and social needs for a service, such as ambulatory medical care. No single technique is relied upon for making this estimate, but data are integrated from many sources. Empirical studies are made on the rate of utilization of ambulatory care by a specific population, in the absence of economic constraints on patients or inhibiting factors such as long waiting times due to an insufficient supply of doctors. Such studies have been made in both urban and rural settings, where transportation and the attitudes and knowledge of people would vary. Clinical examinations are also made on a sample of people in order to detect "unexpressed need." Such studies have been done in Poland, in the USSR, in Czechoslovakia, and in other Socialist countries, and their findings are exchanged at international meetings.

Technical judgments are also based on current statistics on health care utilization from the provinces throughout Poland. There are, of course, variations in local rates, which are studied by the MHSW in the light of other information on local health resources and environmental conditions. Committees of experts in different sectors of the health field are convened to examine these data. From these deliberations, estimates are made of the ultimate needs for ambulatory medical care. These, in turn, are converted into requirements for numbers of primary care doctors, based on the average number of patients seen per hour by personnel judged to be competent.

These estimates, derived from purely technical analyses, are only the first step in the planning process. Consideration must also be given to the nation's economic potential for training the doctors required—that is, the capacity of Poland's ten medical academies. Since the deficiencies in 1946 were obvious, the five prewar medical schools were soon doubled, each school being located at a place enabling it to serve as the technical center for health services in a region (averaging now about five provinces for each of the ten regional academies). The availability of qualified teachers, adequate school buildings and equipment, and so on must be considered before each academy can be assigned the quota of doctors it will be expected to train.

Based on the requests from the MHSW, the National Commission for Planning carries out the necessary economic analyses of the expenditures that would be necessary for health and all other purposes, in relation to the nation's income from all sources. This commission performs a staff function for the Council of State, which represents all of the ministries. With continual statistical studies of the earnings from each sector of the economy, the commission makes recommendations on the allocation of monies, through the Ministry of Finance, to each sector. A department of social policy within the planning commission has responsibility for the health services. As in countries of all types, one hears the technical officials of this department remark how "the goals and norms proposed for the health services are always higher than the nation's capacity."

Having received statements of these ideal goals and the desired current norms from the MHSW, the National Commission for Planning must indicate economic constraints and recommend a reasonable rate for approaching long-range goals. In the light of the nation's productive capacity, it estimates whether a goal in preparing doctors (or other resources) can be reasonably reached in 20 years, 10 years, or sooner. This enables the MHSW to formulate tentative norms for the next year, so that local health authorities can be guided in the preparation of their budgets. As new experience is gained, these norms are revised.

The semifinal decisions on health planning goals and norms, with the financial outlays required, are political. These are made by the Council of State, where decisions are reached by all of the ministers on the allocation of resources to the health field, in relation to the competing needs for industrial investment, housing, agriculture, military affairs, and all the rest. These priority decisions are necessarily influenced by political judgments on Poland's overall situation, domestically and internationally. The final votes on national budgets are made by the *Seym* (parliament), but these rarely differ from the Council of State recommendations because the same political party predominates. (Such uniformity between executive and legislative branches of government, incidentally, characterizes Western European governments as well, until an election changes the composition of parliament. The prime minister and his cabinet are equivalent to the executive branch in the United States; these officials are chosen from the elected members of the party or coalition of parties with the majority of seats in the parliament.)

Within the health sector, there is leeway for the MHSW to vary allocations among different programs. The relative emphasis on ambulatory care in relation to hospitalization, for example, may be modified, with corresponding changes in the norms applied to each subsector. Furthermore, there is some give-and-take between the MHSW and its peripheral units for implementation of the national health plan. On the basis of local developments, for example, the quota for doctors to be prepared by a particular medical academy may be altered, or more funds may be assigned to alcoholism control programs and less to hospital surgery than originally intended.

There are obviously complex interdependencies among these technical, economic, and political inputs into the health planning process in Poland. Things are often not as cut-and-dried as this brief description may suggest. A sudden change in the political situation, international or domestic, may lead to modified plans for health service and every other field. Shortfalls in one sector—for example, steel production—will inevitably affect the attainment of goals in health facility construction; new decisions would then have to be made on the basis of relative priorities of hospitals and primary care centers, or of construction in one geographic region or another.

Through frequent publication of goals and norms by the MHSW, provincial health administrators throughout Poland are guided in their planning efforts. Planning is not a task separated from the functions of local health programs, as it is in the United States (note the provisions of the National Health Planning and Resources Development Act, P.L. 93–641). On the basis of national norms, budgets are prepared first at the ZOZ level; these are submitted to the provincial health department and then to the MHSW. In the highly pluralistic U.S. setting, such a simple process would scarcely be possible. There is an important time dimension, of course, in all health planning. Poland's health plans, like every other country's, are not always carried out perfectly, but the achievements of the last 30 years have been impressive.

LESSONS FOR THE UNITED STATES

There are lessons to be learned by the United States from Poland's methods of formulating and implementing national health policy. Our two societies are built on very different ideological foundations, and if we consider health policy globally there may be little to transmit in either direction. But if we consider special facets of the health field, there are, in my view, many lessons to learn from Polish policy and experience. I should like to cite a few examples.

1. The integrated delivery of primary health care, both preventive and therapeutic, is effective and economical. Every person, adult and child, has access to a primary physician near his home, and necessary referrals are then made as needed.

2. Continuing education of doctors and other health personnel is so widely and systematically provi.'ed, with incentives offered for participation, that nearly every health care provider is stimulated to keep abreast of his or her field. Educational institutions, being within the health service establishment, offer such education, along with quality surveillance of services, as part of their regular functions.

3. With specialists and all other doctors paid by salaries—which vary in accordance with their training, competence, and responsibility—in both polyclinics and hospitals, there are no incentives for unwarranted surgical operations or other excessive and costly services. Since all doctors work in teams, there is daily peer review built into the system (rather than onerous and posthoc review by Professional Standards Review Organizations) to protect patients against perfunctory care. This pattern of organized in-hospital specialty service is not unique to Poland, but characterizes most Western European nations as well.

4. With the majority of Polish doctors being devoted to primary care, there is no need for doctor substitutes of limited training to carry out this crucial function. In the desperate postwar years of doctor shortage, Poland trained *feldshers*, on the Russian model, to help meet the enormous needs of the people, but this was regarded as a temporary expediency. By 1958, the training of new *feldshers* was terminated—just about the time that the United States began training physicians' assistants and nurse-practitioners for primary care, mainly to work in underserved areas (or, more cogently, areas where doctors did not wish to go). The existing *feldshers* were converted to sanitary inspectors, ambulance attendants, health educators, nurses, or other true health auxiliaries, and the brighter among them were encouraged to attend medical school and become physicians.

5. Health services are regarded as a public benefit to which everyone is entitled without charge. The main limitation is the nation's capacity to produce personnel and facilities to meet the needs. Yet a private sector has never been banned, and a certain degree of inequity, based on an individual's ability to pay,

will be permitted until the public services are strengthened further. This strengthening is guided by judgments on the relative needs of different sectors in the total society, not by the dynamics of individual self-interest (that is, the marketplace).

These are just a few examples of lessons the United States might learn from Poland. In technological developments — such as drug production, hospital design, diagnostic tests and immunizations — Poland has obviously learned a great deal from the United States and other countries. Despite the obvious differences, it seems that the U.S. health service is moving in a direction similar to that of Poland, although at a very much slower pace and with numerous variations in detail. If so, the reasons are probably to be found less in the transmission of Polish ideas across the Atlantic Ocean than in the forces that seem to be changing the shape of health care systems in all countries. They are arising from the demands of people to make equal access to health care a basic human right.

19

Health Development and Political Policy in Cuba

The Cuban Revolution of 1959 brought the first Socialist political and economic structure to a developing country in Latin America. The health care system was completely changed, based mainly on the technical advice of consultants from Czechoslovakia. During its first two decades, the health system developed in response to the special conditions of Cuban society.

The usually severe deficiencies of health services in developing countries are customarily attributed to the general poverty of the nations and their consequent lack of resources. The most frequent explanation, in other words, is economic. Without general economic development, the conventional wisdom suggests, poor countries could not possibly afford improved health care.[1]

While economic determinants doubtless play a basic part everywhere in the availability of health services, the progress made in at least one developing country, Cuba, demonstrates strikingly the decisive influence of political policymaking, in spite of economic handicaps. Take note of the data presented in table 19.1.[2] It is evident that among eight Latin American countries, with per capita wealth only

This chapter is an adapted and substantially revised version of "Health Development and Political Policy: The Lesson of Cuba," *Journal of Health Politics, Policy and Law* 4(1980):570–80, that was based on a 1971 field study in Cuba sponsored by the Pan American Health Organization, and on a second such study in 1977, so changes could be observed.

Table 19.1   Economic Levels and Health: Infant Mortality Rate and Life Expectancy, by Per Capita GNP, for Eight Latin American Countries, 1973

Country	GNP Per Capita ($U.S.)	Infant Deaths Per 1,000 Live Births	Life Expectancy (years)
Brazil	460	110	61.4
Peru	480	67	55.7
Cuba	510	28	72.3
Costa Rica	590	56	68.2
Mexico	700	63	63.2
Jamaica	720	27	69.5
Panama	820	34	66.5
Venezuela	1060	52	64.7

Source: World Bank, *Health: Sector Policy Paper* (Washington, D.C., 1975), 72–73.

slightly below or substantially greater than that of Cuba, the record of Cuban health status—according to the two most widely used mortality indexes—is impressively better. What could account for so striking a contrast among developing countries, all in the same northern region of Latin America?

LATIN AMERICAN HEALTH SERVICES

The drastically inequitable distribution of health services, not to mention general standards of living, in Latin American countries is well known.[3] The vast majority of the population in almost all of these countries is impoverished families, in poor housing, with widespread malnutrition, chronic underemployment, and very limited accessibility to modern health services. Large proportions of rural populations are served only by traditional healers or receive no health services at all.

Average per capita GNP (in 1973) was $810 (U.S.) for all South American countries and $450 for countries in Central America and the Carribbean region, compared with $4,410 in the European Economic Community countries and $6,155 in the United States.[4] The enormously lower per capita GNPs of the Latin American countries reflect the conditions of 80 to 90 percent of the people; the vastly better living standards enjoyed by the remaining minority have only a relatively small impact on national health indexes.

Social security programs have brought a much higher level of health services to industrial and governmental workers in most Latin American countries, but these workers typically constitute only small percentages of national populations.[5] Since most Latin American families are engaged in agriculture or marginal forms of other employment, they are typically not entitled to social security benefits.

Taxation in most Latin American countries is mild in its impact on the small upper crust of wealthy families, and governments are notoriously ineffective in collecting even the modest taxes due.[6] Governments depend heavily on revenues collected from import and export taxes, sales taxes, and other indirect means, rather than from income taxes. The public sector as a whole is relatively weak, therefore, and health agencies rarely get more than 5 to 10 percent of public revenues for health promotion purposes.

CUBAN HEALTH SERVICES

In sharp contrast to this general Latin American picture is the system of health services and the general structure of social conditions that have developed in Cuba since its revolution in January 1959. In fewer than 20 years, a society has been built in which equitable distribution of the necessities for a healthy life has been virtually achieved. Meat, eggs, milk, and several other protein-rich foods are rationed, and prices are controlled so that lower income persons—and there are still differences in family income—can receive their fair shares. Elementary school attendance is now universal (unknown in any other Latin American country), and, in addition to basic education, every primary school child is assured a liter of milk per day.[7] Other priority groups for essential foods are pregnant women, the aged, and the sick.[8]

Unemployment has been entirely eliminated; in fact, there is, a shortage of labor. This is one reason why family planning (birth control) is not actively promoted, although contraceptive service is freely available to any family on request. Modern housing is still inadequate, but new dwellings (typically in apartment buildings) are being rapidly constructed, especially in the smaller towns, rural areas, and the suburbs of Havana and other major cities. One does not see the dismal slums surrounding Havana that characterize Caracas, Lima, Rio de Janeiro, and virtually every other major city of Latin America.

The achievements have been most remarkable regarding personal health services. The island is blanketed with a network of 345 polyclinics and 140 rural medical posts staffed with teams of physicians, nurses, and allied health workers. Primary health care is accessible, with only a short travel time, to virtually everyone. An indication of the use of these ambulatory services is the rise from 2.0 medical consultations (visits) per person per year in 1963 to 4.8 in 1975[9]—a rate not very different from that in the United States and much higher than that in other Latin American countries. The ambulatory units are backed up by 257 hospitals, yielding a ratio of 5.0 beds per 1,000. Of all childbirths (with a birthrate down to 19.9 per 1,000 in 1976 from 35.1 in 1963), over 98 percent occur in hospitals—an achievement not matched by any other Latin American country. The national Psychiatric Hospital has been converted to a model rehabilitative institution, in sharp contrast both to its previous squalor and to the sordid mental facilities one sees in other developing (and even some affluent) countries. Resources, both manpower and facilities, have been almost equalized between urban and rural areas.[10]

The crucial resources for personal health services are health personnel—physicians and others. It is widely known that soon after the revolution there was a massive departure of Cuban physicians, who had numbered 6,300 in 1958; the exodus is variously estimated at 40 to 60 percent of these.[11] The flight of doctors and other upper-class persons or families after a revolution is not unique to Cuba (it followed the revolution in the United States in 1776, in Russia in 1917, and in China in 1949). The striking feature about Cuba was the official political policy, which permitted these departures without obstruction. Despite the handicaps created thereby, the ranks of medicine could be rebuilt without internal opposition. Exactly this was done; medical schools were increased from one to three, and their output was greatly enlarged. In 1976, there were nearly 11,000 doctors for a population of 9,464,000, or a ratio of about one doctor per 870 persons—much better than before the revolution. Similar increases were achieved in the numbers of nurses, assistant nurses, dentists, technicians, and other health workers. As in other Socialist countries, however, greater emphasis is given to the expanded output of physicians, about 50 percent of whom are women.

Changes in Cuba's Health Services: 1971–77

Changes that occurred in the Cuban health services in the last half-dozen years offer striking reflections of the influence of political policy on health affairs. I studied the abundant literature about Cuban health care that appeared within the first decade after the revolution,[12] and made my first visit to Cuba in September 1971. This visit was under WHO auspices, and it resulted in numerous observations.[13] In December 1977, at the invitation of the Cuban government, I made a second visit, and several new developments were noteworthy.[14]

1. Administration of the health services (as of other community activities) has become much more decentralized. The former six political provinces (eight health provinces) have been divided to 14. The former 39 health regions were abolished and replaced by 169 municipalities (averaging 12 per province), to which substantial responsibilities are delegated for health service, as for other public affairs.

2. Elections at the municipal level have been introduced, creating municipal assemblies with three delegates per 5,000 population. From these bodies, representatives are elected to provincial assemblies, and, from these, representatives are elected to a National Assembly. At each echelon, the assembly chooses an Executive Council (mainly full-time officials) responsible for day-to-day functions. These councils, for example, appoint municipal and provincial directors of public health and are responsible for providing the health services; as representatives chosen by the people, they invite expression of any grievances and set about to correct them—including the discharge or disciplining of health personnel, if deemed necessary.

3. Availability of primary health care has come to receive much greater emphasis than formerly. This was accomplished not only by expanded staffing of the polyclinics (as more personnel were trained), but by introduction of a policy of "sectorization." Under this, each doctor in the basic polyclinic teams (general internist, pediatrician, obstetrician-gynecologist, and dentist) is responsible for the health care of the population in his geographic sector of 4,000 to 6,000 people. (If a patient is dissatisfied with his sector doctor—said to be rare—he may change to the care of another team.) With about 25,000 to 35,000 people served by each polyclinic, there are five to seven teams in each facility covering the populations of their respective sectors. (Not all sector teams, however, are as yet completely staffed.)

   To heighten the appreciation of future Cuban doctors for primary care, each municipality contains at least one teaching polyclinic, where medical student and intern training parallels conventional training on hospital wards.

4. Medical and dental education have been transferred from the supervision of the Ministry of Education to that of the Ministry of Health (MINSAP), which was formerly responsible for training only allied or middle-level personnel. The new policy is intended to render the content of medical and dental education

more sensitive to the needs of the population, as perceived by the health authorities. The MINSAP administrative structure, furthermore, has been reorganized to be more appropriate to its widened responsibilities—not only in professional education, but also in pharmaceutical production and distribution, in health resource planning, and in international relations.

The latter function includes assignment of medical and allied personnel to some 20 other developing countries—a striking contrast to the brain drain of physicians and nurses from various developing countries (Philippines, Iran, India, South Korea, and so on) to the United States. This foreign medical aid includes dispatch of both civilian and military physicians to recently "liberated" countries of Africa, such as Angola and Ethiopia.

5. New emphasis is being given to chronic disease control, as communicable diseases have been reduced and Cuba's health picture has come to resemble that of a developed country— with heart disease, cancer, and stroke now constituting the top causes of death. Accordingly, a policy of "dispensarization," through which all chronically ill persons are systematically monitored by their sector physician, has been introduced. There is heightened research on chronic diseases through designated research institutes and enhanced health education on the hazards of cigarette smoking, obesity, and other factors contributing to chronic, noncommunicable disorders.

It is noteworthy that all these recent changes in Cuban health service practice involve actions influenced by political considerations or the observations of policymakers on changing priority needs. Except for the quantitative expansion in resources (personnel and facilities), which has made possible the increased rates of utilization of health services (both ambulatory and hospital care), the recent changes have depended not so much on economic growth as on social policy decisions. But even the continued expansion of personnel and facilities, which must indeed depend on economic investment, can be traced essentially to political decisions, which should now be explored.

Investment and Expenditures on Health

Data on the total expenditures for health services (counting both public and private sectors) in developing countries are rarely available. The pioneer studies in this field, done under WHO auspices, were carried out in the 1950s and 1960s, and they contained information on only four developing countries (Chile, Sri Lanka, Kenya, and Tanganyika).[15] In these studies, it was found that in developing (poor) countries total health expenditures were not only relatively small, they were also a lower percentage of the GNP than in affluent countries. Moreover, the information on expenditures by private households tended to be incomplete, so the proportion reported to come from public sources was correspondingly inaccurate.

In more recent years, some special studies on *total* public and private health expenditures in developing countries have been made. These suggest that (1) expenditures in the private sector tend to be relatively high and (2) consequently, the aggregate health expenditures are larger, both absolutely and as a percentage of GNP, than previously realized. Thus, piecing together data from diverse sources, I found that, in one Central American country in 1976, about 5.5 percent of GNP was devoted to health and that some 52 percent of this was derived from private spending; the latter went about half for the benefit of modern medical services to a very small percentage of upper-class families and about half for self-medication of dubious value undertaken by the poor.[16]

A careful study in South Korea in 1976, based on a household survey and other sources, found that 2.7 percent of GNP was spent for health purposes, and an astonishing 84 percent of this was derived from personal household expenditures.[17] A preliminary study of Colombia, deriving data from several sources for 1970 and 1971, suggested that about 50 percent of health expenditures came from the private sector.[18] In 1968, a study in Chile found that, in spite of that country's national health service, 57 percent of all health expenditures came from the private sector.[19] Estimates made in a recent WHO study of Thailand produced data indicating that about 2.5 percent of GNP went for health purposes in 1974, and 75 percent of this was spent through the private sector.[20]

Thus, in spite of the widely broadcast efforts of governments in many developing countries to undertake public programs of personal health care for the great majority of their populations who are very poor, evidently only a discouragingly small share of the financial sources devoted to health has been tapped. The resulting inequities in the receipt of health services are obvious. These imbalances may be due, not so much to deliberate political policy decisions as to the failure of governments to intervene affirmatively with free market dynamics in the health services. Timid governmental behavior would seem to lead inevitably to a robust private health sector, with all its inequities and obstructions to comprehensive health planning.

Against this background, some rough estimates of health expenditures may be offered for Cuba. While not available from published sources, the estimate of a high Cuban official was that overall health expenditures from all sources in 1976 were 57 pesos per person (one peso equals $1.24 U.S.); for the population of 9.4 million, this would amount to 535 million pesos per year.[21] Official government expenditures on health were (in pesos) 330 million for MINSAP health activities, 30 million for construction of health facilities, and 97 million for production and distribution of drugs.

This would leave 78 million pesos derived from nonpublic sources, such as the payments made by patients for a fraction of the cost of drugs in government pharmacies and personal expenditures for the small sector of private health service (mainly dental restorative care) remaining in Cuba. Roughly, the proportions are 85 percent of health expenditures from public sources and 15 percent from private — in striking contrast to the breakdowns noted above for non-Socialist developing countries.

To make estimates of the proportion of GNP in Cuba devoted to health is difficult, because the national accounts procedures in this Socialist country do not consider services (including health care) as contributing to the GNP, only physical commodities. In 1970, however, MINSAP expenditures constituted about 10 percent of total government expenditures.[22] In a Socialist economy, where nearly all production is governmental, this would be expected to be close to the percentage of total GNP (as conventionally calculated) devoted to health services. If approximately so, this proportion (10 percent) would be much higher than that devoted to health in other developing or even affluent countries. (The United States, for example, in 1976 devoted 8.6 percent of its GNP to health purposes.)

Priority for Health Services

Whatever may be the correct financial figures and proportions, it is clear that Cuban social policy gives high priority to health services as well as to education. Considering its moderate overall level of economic development, the availability of health services to the general population of the country is remarkably greater than is found in any other Latin American nation, including those like Venezuela, Argentina, and Chile, which have much greater national wealth, not to mention those like Bolivia or Paraguay which have lesser wealth. The question is: How could an infant mortality rate of 22.8 per 1,000 live births, a tuberculosis death rate of only 2.7 per 100,000, a crude death rate of 5.6 per 1,000, and a life expectancy at birth of 72.3 years be achieved in the 1970s—health records better than those of any other country of Latin America, most of which are of higher per capita wealth.[23,24] Even before the Socialist revolution, one must realize that Cuba's health record (e.g. 1950–55) was not among the poorest in Latin America; its life expectancy was exceeded only by Argentina, Panama, and Uruguay.[25] Yet by the mid-1970s, Cuba's life expectancy exceeded that of even these three countries. More important, Cuba's achievements were made in a period of extreme hostility from the United States (embargoes, blockades, even invasions) and several other countries—handicaps not faced by other Latin American countries (until the guerrilla rebellions in Central America of the 1980s).

The answer must be found simply in the political decision-making process, in its broadest sense. Faced with serious external threats during its early years, as well as with actual attempts at foreign invasion, the Cuban political leadership decided that the survival of the revolution depended on the full and devoted support of the people. This could be won by providing the people, especially the majority in rural areas, with important and appreciable benefits they had never had before. Education for all children, personal health services for everyone, and better housing as rapidly as it could be built were such benefits—benefits that could be felt promptly by virtually every family. Deprivation of freedom of the press, termination of free elections, and leadership from a single, small political party built on the Leninist model were acceptable losses for the mass of the people, in return for these gains in their material standard of living. Religious freedom, deeply meaningful to some, was not destroyed; the churches remain open, although they are attended mainly by aged persons.

With the blockade imposed by the United States in 1960 and the 1963 embargo against trade, the Cuban Revolution was able to survive only because of the deliberate and massive support of the Soviet Union and other Socialist countries of Eastern Europe. (One may see the analogy to Israel, surrounded by enemy nations and surviving thanks largely to massive assistance from the United States.) This is not to deny the heroic and disciplined performance of the Cuban people under the leadership of Fidel Castro and the Cuban Communist party, but simply to recognize the basic facts.

Much of the aid to Cuba from the Soviet Union and allied countries has been indirect but definite material subsidy. In recent years, for example, when the world price of sugar (overwhelmingly Cuba's major source of income) fell to less than $0.10 per pound, the USSR continued to purchase most of her output at $0.36 per pound. Likewise, when the world price of oil (Cuba's major source of energy) rose to about $30 per barrel, the USSR continued to sell Cuba Soviet oil at $10 per barrel.[26] Can there be any surprise at Cuba's dispatch of troops (along with medical personnel) to Angola and Ethiopia, as well as its dispatch of technical experts to Mozambique, Tanzania, and elsewhere without "orders from Moscow"? Soviet assistance has clearly made the Cuban government and average citizen feel part of a global movement toward socialism. At the same time, there are signs that Soviet bounty has permitted a certain laxness in cost considerations, and one is often told that more rigorous cost accounting is required in the future (for the health services, among others).

With the highly permissive attitude toward departure of dissident physicians and other upper- and middle-class persons, as well as the gradualist approach toward expropriation of land and private enterprises, there has remained in Cuba no significant opposition to national policy. At the same time, there grew up naturally a new generation of young workers, farmers, and intellectuals who felt they were participating in the construction of a new and different society. Everywhere the visitor is struck with the relative youth and enthusiasm of persons in leadership positions—no less in the health services than in other fields. The young physician does not complain at being paid 250 pesos per month, a salary only slightly above that of the skilled manual worker. With seniority and further training, his or her monthly earnings may rise to about 425 pesos, but not to the salary levels of prerevolutionary doctors, who were rewarded for remaining in Cuba with salaries of 600 pesos per month or sometimes more.

Municipal elections were introduced in 1976 and with them a pyramidal structure of municipal, provincial, and national assemblies. Anyone may be nominated, but election requires a majority of the total vote, so there are often runoff elections. Candidates are not required to be Communist party members, but, since party members are the visible activists in local affairs, they constitute a large proportion of assembly members, especially members of the three echelons of Executive Councils. The year 1976 was known in Cuba as the "Year of Institutionalization" because, as demonstrated by the introduction of elections, the movement to socialism was firmly established and the national leadership felt secure enough to permit popular voting. This policy is called *Poder Popular*, or People's Power.[27] This community participation permeates the health services as much as all other social sectors.

CONCLUSION

Developments in health services and the health status of the Cuban population since the revolution are a vivid demonstration of the preeminent importance of political decisions in the determination of health care resources, nutrition, education, housing, and so on. By typical criteria of economic development such as per capita GNP, Cuba is a poor country. It is in the same general class as scores of other developing but non-Socialist countries, where conventional wisdom suggests that the nation cannot afford better health care coverage.

Despite its modest economic status, Cuba has placed a high priority on health services, both therapeutic and preventive, and on nutrition and education, which likewise have major impacts on health. To a substantial extent, this has been made possible by material support from the Soviet Union and other Socialist countries. This is not essentially different from the foreign aid programs the United States and other capitalist nations have set up for developing countries espousing free enterprise, particularly for those countries aggressively opposing socialism. Whatever the explanation, the foundations of Cuba's high priority for the health sector are clearly more political than economic. Observation of Cuban accomplishments makes one hesitate to accept the severe health deficiencies of most developing countries as an inevitable consequence of poverty and the associated lack of resources.

NOTES

1. G. Myrdal, *Beyond the Welfare State: Economic Planning and Its International Implications* (New Haven: Yale University Press, 1960).
2. World Bank, *Health: Sector Policy Paper* (Washington, D.C., 1975), 72–73.
3. M. I. Roemer, "Organizational Issues Relating to Medical Priorities in Latin America," *Social Science and Medicine* 9(1975): 93–96.
4. United Nations Conference on Trade and Development, *Handbook of International Trade and Development Statistics* (Geneva, 1976), 333–34.
5. M. I. Roemer, "Development of Medical Services under Social Security in Latin America," *International Labour Review* 108 (July 1973):1–23.
6. B. Ward. *The Rich Nations and the Poor Nations* (New York: Norton & Co., 1962).
7. L. S. Stavrianos, "Cuba: Update on a Revolution," *The Nation,* 5 March 1977, 270–74.
8. Ministerio de Salud Publica, *Informe Anual 1976* (Havana: el Ministerio, Centro Nacional de Informacion de Ciencias Medicas, 1977).
9. Ibid., 25.
10. Organizacion Panamericana de la Salud, *Informe de Ministerio de Salud Publica de Cuba,* IV Reunion Especial de Ministros de las Americas (Washington, D.C., 1977).
11. M. I. Roemer, *Cuban Health Services and Resources* (Washington, D. C: Pan American Health Organization, 1976).

12. Editorial de Ciencias Sociales, *Diez Años de Revolucion en Salud Publica* (Havana: Instituto del Libro, 1969); Ministerio de Salud Publica, *Informe sobre los Servicios Generales de Salud de la Republica de Cuba* (Havana, 1965); _____, *Salud Publica en Cifras 1970* (Havana, 1971); C. P. Roberts and M. Harmour, eds. *Cuba 1968: Supplement to the Statistical Abstract of Latin America* (Los Angeles: University of California, Latin America Center, 1970); World Health Organization, *Fourth Report of the World Health Situation 1965–1968* (Geneva, 1971), 133–37; F. Rojas O., "La Red Hospitalaria del Ministerio de Salud Publica en el Periodo 1958–1969," *Revista Cubana de Medicina 10* (Enero-Febrero 1971):3–42; _____, "El Policlinico y la Asistencia a Pacientes Ambulatorios en Cuba," *Revista Cubana de Medicina 10* (Marzo-Abril 1971):207–25; V. Navarro, "Health, Health Services, and Health Planning in Cuba," *International Journal of Health Services 2* (1972):397–432.

13. Roemer, *Cuban Health Services.*

14. _____, "Progress in Cuban Health Services," report to the Pan American Health Organization, Washington, D.C., December 1977.

15. B. Abel-Smith, *An International Study of Health Expenditure and Its Relevance for Health Planning,* public health paper no. 32 (Geneva: World Health Organization, 1967).

16. See chapter 4 in this book.

17. C. K. Park, *Financing Health Care Services in Korea* (Seoul: Korea Development Institute, 1977).

18. D. K. Zschock, R. L. Robertson, and J. A. Daly, *Health Sector Financing in Latin America: Conceptual Framework and Case Studies* (Washington, D. C.: Department of Health, Education, and Welfare, Office of International Health, 1976).

19. T. L. Hall and S. Diaz P., "Social Security and Health Care Patterns in Chile," *International Journal of Health Services* 1(1971):342–77.

20. World Health Organization. "Information on Financing Health Services in the South-East Asia Region" (New Delhi, 1977).

21. J. A. Guttierrez Muniz, Minister of Health, Government of Cuba, personal communication, December 1977.

22. Roemer, *Cuban Health Services,* 63.

23. Ministerio, *Informe Anual 1976.*

24. Pan American Health Organization, *Health Conditions in the Americas, 1969–72* (Washington, D. C., 1974), 13.

25. United Nations, Department of Economic and Social Affairs, *World Population Trends and Prospects by Country, 1950–2000* (New York, 1982).

26. D. Joly, country representative of the World Health Organization in Havana, personal communication, December 1977.

27. Comité Central del Partido Comunista de Cuba, *Plataforma Programatica del Partido Comunista de Cuba* (Havana, 1976).

20

Health Services in the People's Republic of China

The Liberation of China, as the Chinese call the change of power and birth of the People's Republic in 1949, was surely one of the crucial events of the twentieth century. The largest nation on earth became Socialist. Even in the few decades since 1949, several major political changes have occurred; each of these has been associated with certain modifications in the health care system. This chapter describes only the main features of that system and how they have developed.

In 1949, China, the most populous nation on earth, had a Socialist revolution and became the People's Republic of China. The system of health services that has developed in these first three decades of the People's Republic of China probably demonstrates the dependence of health policies on larger social and political events more dramatically than does the health care situation in any other country.

HISTORY

China has one of the oldest civilizations on earth, but most of its thousands of years were a story of emperors and conquests, of enormous differences between social classes, of magnificent glory for the

---

Based on a field visit to China in 1975, along with information from several books on China's health services published in recent years (see the bibliography at the end of this chapter).

rulers and misery, starvation, and slavery for the masses. Westerners know of feudalism in Europe, but in China the same kind of society meant even greater suffering for the millions of impoverished peasants. To most people of the West (Europe and the United States), China was "the mysterious Orient." Only in the nineteenth century were coastal cities like Shanghai settled and controlled by Western powers, as footholds for trade with the great unknown interior. Gradually a class of Chinese merchants and small entrepreneurs arose; in 1911, under the leadership of a great intellectual, Dr. Sun Yat-sen, they launched a bourgeois-capitalist revolution against the feudal landlords, the foreign colonists, and the Manchu dynasty. The Republic of China was born.

A limited form of parliamentary government took shape, known as the Kuomintang and representing largely the newer entrepreneurial classes. It took the invasion by Japan in 1930, however, to unify the country under the leadership of General Chiang Kai-shek. Meanwhile, in Russia, the 1917 Revolution had occurred. During the 1920s, its ideas spread to a small communist movement in Shanghai. Unlike the Russian Marxists, the Chinese drew their main strength from the oppressed peasants. Eventually, under the leadership of extremely hard-working and dedicated revolutionaries, such as Mao Tse-tung and Chou En-lai, the Chinese Communists gained control of territories in the northwest, in and around the Province of Hunan. A Chinese Red Army was formed mainly from peasants, who were won over to the Communist cause not by theoretical writings, but by land distribution, free education, and other reforms. The Red Army devoted its main energies to battling the Japanese in the northeast (called by them Manchuria), but the Kuomintang armies under Chiang Kai-shek seemed to be more concerned with fighting the Chinese Communists.

After the defeat of Japan by the Western Allies and the Soviet Union in 1945, the struggle between the Kuomintang and Communist forces became intense. Because of their appeal to the landless peasants, the Red Army grew steadily in strength; by 1949 it had gained control of nearly all of mainland China. Much military assistance had come from the Soviet Union. Chiang Kai-shek and thousands of his followers (with aid from the United States) escaped to the Chinese island of Taiwan (also called Formosa), which they declared to be the Republic of China. By 1949, the cold war between the Western capitalist countries and the Soviet Union and its Socialist allies was under way. Therefore, the Republic of China (Taiwan) was promptly recognized as the "true" China—it occupied the seat of China in the United Nations, for example—and the Asian mainland, with its hundreds of millions of Chinese people, was essentially ignored. After the trauma of World War II, another war was not going to be mounted in Asia, but Taiwan became heavily armed as an independent nation. From the viewpoint of the new government in Peking, the mainland, with its 21 provinces, had been liberated as the People's Republic of China, while the 22nd province, Taiwan, remained to be liberated.

In preliberation China, modern health services were virtually nonexistent outside the main cities. Vital statistics are lacking for the vast rural population, but even in Peking the crude deathrate was reported in 1949 to be 14.1 per 1,000 persons. Tuberculosis was rampant, along with extreme malnutrition. Every few years the outside world read of famines causing millions of deaths in China. Schistosomiasis, filariasis, typhoid fever, cholera, and small pox were endemic, and no one knows the rate of infant mortality from diarrhea, pneumonia, or other causes.

Under the Kuomintang, some development of health resources had occurred in the main cities. The Peking Union Medical College, training physicians on the Western model, had been founded by the Rockefeller Foundation in 1921. By 1949, there were estimated to be about 12,000 modern doctors in China—for the population then of 450 million, that was a ratio of 1 to 35,000—but they were practically all concentrated in the cities. Insofar as the rural population had access to any health care, it was from traditional practitioners of Chinese medicine and was based on theories laid down 2,000 to 3,000 years ago. Urban health facilities also existed; in the 22 provincial capitals there were some 150 hospitals in 1946 (the number of beds is not known). At the county seats there were 1,775 health centers, each serving an average of 250,000 people. In some smaller towns there were little clinics, with beds, operated by private groups or foreign religious missions; there were 307 of these clinics in 1946.

THE PERIOD OF
CHINESE-SOVIET COLLABORATION

The first ten years after liberation were, of course, extremely difficult, as the Communist government attempted to rebuild industry and agriculture after the devastation of 19 years of war (1930–49). In this first decade of the People's Republic (1949–59), a great deal of technical advice was offered by and welcomed from the Soviet Union. In the health field, this meant the training of large numbers of medical assistants (like the Soviet *feldshers*), the unification of authority under a central ministry of health, and the construction of hundreds of hospitals and health centers.

The organized health services for industrial workers in the cities, which were started under the Kuomintang—that is, supported by insurance in each establishment but employing their own doctors and using their own separate facilities—were enlarged. For the worker, the complete costs of medical care were covered; for his or her dependents, about half the costs were covered. In the vast rural areas, where 80 percent of the population lived, the system was different. General hospitals were built in hundreds of counties, and hospitals in the provincial capitals were expanded.

At the local level, the entire health structure was built within the network of collectivized farms, or communes, into which Chinese agriculture had been organized. Efforts were made to establish a health center, staffed by at least one trained doctor plus auxiliary personnel, in each of the approximately 25,000 communes. Most health centers maintained ten to 20 beds for emergency cases, pending their transfer to a hospital. The population of communes varied greatly in size, but most had between 10,000 and 50,000 people—virtually the size of a rural county in the United States. Many of these commune health centers, however, were not well staffed, and below this level there was little organized health care.

Between 1949 and 1957, some 860 new hospitals (with 100 to 350 beds each) were built. It has been estimated that by 1965, all 2,200 counties had at least one general hospital. Under Soviet influence, there was a massive expansion in the output of Soviet-style doctors, reaching 150,000 by 1966 (a ratio of one to 5,000 people). Since many of these doctors were posted at county hospitals and health centers, rural coverage was greatly improved. Campaigns were also started against schistosomiasis, by killing snails in the irrigation canals, and infants were immunized. Middle medical personnel were also trained—about 150,000 medical assistants (*feldshers*) and nurses between 1949 and 1952, plus another 340,000 between 1958 and 1970. These personnel were the principal staffs of county hospitals and health centers.

Around 1959–60, a great turning point occurred in Chinese political ideology. For many reasons, the Chinese became increasingly dissatisfied with the leadership of the Soviet Union. They did not like the emphasis on building up industry, highly centralized control, and a low priority for agriculture. Political antagonism also emerged between Joseph Stalin and Mao Tse-tung. By 1960–61, the schism between these two great Socialist powers became open, and the USSR withdrew all its technicians and advisers. China soon came to look upon the Soviet Union, along with the United States, as its great enemy. This huge nation of some 600 million people was now on its own.

In spite of the changes occurring after the Chinese-Soviet schism, one cannot ignore the progress made during the period of collaboration. Thousands of health personnel had been trained, health facilities had been constructed, public health campaigns had been launched, and the basic structure for rural health services in communes had been developed. Outside the industrial health insurance programs, the county-level health services were financed primarily by the central government. They were not free, however; patients had to pay small fees to help cover the costs.

After the departure of the Soviet Union, China set out to develop its own brand of socialism. Essentially this meant a much higher priority for agriculture, as opposed to industry, and extensive decentralization of authority. In order to motivate agricultural people to produce more food, the slogan "local self-reliance" was formulated and far greater authority was vested in the communes. There is little doubt that assigning top priority to agriculture led to greatly improved nutrition, which has been a major factor in the overall improvement of the health of the Chinese. The Communist party machinery continued to operate throughout the nation and to convey messages from Peking to the periphery, but the implementation of policies was up to each local unit, mainly the communes. Certain bureaucratic tendencies evidently developed in the party framework, and these led to another crucial change of course in 1965.

THE GREAT PROLETARIAN CULTURAL REVOLUTION

Starting with university students in Peking, opposition arose against the Communist party bureaucracy. Calling themselves Red Guards, these angry young people rebelled against what they regarded as the special privileges of not only party officials, but virtually all persons in authority. Chairman Mao Tse-tung, who had his own disagreements with the hangovers of Soviet influence in the party bureaucracy, encouraged the rebellious youth. He told them to "storm the party headquarters" and remove the leaders who were said to be taking China along a capitalist path. The turbulent years from 1965 to 1970 (and perhaps later) became known as the Great Proletarian Cultural Revolution, though subsequent information revealed turmoil on more than a cultural level. Universities closed down, industrial production was massively disrupted, and the whole structure of government was decimated. Progress was apparently not disrupted in agriculture, however. This was the period when, to counteract elitism, urban professionals, intellectuals, and university students were required to periodically do agricultural and other manual labor.

The Cultural Revolution had enormous impact on the health services of China. In 1965, Mao openly condemned the Ministry of Public Health, regarding it presumably as still being influenced by Soviet policies. He is quoted as saying:

> The Ministry of Public Health only works for 15 percent of the population. It is not a people's ministry and should be called the "urban public health ministry." . . . We should keep in the cities those doctors who have been out of school a year or two and are lacking in ability. The remainder should be sent to the countryside.

In response to this attack, two major policy changes were launched around 1966: the training of vast numbers of peasants as rural "barefoot doctors" and the integration of Western and traditional medicine.

To understand the place of the now-renowned barefoot doctors, one must take note of the jurisdictional levels of Chinese Socialist society. As of about 1970, China had 22 provinces (plus certain autonomous regions and separate cities), averaging some 35 million people each. The provinces and regions are divided into counties, averaging 100 each, or about 2,200 in all; thus, a typical county would have a population of about 350,000. Rural counties (the vast majority) are composed of large agricultural communes with about 12 per county containing 10,000 to 50,000 people each. There are over 25,000 communes. The commune, while basically an economic entity for production, functions also as a unit of local government.

Even the commune has too large a population for efficient agricultural production in China, so it is further subdivided into "production brigades"; these have about 1,500 adults each. (In the cities, equivalent jurisdictions are called "lanes," or neighborhoods, and have about 2,000 adults.) For specific tasks, production brigades are composed of several "production teams," composed of between 50 and 300 adult workers. It is at the level of the production brigade that China's barefoot doctor is selected and serves. Most often the person chosen for this role is a young man or woman who continues to work part of the time in the fields and part-time in a small health post. He or she is paid by the brigade (not by the county or central government) on the basis of "work-points," in the same way that other brigade members are paid for farm labor.

Because of the decentralization of authority and the principle of local self-reliance, there are great variations in the schedules for training barefoot doctors. Most frequently, the training lasts three to six months and takes place at the commune health center or a county hospital. Instruction is highly practical and is based mainly, but not exclusively, on current scientific concepts. Part of the training, however, is based on traditional Chinese medicine, including the use of medicinal herbs and acupuncture. Major emphasis is put on preventive service, including immunizations and promotion of environmental sanitation. The use of drugs (including antibiotics) for treating common ailments is taught, as well as the dispensing of contraceptive pills. Female barefoot doctors are taught about preventive maternal and child health care, including hygienic handling of childbirths in the home. An important aspect of the training is continuing education, which must be taken for about one month every year. A patient whom the barefoot doctor does not feel capable of handling is supposed to be referred to the commune health center or a county hospital.

Barefoot doctors are taught not only by the staff of health centers and county hospitals, but also by specialists from provincial hospitals who are undertaking their rural service. So widespread had this program become, that in 1982 the WHO estimated that 1.5 million barefoot doctors, plus another 3 million health aides (who are given a little on-the-job training at the production brigade health post), had been trained.

The second principal health policy launched with the Cultural Revolution was the combination of traditional and modern medicine. Even with the enormously increased output of Western-type doctors in the first 15 years of People's China, the majority of the rural millions could not be reached. After Mao's criticism, therefore, the policy was changed from ignoring traditional practitioners, who were essentially in private practice everywhere, to bringing them into the official system. In 1960 there were an estimated 300,000 traditional doctors—far more than Western doctors. Soon after 1966, one or more traditional doctors was appointed to the staff of every health facility. The patient was given a choice of which type of doctor he wished to see, and sometimes he could see both. Furthermore, the policy was to encourage consultation between the two types of doctors.

The principles of traditional Chinese medicine were also taught in the curriculums of the approximately 110 regular medical schools. These and other health professional schools are linked to hospitals and come under the administrative authority of the Ministry of Health (rather than the Ministry of Education), as in other Socialist nations. Likewise, essentials of modern scientific medicine—particularly prevention of communicable diseases—are taught in the smaller number of schools devoted mainly to traditional medicine. Research institutes are attempting to test systematically the therapeutic value of various traditional medications, separating those found to be effective from the others.

1971 AND AFTER

The political factors that led the United States to modify its hostile attitude toward China in 1971 need not concern us here, but this action undoubtedly had great influence on China's relationship to the entire world. A few months after the Nixon visit to Peking and the Shanghai Communiqué, the People's Republic of China was welcomed into the United Nations, to replace Taiwan in occupying the seat of China in the General Assembly and the Security Council. In 1972, similar action was taken in the World Health Organization. After more than 20 years of isolation from the world community, several developments in Chinese health services had a sensational impact on worldwide concepts of health policy, of which a few warrant special mention. Some were conceptual, others highly practical.

Nothing was more impressive than the central principle on which China's health service (like so many other sectors) was built: serve the people. This meant many things, but in contrast to policies in most of the Western world, it meant that health care was not a commodity to be bought and sold in a market. It was to be provided to those who needed it. This did not, however, mean for the present that all health care was free of charge. China was still a very poor country and did not yet have the resources to provide complete health service to all. Small fees were charged, but no one was turned away for lack of money. More important, the fees paid never went to the individual provider, but only to the institution or organization running the service. Health care was not a matter for private profit.

In sharp contrast to most of Western medicine, the major emphasis in China was put on primary health care—not sophisticated services for the few, but basic and essential services for the many. To achieve this emphasis demanded a fresh, innovative approach. Preventive and ambulatory care were emphasized more than hospitals. Practice was put ahead of theory in the training of all health personnel, including physicians. During the Cultural Revolution, medical school education was reduced from six to only three years (although it was later changed back to six years).

The policy of local self-reliance and priority for the rural areas inevitably meant that there would be great differences in the level of health services developed in different areas of the country. If a commune suffered great adversity (for example, from drought or flooding), it might receive special assistance from the central government. Most communes have organized cooperative medical funds to which everyone contributes. Fees are paid from these funds to a hospital or health center to which a commune member is sent for care, but the amount of the fee will vary depending on the affluence of the commune.

The general population is mobilized for many disease-control campaigns, for example, elimination of the snail vectors of schistosomiasis, or other pests, such as mosquitoes, flies, and bedbugs. In addition to organized pest-control programs, each individual is encouraged to cooperate. Children, for example, are given small rewards for filling a container with swatted flies.

In 1976, the inspiring leader of the Liberation of China, Mao Tsetung, died. The people who came to power represented a faction of the Communist party that was oriented toward rapid industrial development. A movement was started to eliminate "ultraleftist" influences from the party by identifying a "gang of four" (including Mao's widow), who were accused of many disruptions in orderly work and restrictions on the freedom of the people. To increase incentives for higher productivity, a greater share of the earnings of each enterprise was permitted to be retained locally, raising the earnings of the workers. The importance attached to political education was reduced; intellectuals and professional personnel were no longer required to do manual work periodically. Admission to universities, including medical schools, was no longer based on the decision of community people, but rather on competitive examinations.

The strategy after 1976 was summarized as the "four modernizations"; these had been proposed by Chou En-lai in 1975, but the new leadership gave them greater prominence. The four modernization goals call for improvements in agriculture, industrial development, national defense, and science and technology. Regarding industry, greater attention was to be given to the production of consumer goods, to raise the standard of living of the people.

Nevertheless, the basic principles of China's health care system, formulated at the First National Health Conference in 1950, seem to be still applied. These principles are (1) serve the workers, peasants, and soldiers; (2) put prevention first; (3) unite traditional Chinese and Western medicine; and (4) integrate health work with mass movements. The various policy developments noted above may all be linked to one or another of these principles.

The first principle requires that health service be established as an entitlement of everyone. Hence, the private practice of medicine or other fields was eliminated. All the health personnel are employed in some social framework. Even though services must be paid for, the practitioner does not get fees. Identification of the great needs of peasants, of course, required the shift of priorities in the 1960s to the rural areas. Most observers are agreed that, even though the technical content of service may be modest, some sort of health care has been made available to the entire population.

Putting prevention first is seen in the services for which barefoot doctors (and their urban counterparts, "red medical workers") are trained. Immunizations, environmental sanitation, and the education of people about good hygiene are emphasized. Major priority also goes to family planning. Immediately after liberation, China was opposed to birth control as a capitalist approach to the solution of social problems. Then, when it became clear that rapid population growth was impeding economic development, the policy changed. Contraceptive pills were manufactured domestically, and they are widely dispensed. An ideal of two-child (and later one-child) families was widely promoted, and barefoot doctors are expected to monitor every family. If a third child is on the way, an abortion is encouraged and provided. In the 1980s the movement toward only one child to a family was even backed up by certain economic penalties for more than one.

The combination of traditional and Western medicine is seen throughout the health care system, in hospitals, health centers, medical schools, and so on. This policy was useful not only for making possible a vast expansion of health manpower, but also for the elimination of private practice. Including traditional doctors in the official system meant that they became subject to organizational controls. It also meant that they would learn about the use of clearly valuable Western measures, such as immunizations and antibiotics.

The integration of health work with mass movements is observable in the campaigns against the four pests (mosquitoes, flies, bedbugs, and rats). It is also reflected in the promulgation of methods for maintaining a sanitary environment. For centuries, China has used human excreta ("night soil") as a major agricultural fertilizer; today the policy in rural areas is to collect this waste in special tanks in which pathogenic organisms are destroyed. More broadly speaking, the system of health care is built into the economic structure of the whole society. Thus, the barefoot doctors in communes are employed and paid in the same way as agricultural workers, by work points. As noted earlier, industrial workers are insured for medical care costs through their enterprises; their dependents are insured for 50 percent of medical expenses. Government employees have similar health insurance protection.

Compared with the health care system of the USSR, China's is much more flexible and subject to local variations. In the cities, people may seek medical care at any facility they choose; they are not expected to use only the one in their local district. The training of barefoot doctors is not nationally standardized, but varies widely in different places. (Attempts to standardize their training arose in 1981.) Likewise, barefoot doctors are supervised in various ways by physicians in commune health centers, in county hospitals, or elsewhere. Since about 1980, the training of barefoot doctors has been prolonged and strengthened.

In the 1980s, as the new post-Mao leadership became consolidated, the four modernizations were pursued with mounting vigor. To increase production, industrial workers were given incentive pay for greater output. On the communes, families were permitted to cultivate agricultural plots of their own, selling the produce in a private market. Even the barefoot doctors in some communes were permitted to engage in a type of private practice, selling the drugs they dispensed and earning a profit. Incentives have accordingly been shifting from preventive to curative health services. Intensification of industrial development in the main cities has naturally magnified environmental pollution. Inevitably, changes in the dominant political ideology of China, as in other countries, affects health conditions and policies in the national health care system. Problems that may then be generated will doubtless stimulate further changes and reforms.

ACHIEVEMENTS IN HEALTH

In great contrast to preliberation conditions, the health of the Chinese people is enormously improved. In both the cities and rural areas the cleanliness is remarkable. Children everywhere appear to be well-nourished and happy. One does not see beggars or prostitutes in the streets, such as still prevail in India. Venereal disease has been virtually eliminated.

Smallpox, cholera, and plague have all disappeared. Tuberculosis has been reduced to one-fifth of its former prevalence. Malaria has been greatly reduced, although not yet eliminated. Schistosomiasis remains in only a few rural areas. The birthrate has been phenomenally lowered — to under ten per 1,000 in large cities. By all reports, opium addiction, which was extensive in old China, has been wiped out. China has not yet developed a reporting and statistical system to yield information on nationwide health status, but in large cities like Shanghai life expectancy is said to be 70 years. Infant mortality in Shanghai is reported to be as low as that in Sweden. The major causes of death are now cancer and heart disease, as they are in the United States. Nutritional status has been vastly improved.

The greatest overall achievement of China in the health sector has doubtless been to make primary health care accessible to the total population. In spite of the flexibility in their implementation, overall policies, such as the training and use of barefoot doctors or the combination of modern and traditional medicine, are followed throughout this very large nation. The mechanism for this implementation is the framework of the Communist party. With its headquarters in Peking, the party has an organized network in every province, county, and commune. Health care is subject to controls and surveillance, like everything else. As in other Socialist countries, even with very different fundamental socioeconomic structures, health service is appreciated as a basic requirement for general progress. Good health is regarded as a necessary condition for both work and happiness in the population.

REFERENCES

Horn, J. S., *Away with All Pests: An English Surgeon in People's China, 1954–1969* (New York: Monthly Review, 1971).

Lampton, D. M., *The Politics of Medicine in China* (Boulder, Col.: Westview Press, 1977).

Quinn, J. R., ed., *Medicine and Public Health in the People's Republic of China* (Washington, D.C.: Department of Health, Education, and Welfare, Fogarty International Center, 1972).

Sidel, R., and Sidel, V. W., *The Health of China* (Boston: Beacon Press, 1982).

Sidel, V. W., and Sidel, R., *Serve the People: Observations on Medicine in the People's Republic of China* (New York: Josiah Macy, Jr. Foundation, 1973).

Wegman, M. E.; Ki, T. Y.; and Purcell, E. G., *Public Health in the People's Republic of China* (New York: Josiah Macy, Jr. Foundation, 1973).

Part Five

General Health
Policy Issues

21

Organized Ambulatory Health Care— Its Origins and Worldwide Development

Throughout this book, references have been made to clinics, polyclinics, health centers, and other forms of organization of health services for the ambulatory or nonhospitalized patient. This chapter will trace the origins of these arrangements and review the current characteristics of ambulatory care organization throughout the world.

The rise of organized arrangements for providing ambulatory health care, compared to the social actions generating hospitals and community preventive services, is a relatively recent phenomenon. Just as the needs of the poor stimulated the founding of hospitals in the early Middle Ages, medical service to the poor stimulated the efforts to provide ambulatory care outside the premises of the individual physician or apothecary.

THE EARLY DISPENSARIES

Hospitals of a sort had provided bed care for wounded soldiers and sick slaves in ancient Rome, but the precursors of the modern hospital are usually considered to be the charitable institutions for the poor in European cities of the eleventh and twelfth centuries.[1] These early Christian hospitals saw their mission as succoring the impoverished

Based on excerpts from M.I. Roemer, *Ambulatory Health Services in America: Past, Present, and Future* (Rockville, Md.: Aspen Systems Corporation, 1981), 15–28, 410–19.

person who was seriously sick and needed shelter, a bed, food, and care. "Care" called for ministrations to the patient's soul as well as to his or her body. It was several centuries, however, before these hospitals considered it appropriate to give attention to outpatients (those not requiring bed care) as well as to inpatients.[2]

The earliest systematic effort to provide medical attention to the ambulatory sick poor has been attributed by René Sand, the Belgian scholar, to a French doctor, Théophraste Renaudot, who founded a free consultation service in Paris in 1630.[3] Renaudot was wealthy, and, not being with the Roman Catholic majority that controlled the hospitals, he established his service in a separate building that he either owned or rented. He assembled 20 doctors to give out-of-hospital consultation to the sick poor, either directly or by correspondence. As is so often true of social innovators, Renaudot was from an ethnic minority, the French Huguenots (Protestants), who were discriminated against because of their faith. Not surprisingly, therefore, his actions were opposed by the leading doctors of the day, including the faculty of medicine of the University of Paris.

Many poor people in Paris used this free consultation service, and it became increasingly popular, attracting donations from other philanthropists. (The doctors were not paid, but funds were nonetheless needed to purchase medications for the poor.) The opposition to Renaudot's service was ineffective; in fact, goaded by its success, the faculty of medicine organized its own ambulatory consultation service for the poor in the late 1630s.

The medical faculty service was offered two mornings a week, preceded by a Catholic mass. In 1641, the dispensing of drugs was added, hence the name dispensary. In 1644, with the death of many of the patrons of the original Renaudot dispensary, parliament ordered this pioneer unit closed. By then, however, the idea had become established, and it was adopted in other cities of France. In 1707, King Louis XIV (not renowned for his generosity to the poor) ordered that a free ambulatory care dispensary be established at every French medical school. The prestigious medical faculty physicians received no pay for this work; their earnings came from charges to their upper-class patients, who were usually treated at home. The ambulatory sick poor, moreover, served as useful teaching cases for medical students, just as they do today.

In England, a similar development occurred somewhat later. The sick poor would go directly to apothecaries for care, without benefit of medical advice, even as today the corner drugstore often serves as the poor person's doctor. Hospitals, as on the Continent, only treated poor in-patients needing bed care. In 1675, in the Royal College of Physicians of London, a plan was proposed to provide a free consultation service to the poor.[4] The college asked the Society of Apothecaries to cooperate by providing drugs at low prices that the poor could afford, but agreement could not be reached. In 1687, the Royal College of Physicians resolved that all members should give free advice to the poor within London and for seven miles around, but no provisions were made for drugs or for definite times and places for the service. It was not until 1696 that the college, in response to a plea from the Common Council of the City of London, decided to provide at its own expense (each doctor contributed £10 to start the scheme) a repository of drugs. These would be dispensed free to the poor at the headquarters of the college.

Opposition continued, however, not only from the apothecaries, but also from some physicians, who objected to losing any patronage, even that of the poor. In 1725, therefore, the college dispensary was closed. It was not until 1770 that the dispensary idea once more gained support. After 1775, dispensaries grew rapidly in London and the English countryside. They were still separate from hospitals. Each dispensary had a board of governors composed of wealthy persons who financed the charity. For entitlement to care, poor patients were often expected to produce an introductory letter from one of the governors. By the late eighteenth century, however, doctors were busier with private patients, and it became necessary to pay them salaries (£50 per year in 1783, and £100 in 1786) to attract them to dispensary work. After 1800, many of the London dispensaries offered smallpox vaccinations to supplement ambulatory services.

The idea of the dispensary as a freestanding place for treatment of the ambulatory poor spread to the New World soon after the American Revolution. The first dispensary was established in 1786 in Philadelphia, the same city where the first U.S. hospital had been founded in 1751.[5] The two institutions, however, were not related. A dispensary was set up in New York City in 1791, in Boston in 1796, and in Baltimore in 1800.

Dispensaries grew slowly at first, with no additional ones until 1816, when managers of the Philadelphia dispensary set up two satellite units as the city spread north and south. Between 1827 and 1852, four new dispensaries were set up in New York. By 1874, there were 29 dispensaries in New York, and by 1877 there were 33 in Philadelphia. Dispensary use also increased; records in New York show a total of 134,000 patients served in 1860, and the number rose to 876,000 by 1900.

These early U.S. dispensaries had certain features in common. All of them were intended to serve the urban poor who did not require inpatient hospital care. All had a central building, with the exception of the Boston dispensary, which had none until the 1850s. There was usually one full-time person in charge, an apothecary or a physician, who performed minor surgery, gave smallpox vaccinations, extracted teeth, and prescribed medications. By the middle of the nineteenth century, the larger dispensaries had both a physician and a pharmacist. Young physicians were appointed to visit sick patients at home. Such "district visiting" was, in fact, the principal function of the Philadelphia dispensary when it was started in 1786, and it remained the sole activity of the famous Boston dispensary until 1856. After they were well established, the dispensaries appointed community practitioners as attending staff for certain scheduled times.

Financial support of the early dispensaries was meager. They were dependent mainly on private donations, which were principally used for the purchase of drugs. Physicians ordinarily volunteered their services. The dispensaries in New York were an exception; they received subsidies from the city and state governments. The Boston and the Philadelphia dispensaries gradually accumulated some endowment funds. Often, earnings would be derived by renting space in the dispensary building to commercial tenants.

Throughout the nineteenth century, first in Europe and later in the United States, health care movements of three other types became increasingly prominent. First, hospitals gradually became recognized as facilities for safe and scientific medical care for everyone, rather than as places of refuge for the poor; in the larger cities they added departments for out patients. Second, public health agencies expanded, especially with the rise of bacteriology after the 1870s, and clinics were developed for preventive surveillance of babies, for tuberculosis control, and for other preventive purposes. Third, physicians were trained in much greater numbers than before, and private medical practice spread everywhere.

All three of these movements gained momentum after the turn of the twentieth century, gradually taking over the functions of the dispensaries. After World War I, hospitals, public health agencies, and private medical practice continued to flourish, but the idea of the dispensary as a place for general ambulatory care of the poor did not die completely. The dispensary was replaced by another type of facility, linked mainly to local government and the public health movement— the health center.

THE RISE OF HEALTH CENTERS

Several social currents contributed to the development of the health center. The first official formulation of the concept was in Great

Britain in 1920. In that year, the Consultative Council on Medical and Allied Services, set up as a link between the Ministry of Health and the private medical profession, issued its historic *Interim Report on Future Provision of Medical and Allied Services.*[6] This called for provision of primary health care by teams of physicians and allied personnel based in primary health centers. It proposed that a network of such facilities should cover the entire nation and serve the whole population, not just the poor. In the language of this report (better known as the Dawson Report, from the name of the council's chairman), the health center would be "an institution equipped for services of curative and preventive medicine to be conducted by the general practitioners of that district, in conjunction with an efficient nursing service and with the aid of visiting consultants and specialists." The physicians would remain in private practice, but the close association with government nurses and other allied personnel would presumably strengthen the quality and effectiveness of their services.

As Vicente Navarro has pointed out, the council was established in response to the demands of the British Labour party for a "new social order."[7] This was just after the success of the Bolshevik Revolution in Russia, and a State Medical Services Association, on behalf of the Labour party, was demanding that all health facilities be nationalized and all medical personnel become salaried civil servants. The recommendations of the Dawson Report were a relatively moderate response to these demands. (The State Medical Services Association later became the Socialist Medical Association, which still exists in Great Britain.)

Nevertheless, even these relatively moderate proposals were too radical for implementation by the government in the face of opposition from private physicians and the declining militancy of the Labour party. It was not until the Labour proposals after World War II, which resulted in the national health service in 1948, that the issue of health centers as the customary locale for primary care was revived. Once again, the government, even though under Labour party control, did not press the idea too vigorously. Viscount Dawson of Penn himself, writing in 1942, stated that a trend:

> . . . more and more apparent during the last 25 years, is the need for greater institutional provision. The increase of knowledge, and with that the development of teamwork, has made this inevitable. The doctor works best where equipment and ancillary services are available, and side by side with his fellows. Further, such institutional provision is economical of both time and cost and makes a health service available for all citizens. In short, the tendency is for the centre of gravity of practice to shift away from the [patient's] home to organized surgeries, clinics,

health centres, and hospitals, and these would . . . constitute a coordinated scheme of service. . . .[8]

Finally, in the 1960s the health center idea took on new life in Great Britain; hundreds were built throughout England and Scotland, and GPs located their surgeries in them, side by side with government visiting nurses, social workers, technicians, and other allied personnel.[9] Concepts of regionalized hierarchies of primary, secondary, and tertiary services, also proposed in the Dawson Report, were embodied in the national health service.

While it took more than 40 years for the health center idea to be implemented in Great Britain, a modified version of it was introduced in 1926 in Ceylon (now Sri Lanka), a British colony at the time.[10] The crucial modification, however, was the major focus on preventive services. Patients needing treatment were referred to a hospital outpatient department. This idea of health centers as facilities limited to preventive services, though a broad range of them, was promoted in the developing countries by the Rockefeller Foundation in the 1930s and 1940s. There were valid reasons for this stress on prevention in a period when the treatment of diseases that were preventable absorbed most of the efforts of developing countries. By the 1950s, however, the value of combining prevention with primary treatment of the sick became recognized almost everywhere.[11]

In 1920, the year of the Dawson Report, the New York State Commissioner of Health, Herman Biggs, proposed a network of health centers to serve the rural population (not solely the poor) with both preventive and curative services. While the emphasis was to be on health promotion and prevention, the Biggs ambulatory care facilities were to be comprehensive in scope.[12] In the atmosphere of post-World War I conservatism, the idea was vigorously opposed by the private medical profession and was not implemented. A similar proposal, restricted to serving the poor, was made in 1919 by the health officer of Los Angeles County, J. L. Pomeroy. It, too, failed to be implemented.[13] In place of the comprehensive primary care facilities originally advocated by Pomeroy, district health centers were developed for basic preventive services. Patients needing medical treatment were referred to private physicians.

If one thinks of health centers as ambulatory care facilities limited to the provision of a full range of preventive services, their origins in the United States can be traced to an earlier period. Such facilities were offshoots, in a sense, of settlement houses for the poor, which originated in large city slum districts in the 1890s.[14] These facilities attempted to bring together various educational, social work, and recreational services that would be helpful to largely immigrant, low-income families. Around 1910, a movement developed to integrate various organized ambulatory health services—for child health, tuberculosis, immunization, feeding the poor—that had begun to spring up under both public and private auspices. Even limiting health center functions to purely preventive services, which were not competitive with private medical practice, did not shield these early U.S. health centers from attack by conservatives.

By the Great Depression of the 1930s, the concept of the health center as a locale for coordinating numerous different public and private agencies in an area had begun to wane. Agencies depending on charitable donations lost their philanthropic patrons. The medical profession, hit hard by the loss of many of its private paying patients, became increasingly suspicious of any organized community facility that might openly or covertly become competitive. The immigrant population, which had provided a natural neighborhood grouping for the charitable services of multiple agencies, was no longer so geographically concentrated.

As a result, like the dispensary movement in an earlier period, the health center movement lost its missionary zeal. Structures known as health centers continued to be built in the United States, but they became essentially facilities for housing official public health agencies, that is, branches of the health department in large metropolitan cities or the central headquarters of health departments in rural counties.[15] Except for venereal disease and tuberculosis clinics, which provided treatment to prevent contagion, any vestige of medical care, even for the poor, was eliminated. Treatment was appropriate only in the outpatient department of hospitals, where an admission clerk or social worker had to make certain of the patient's indigence; for those who could afford to pay, a private physician was the only resource.

This strictly preventive and public health agency definition of the health center prevailed well into the 1960s. Not until the riots of ethnic minorities in large city slums during the mid-1960s was the comprehensive (preventive and curative) neighborhood health center revived. With the rediscovery of poverty in the midst of urban affluence, the organized provision of general ambulatory health care again became an accepted concept in America.[16]

HEALTH CENTERS TODAY

Internationally, the idea of the health center as a facility for providing comprehensive ambulatory health services has had much greater vitality since the 1920s. It has been implemented to some extent in virtually every nation.

In the Socialist countries, now constituting about one-third of the world's population, organized health centers have become almost the exclusive mode for delivery of ambulatory care, integrating personal preventive and treatment services. In virtually all the developing countries of Asia, Africa, and Latin America, health centers have also become the dominant means of providing modern ambulatory health services, not only by ministries of health but also by social security and other agencies serving various segments of the population. In the industrialized and capitalist countries of Western Europe and elsewhere (for example, Japan and Australia), health centers, while not yet predominant, have been rapidly increasing in importance.[17] The major highlights of the delivery of ambulatory health care in these three broad groups of countries are of interest. (There are numerous variations within each grouping.)

Health Centers in Socialist Countries

Soon after the Russian Revolution of 1917, the ruling political party declared that health service should be a government responsibility, freely accessible to all without charge.[18] This would be done by greatly expanding the training of doctors and allied health workers, all of whom would be engaged as civil servants. Prevention and treatment would be integrated, with emphasis on prevention. Ambulatory services would be provided by teams of salaried doctors, nurses, and other personnel working at health centers, often called polyclinics, conveniently located throughout cities and rural areas.

This ideal plan was not implemented overnight. The years following World War I and the revolution were turbulent, and the first five-year plan—the subsequent hallmark of Socialist economic and social development—did not get under way until 1928. The major efforts of the early years were directed toward a massive increase in the output of medical personnel, construction of health centers and hospitals, a buildup of the chemical industry (to produce drugs, among other products), and establishment of a governmental framework for administration of the whole system.[19]

The pattern of ambulatory care delivery that emerged varies between cities and rural areas and is by no means identical everywhere in the USSR. Its essential features, however, are as follows:[20] for each local area of 10,000 to 50,000 people (varying with population density) there is an ambulatory care center. The basic team for primary care consists of an internist or general practitioner, a pediatrician, an obstetrician-gynecologist, a dentist, nurses, and numerous allied personnel. Because this primary care team is composed of several specialists working together, the facility is often called a polyclinic, rather than a health center. Each primary care team serves a population of about 4,000 persons in the adjacent area; thus, a polyclinic serving a district with 40,000 persons would have ten teams. Backing up these primary care teams are secondary care specialists, such as ophthalmologists, neurologists, and orthopedic surgeons, at hospitals or, in metropolitan areas, at specialized polyclinics. Patients are referred to these secondary facilities as necessary; however, simple laboratory tests or procedures can be performed at the primary care unit.

No charges are levied for any service at the polyclinic or hospital. For certain prescribed drugs, which may be bought in governmental pharmacies, there are small charges, but these are waived for pensioners, military veterans, persons with serious chronic disorders, and so on. Larger factories and mines also have polyclinics, which may be used by the workers in addition to their neighborhood polyclinic. Persons with chronic diseases or at special risk of disease for any reason are summoned back for periodic examinations and care, a process known as dispensarization. Much attention is given to health education, immunizations, and environmental hygiene. Every new medical graduate must spend three years at a rural post, after which he or she (most Soviet physicians are women) is free to go wherever there is a position open. Private practice has never been prohibited in the USSR, and a little of it exists; but the number of patients willing to pay private fees when extensive services are available free is very small.

The essential framework of the Soviet health care system was emulated in the other countries of Eastern Europe, which became Socialist after World War II.[21] These vary in accordance with certain national traditions. In Poland, for example, where a very strong tradition of independence characterized the peasantry, the rural people were not fully covered by the national system until 1972, some 25 years after the birth of the Polish People's Republic.[22] In Czechoslovakia, the medical schools have remained within the universities and under the general supervision of the Ministry of Education, although in the Soviet Union the schools of medicine, as well as all other programs for training health personnel, are integrated with the health services under the Ministry of Health.

The People's Republic of China, established in 1949, emulated the Soviet model for its first dozen years or so; then in 1962 China departed sharply from the Soviet-led group of nations. Its health care system moved away from a centralized hierarchical framework and put its major stress on local self-reliance.[23] Ambulatory care remained organized, but most local units were much smaller. The vast rural population was organized into communes for collective agricultural production; these had from 10,000 to 50,000 people. In most communes, there is a health center for ambulatory care that also has a few beds; the staff includes at least one modern physician. The basic primary care unit, however, is the health post, which is located in a production brigade of about 1,500 adults. The health post is staffed mainly by the barefoot doctor, a peasant who has been trained for only a few months to give preventive services (including family planning) and to treat common ailments. Difficult cases are referred to the commune health center or to a county hospital (several communes compose a county).

In the health centers, in addition to one modern physician, there are usually doctors of traditional Chinese medicine, nursing assistants, sanitarians, and others. One of the important ways in which China differs from the USSR is in its effort to integrate the delivery of traditional and Western medicine. Another difference is that, at the most local level, health care is not a responsibility of the Ministry of Health, but rather of the commune.[24] Thus, the cost of operating the barefoot doctor's clinic is borne by the commune (out of its earnings from the sale of agricultural products), and small fees are also payable by the local people who come for care.

Still another model has been implemented in Cuba, which underwent its political and economic transformation to socialism after 1959. In spite of its predominantly rural and agricultural character, the Cuban health care system was modeled not on China's system, but on that of the Soviet Union. Thus, there is a definite hierarchical framework, starting at the level of the local health area of 25,000 to 35,000 people served by a polyclinic.[25] For several years the next level was the health region, of which there were 39, but in the early 1970s this was changed to a smaller unit, the municipality. Above the 169 municipalities, there are 14 health provinces; these, in turn, are directed by the Ministry of Health in Havana. Cuba has been able to train relatively large numbers of doctors to staff its polyclinics and hospitals, along essentially the same lines as the USSR. No charges are made for polyclinic or hospital services.

Health Centers in Developing Countries

The many developing countries are much more varied than the world's Socialist countries, but they have in common a relatively small degree of industrialization, economic dependence on agriculture or natural extractive production (mining or petroleum), and the poverty and low level of literacy of their populations. One can distinguish the most severely underdeveloped countries of sub-Saharan Africa and parts of Asia, where the per capita GNP is typically under $400 (U.S.) per year, from the more transitional developing countries of Latin America and the Middle East, with per capita GNPs of $400 to about $3,000 per year.[26]

In both these types of less developed countries (LDCs), the organized health center and the more peripheral health posts, or health stations, play a substantial role in the delivery of ambulatory health care. In the more severely underdeveloped countries of Africa and Asia, collective economic support of health services is weak, so most of the money spent for health purposes comes from private households. Thus in Ghana, a former British (Gold Coast) colony of western Africa, the World Bank estimates 4 percent of GNP to be devoted to health purposes; of this, however, 73 percent is derived from personal household expenditures and only 27 percent from all government sources.[27] In Thailand, with a per capita GNP of $420, the relationships are similar; this monarchy in Southeast Asia, never a colony, spent in 1977 about 4.16 percent of its GNP on health. Of this amount, however, 65 percent came from private household expenditures, 33 percent from the government, and only the trifling remainder from voluntary agencies or foreign aid.[28] These large private sector proportions, illustrated by countries such as Ghana and Thailand, reflect not only the substantial expenditures of the small upper class for private medical care, but also the numerous small expenditures of the masses of poor people on self-medication, traditional healers, and even care by private doctors.

Insofar as the governments of these poorest LDCs provide modern ambulatory health services, it is through various clinics—rural and urban health centers and rural health posts. The staffs of these ambulatory care centers are principally made up of middle-level health personnel—health officers, medical assistants, village health workers, and other auxiliaries. The handful of trained physicians located outside the main cities is either in government hospitals or in private practice. Government health facilities for both ambulatory and inpatient care may even require small fees from all but the most destitute patients. The planning of all these countries calls for gradual extension of national population coverage with a regionalized network of health centers—very simple at the rural periphery, with increasingly specialized and better trained staff as one moves toward the larger towns and provincial capitals. The model laid out in India in 1946 (in the Bhore Commission Report) and again in 1962 (in the Mudaliar Report) is being adopted, at least in theory, in most of these LDCs.[29] In practice, of course, plans often remain only partially fulfilled.

The more transitional LDCs might be illustrated by Lebanon and Egypt in the Middle East or by Mexico and Peru in Latin America. In all these countries, while a substantial private sector persists, major steps have been taken by government to extend ambulatory health services by means of a network of organized health centers throughout the country. Thus, in Lebanon, with a GNP of $1,070 in 1978, there are scores of primary care centers (health centers and dispensaries) offering general preventive and treatment services to the rural population.[30] In addition, in the main cities, where a certain amount of industry has developed, a small program of medical care under social security financing has been started for industrial workers and government employees. Social security funds are not used to pay private medical fees, however, but to support special clinics staffed with salaried doctors and serving insured persons.

In Latin American countries, the patterns of organized ambulatory care are similar, although somewhat more highly developed. Thus, in Mexico (with a per capita GNP of $1,120), the Ministry of Health and Social Assistance operates hundreds of health centers, staffed with both doctors and auxiliary personnel, to serve the rural population.[31] The Mexican Institute of Social Security, which started in 1942 in the national capital, has gradually extended its coverage through an impressive network of health centers and hospitals staffed with salaried doctors and allied personnel. In addition, there are similar organized health care facilities for government employees, petroleum workers, and railroad workers. Altogether, about one-half of the Mexican population was eligible in 1980 for the relatively well-developed health services of the overall social security system.[32]

It is noteworthy that these somewhat more prosperous LDCs of Latin America and the Middle East, in launching social insurance programs for the segments of their populations with regular wages or salaries (typically a minority), have not emulated the European pattern of simply reimbursing private practitioners. The market for private practice earnings has been so small and the social insurance device has been so effective in raising funds that many physicians are pleased to accept employment (usually two to four hours per day) in organized facilities for both ambulatory and hospital care. This pattern has been adopted throughout these developing countries because it is more economical and because it is more amenable to planning and regulation than is the pattern of private medical practice.[33]

In a word, the health problems of the developing countries have been stimulating efforts to provide health services along organized lines. The burden of preventable infectious disease, as well as all types of disease and injury for which effective treatment is known but not applied, is still enormous.[34] But through international health activities, biomedical and organizational knowledge is being rapidly spread to all countries. The faulty strategies of the era of imperialism, when European technologies were mechanically transplanted to the colonies without regard to the real needs of their populations, are being replaced by far more democratic and objective concepts of technology transfer. Scientific knowledge is being transmitted, but with the recognition that its mode of application must be determined by the people of each country.[35] Accordingly, it is not surprising that ambulatory health services of all types in the developing countries are becoming increasingly organized, both in their economic support and in their pattern of delivery.[36]

Health Centers in Industrialized Countries

The variability in social structure, including the health services, is probably greatest among the 30 or 40 predominantly industrialized and capitalist countries of the world. Health care systems range from the very individualistic and entrepreneurial, represented by the United States and perhaps Australia and South Africa, to the very socially oriented, represented by countries such as Sweden and Great Britain. In between are the many other welfare states of Western Europe, Canada, Japan, New Zealand, and perhaps Israel.

In almost all of these countries, there are systems of national health care financing that make medical services economically accessible to virtually the entire national populations.[37] The exceptions are the three most individualistic countries: South Africa, Australia, and the United States. In these countries, voluntary health insurance is still the major mechanism for financing medical care for the self-supporting population, while various programs financed through general revenues provide care (with limitations) for the poor. Associated with the national health care financing systems has been a gradual extension of organized clinics to furnish ambulatory services more economically and effectively.

In France, where national health insurance is the financing mechanism and where medical individualism is quite strong, there has nevertheless been a growth of health centers, in which physicians work on salaries. Preventive services are provided at these facilities through financial support from local government, and treatment commands fees from the social insurance program.[38] In Belgium, health centers restrict their functions to prevention (mainly maternal and child health services), but many local health insurance societies have organized polyclinics with an array of specialists working together.[39] These specialists are paid fees by the health insurance program; however, unlike specialists in purely private practice, they cannot demand supplementary personal payments from the patients.

Group medical practice of private physicians has also been growing slowly in Western Europe. Unlike the U.S. pattern, however, most European medical groups consist entirely of GPs, among whom there is some specialization, such as in disorders of children, gynecological problems, or skin diseases.[40] In West Germany, these are designated as communal practices, and about 300 of them were estimated to be functioning in 1970. In Canada, group practice has been growing perhaps more rapidly than it has in the United States, mainly along multispecialty lines. More than one-third of Canadian medical groups, however, consist only of GPs.[41]

Of particular interest in Canada has been the national policy, promoted also by many of the provincial governments, of encouraging the establishment of community health centers. These Canadian health centers are intended to serve anyone who chooses to come to them, not solely the poor. The objective is to bring together GPs and some specialists, along with nurses and other personnel, to provide fairly comprehensive ambulatory care. Local groups of citizens are encouraged to take the lead in organizing these units. The costs of physicians' care would be met by the national insurance program.[42] These facilities have been organized with special enthusiasm in the province of Quebec, where certain citizen groups have looked upon the projects as a rallying point for general political activity.

In Sweden, voluntary health insurance operated by local societies had existed since the nineteenth century. In 1931 it was made mandatory for certain occupational groups, and in 1962 population coverage became universal. Hospitalization for the total population, however, was long financed mainly from general revenues, with only small charges to the insurance funds. In the overall Swedish health care system, hospital service traditionally got the greatest emphasis and absorbed the lion's share of expenditures. In reaction to this, government policy changed in the 1960s to encourage development of health centers for ambulatory medical care; these would function as satellites of the hospitals and would be staffed mainly by GPs with ancillary staff.[43] Because of the strength of Swedish local governments, which must take the initiative for health center construction, progress has been relatively slow. But the planning calls for eventual coverage of the entire country with health centers instead of private medical offices.

In New Zealand, where universal health insurance has been in effect since 1939, there has also been a rising tide of interest in health centers as a setting for improved general medical practice. There has long been a sharp distinction in this country between specialists, who are salaried and hospital-based, and GPs, who have typically practiced from private, individual quarters in the community. In order to strengthen their position, the GPs have actually favored the establishment of health centers in which they could rent space and be assisted by nurses, social workers, and others.[44] Accordingly, the New Zealand Regional Hospital Boards have been authorized to construct these facilities entirely for primary ambulatory care.

Among the industrialized welfare states, perhaps the most significant trend toward widespread use of health centers for primary care of the general population has been in Great Britain. Unlike nearly all the other non-Socialist national health care systems, the British national health service is financed mainly from general revenues, rather than from social insurance collections. The original planning of the NHS called for a network of local ambulatory care facilities along the lines of the 1920 Dawson Report; in the political debate that ushered in the NHS in 1948, however, this feature was dropped.[45] British GPs had opposed health centers as the setting for their practices for fear that they would lead eventually to employment by the government and loss of independence. In the 1960s, however, attitudes changed. To ease the pressures on their professional lives, GPs gradually joined together in small partnerships of two, three, or four. By 1966, it was estimated that only 25 percent of them remained in completely solo practice.[46]

In the 1950s, after the wartime destruction, the British government began building new towns to reduce the congestion in London and other larger cities. These freshly planned communities included health centers, usually providing space for a few GPs, district nurses, social workers, laboratory technicians, and clerks. There was no lack of applications for these new rental quarters; the physicians occupying them remained in private practice, with their capitation lists, as before. By 1968, there were 93 such health centers operated by local and public authorities.[47] By 1971, some 475 health centers were in operation or under construction in Britain, with quarters to accommodate 2,600 practitioners.[48] These facilities housed from one to 22 doctors each, with an average of 5.5.

Thus, in all three major types of countries in the world, one can see movement toward increased organization of the delivery of ambulatory health services. The objective everywhere is to provide a comprehensive range of health care skills that isolated medical practitioners cannot offer. Through teams of personnel of various types, it is expected that services of better quality can be provided in an efficient manner.

It is important to recognize that, almost everywhere, organized ambulatory care centers are intended to serve the entire surrounding population, not exclusively the poor or other selected groups. Even when, as in Latin America, some health centers are limited to insured persons, other such facilities ordinarily serve the noninsured population. This broad scope of eligibility is associated with the basic coverage of populations by systems of national health insurance or other forms of economic support giving universal entitlement to health care. In many impoverished developing countries, where governmental financial support is weak, charges may be collected for health center service from those who can afford to pay. Patients are not turned away on the ground of being too affluent. This connection between systems of financing and patterns of delivering health service is fundamental.

NOTES

1. H. E. Sigerist, "An Outline on the Development of the Hospital," *Bulletin of the Institute of the History of Medicine* 4 (1936):573–81.
2. M. Risley, *House of Healing* (Garden City, N. Y.: Doubleday & Co., 1961).
3. R. Sand, *The Advance to Social Medicine* (London: Staples Press, 1952), 80–82.
4. W. Hartston, "Medical Dispensaries in Eighteenth Century London," *Proceedings of the Royal Society of London* 56 (1963):753–58.
5. C. E. Rosenberg, "Social Class and Medical Care in Nineteenth Century America: The Rise and Fall of the Dispensary," *Journal of the History of Medicine and Allied Sciences* 29 (1974):32–54.
6. England and Wales, Ministry of Health, Consultative Council on Medical and Allied Services, *Interim Report on the Future of Medical and Allied Services* (London: H. M. Stationery Office, 1920).
7. V. Navarro, *Class Struggle, the State, and Medicine: An Historical and Contemporary Analysis of the Medical Sector in Great Britain* (New York: Prodist, 1978), 14–24.
8. Viscount B.Dawson of Penn, "Medicine and the Public Welfare," *Medical Care 2* (1942):322–36.
9. M. Curwen, and B. Brookes, "Health Centres: Facts and Figures," *Lancet 2* (1969):945–48.
10. S. F. Chellappah, and W. P. Jacocks, *A Guide to Health Unit Procedure in Ceylon*, 2nd ed. (Colombo: Ceylon Government Printing Office, 1949).
11. M. I. Roemer, *Evaluation of Community Health Centres*, public health paper no. 48 (Geneva: World Health Organization, 1972), 12–20.
12. M. Terris, "Herman Biggs' Contribution to the Modern Concept of Health Centers," *Bulletin of the Institute of the History of Medicine 20* (1946):387–412.

13. J. L. Pomeroy, "Health Center Development in Los Angeles County," *Journal of the American Medical Association 93* (1929):1546–50.
14. J. Addams et al., *Philanthropy and Social Progress: Seven Essays* (New York: Crowell, 1893).
15. H. E. Handley, *Health Center Buildings* (New York: Commonwealth Fund, 1948).
16. L. Bamberger, "Health Care and Poverty: What Are the Dimensions of the Problem from the Community Point of View?" *Bulletin of the New York Academy of Medicine 42* (1966):1140.
17. M. I. Roemer, "Organized Ambulatory Health Service in International Perspective," *International Journal of Health Services 1* (1971):18–27.
18. H. E. Sigerist, *Socialized Medicine in the Soviet Union* (New York: Norton & Co., 1937).
19. M. G. Field, *Soviet Socialized Medicine: An Introduction* (New York: The Free Press, 1967).
20. I. P. Lidor, A. M. Stochik, and G. F. Tserkorny, *Soviet Public Health and the Organization of Primary Health Care for the Population of the USSR* (Moscow: Mir Publishers, 1978).
21. E. R. Weinerman, *Social Medicine in Eastern Europe* (Cambridge, Mass.: Harvard University Press, 1969).
22. M. I. Roemer, and R. Roemer, *Health Manpower in the Socialist Health Care System of Poland*, DHEW publication HRA 77–85 (Washington, D.C.: Health Resources Administration, 1977), 4.
23. V. W. Sidel, and R. Sidel, *Serve the People—Observations on Medicine in the People's Republic of China* (New York: Josiah Macy, Jr. Foundation, 1973).
24. J. R. Quinn, ed., *Medicine and Public Health in the People's Republic of China* (Washington, D.C.: Department of Health, Education, and Welfare, Fogarty International Center, 1972).
25. M. I. Roemer, "Health Development and Political Policy: The Lesson of Cuba," *Journal of Health Politics, Policy, and Law 4* (1980):570–80.
26. World Bank, *Health: Sector Policy Paper* (Washington, D.C., 1980), 67–70.
27. Ibid., 85.
28. M. I. Roemer, *The Health Care System of Thailand* (New Delhi: World Health Organization, South-East Asia Regional Office, 1981).
29. Government of India, Health Survey and Development Committee, *Report*, 4 vols, (New Delhi, 1946). Also H. S. Takulia et al., *The Health Center Doctor in India* (Baltimore: Johns Hopkins Press, 1967).
30. Department of Health, Education and Welfare, Office of International Health, *Syncrisis: The Dynamics of Health—Lebanon* (Washington, D.C., 1978).
31. M. I. Roemer, *Medical Care in Latin America* (Washington, D.C.: Pan American Union, 1964), 125–68.
32. A. Lopez-Bermudez, national public health consultant, personal communication, Mexico City, July 1980.
33. M. I. Roemer, *The Organization of Medical Care under Social Security: A Study Based on the Experience of Eight Countries* (Geneva: International Labour Office, 1969), 181–226.

34. J. Bryant, *Health and the Developing World* (Ithaca, N.Y.: Cornell University Press, 1969).
35. P. E. Basch, *International Health* (New York: Oxford University Press, 1978).
36. M. I. Roemer, *Comparative National Policies on Health Care* (New York: Marcel Dekker Co., 1977).
37. Social Security Administration, *Social Security Programs Throughout the World, 1979*, SSA publication 78–11805 (Washington, D.C., 1980).
38. M. I. Roemer, *Evaluation of Community Health Centres*, public health paper no. 48 (Geneva: World Health Organization, 1972), 18–19.
39. R. Roemer, and M. I. Roemer, *Health Manpower Policies in the Belgian Health Care System*, DHEW Publication HRA 77–38 (Washington, D.C.: Health Resources Administration, 1977).
40. Canadian Association of Medical Clinics and Medical Group Management Association of Canada, *New Horizons in Health Care: Proceedings, First International Congress of Group Medicine* (Winnipeg, Manitoba: Wallingford Press, 1970).
41. R. Roemer, and M. I. Roemer, *Health Manpower Policy under National Health Insurance—The Canadian Experience*, DHEW Publication HRA 77–37 (Washington, D.C.: Health Resources Administration, 1977).
42. Conference of Health Ministers, Community Health Centre Project, *The Community Health Centre in Canada*, 3 vols. (Ottawa: Information Canada, 1972). Canadian Department of National Health and Welfare, Directorate of Community Health, *Community Health Centres in Canada* (Ottawa, 1974).
43. S. A. Lindgren, "Sweden," in *Health Service Prospects: An International Survey*, I. Douglas-Wilson and G. McLachlan, eds. (London: The Lancet and The Nuffield Provincial Hospitals Trust, 1973), 99–123.
44. C. W. Dixon, "New Zealand," in J. Z. Bowers and E. Purcell, eds., *National Health Services: Their Impact on Medical Education and Their Role in Prevention* (New York: Josiah Macy, Jr. Foundation, 1973), 81–91.
45. A. Lindsey, *Socialized Medicine in England and Wales: The National Health Service 1948–1961* (Chapel Hill: University of North Carolina Press, 1962).
46. Medical Practitioners Union, *Design for Family Doctoring* (London: Medical World, 1967).
47. M. Curwen and B. Brookes, "Health Centres: Facts and Figures," *Lancet* 2 (1969): 945–48.
48. G. Forsyth, "United Kingdom," in *Health Service Prospects*, 1–35.

22

Regionalized Health Services in Seven Countries

In almost all countries, the distribution of populations in rural areas and cities has created problems for the delivery of appropriate medical services. Many countries have tried to overcome these problems by developing their hospitals and other health facilities into regionalized networks. This chapter describes the varied regionalization strategies in seven countries of different types.

In the interests of both quality and economy in health care delivery, most countries of the world are attempting to apply the concept of regionalization. The goal of quality would be reached through assurance that every person receives care appropriate to his needs, wherever he may live. Economy would be achieved through use of resources no more elaborate or expensive than are required by each patient's condition.

THE CONCEPT OF REGIONALIZATION

One must refer to countries *attempting* to apply the concept of regionalization, because the concept is an ideal that no country has yet fully attained. Regionalization attempts to adjust to the steadily ad-

Reprinted, with permission, from *Hospitals*, published by the American Hospital Association, copyright December 16, 1979, Vol. 53, No. 24, 72-82.

vancing technology of medical science, on the one hand, and the irregular settlement of populations, on the other.[1]

Medical technology has become increasingly complex. It is applied through some 50 specialties and subspecialties of medicine and scores of ancillary personnel associated with vast arrays of elaborate equipment. It would be extravagant and unnecessary for every hospital to offer this full range of technology. It is much more reasonable to staff and equip hospitals and other health facilities on the basis of the kinds of services they are expected to provide. Likewise, populations are unevenly distributed in all countries. Hospitals are naturally established in cities, but millions of people live in rural areas. Between the patient and the medical care he may need are various constraints of transportation, costs, and the patterns of practice of various doctors.

The solution proposed for coping with these problems almost everywhere has been the establishment of health facilities in regionalized networks. Thus, throughout a region of perhaps 1 or 2 million persons, there would be several small general hospitals (50 to 100 beds) close to where many people live and capable of handling common conditions—minor injuries, simple infections, normal childbirths, and so on. At the next level would be a smaller number of intermediate hospitals (100 to 300 beds), capable of providing proper service to more difficult cases—serious infections, major abdominal surgery, severe injuries, and so on. At the center of the region, usually in the main city, would be a large medical center (500 to 1,000 beds), sometimes associated with a medical school or research institute. Here would be available the full range of specialties and subspecialties—for brain or cardiac surgery, complex cancer cases, and so on. Some beds in the regional and intermediate hospitals would be reserved for treating local patients.

Movement in this pyramidal structure of hospitals would occur in two directions: (1) transporting certain patients from peripheral to central facilities, and (2) arranging for certain consultant services to pass from the central or intermediate levels to the periphery. Moreover, as a patient in a central facility recovers from the critical phase of his condition, he may be sent back for convalescence to the peripheral facility nearer his home. Regionalization has two main logistical aspects: (1) the building and staffing of hospitals and (2) their subsequent operation. For full realization of the concept, both aspects must be implemented.

Another administrative feature of hospital operations that may benefit from regionalization is the unified provision of certain services for several hospitals in a region. One laboratory may perform certain tests for several hospitals in the region, or there may be a centralized accounting service or laundry. Such shared services are more easily developed if hospitals are coordinated in a regionalization scheme, but they may be launched without it.

REGIONALIZATION IN THE UNITED STATES

In the United States, elements of regionalization have been implemented in selected places, and to some extent the construction aspect has been applied in all the states. The Bingham Associates Fund in Maine and Massachusetts and the Rochester Regional Hospital Council in New York State pioneered the idea in the 1930s and 1940s.[2] Under the Hospital Survey and Construction (Hill-Burton) Act of 1946, federally subsidized hospital construction was intended to be done in accordance with a regionalized master plan. For many reasons, however, regionalization seldom worked.[3] In 1965, a fresh attempt was made to breathe life into the concept through the federal legislation on regional medical programs for heart disease, cancer, and stroke; some progress was made in spreading knowledge from medical teaching centers to peripheral facilities.[4] Categorical medical care programs for American Indians and military veterans have applied the regionalization concept to their designated populations.[5] In recent years, shared services as a means of saving money have been organized in several networks of hospitals under unified sponsorship by religious bodies or by corporate entities.[6]

The enactment in 1976 of the National Health Planning and Resources Development Act, which established Health Systems Agencies in some 210 health service areas throughout the nation, may well be furnishing a new stimulus to regionalization in the United States.[7] Widespread and effective application of the idea, however, will probably not occur until the United States joins the ranks of virtually all the other industrialized countries of the world and supports medical care through some system of national social financing. This may be clarified through examining regionalization in other countries with such financing. The health care policies of Canada, France, Norway, England, Chile, and Poland range from substantial local autonomy in health care financing to strong central control.

CANADA

Somewhat like the workmen's compensation acts in the United States, the social insurance financing of medical care in Canada arose in the provinces. In 1947, the first statute for universal hospital insurance coverage took effect in the prairie province of Saskatshewan.[8] Soon British Columbia followed suit, and by 1957 the advantages of the idea were so widely accepted that the national Hospital Insurance and Diagnostic Services Act became law with very little opposition. This Act provides federal grants for roughly 50 percent of the cost of any provincial hospital insurance program that meets certain standards. In 1962, Saskatchewan enacted the first provincial insurance scheme covering every resident for complete physicians' care. In spite of a traumatic 23-day doctor strike, the program rapidly became a great success with the population, and doctors' incomes in Saskatchewan soon rose from the lowest in the ten Canadian provinces to the highest. It took only four years for a similar proposal, the Canadian Medical Care Act, to become national law (see chapter 13).

Legal responsibility for administering both of these health care insurance programs rests with the provinces, and the role of the national government is essentially to share in the financing, as long as certain minimum standards are met. Since the provinces must provide the other 50 percent from their own tax funds, they have plenty of incentive to promote economy, while maintaining quality standards. In Canada, as in the United States and most other countries, hospitalization absorbed the lion's share of the health dollar, so attention was soon directed toward finding some means of controlling hospital costs. Most important were developing an effective scheme of hospital reimbursement and a process of hospital budget review based on the regionalization concept.

Saskatchewan, as the first province in the field, applied two methods of payment (first a scaled hospital classification system and then a scheme of average per diem payments based on individual budget reviews) before it settled on the method it now uses (and that is used in one form or another by the other provinces). It is prospective global budgeting, through which the provincial government reviews each hospital's operating budget at the start of the year. Then, assuming an occupancy level of 80 to 85 percent, the province pays each institution a fixed amount every two weeks in accordance with the approved budget, regardless of the actual number of patient-days of care and associated procedures provided. If some unexpected event, such as an epidemic, causes exceptionally high occupancy, or if personnel salaries have to be raised in mid-year to fill essential posts, then a supplemental allotment is paid to the hospital. If actual costs turn out to be lower than projected costs, the hospital may keep the surplus.

The crucial step in this process is the governmental budget review, and this is where regionalized planning plays its key role. The provincial health agency, which administers the program, maps out the location, the approved bed capacity, and the appropriate scope of services of each hospital in the province. Thus, for example, a small, 50-bed rural hospital would not be expected to operate a radiation therapy department; moreover, its previous occupancy as well as the population distribution might point to a reasonable capacity of only 40 beds. On the other hand, a hospital classified as an intermediate facility might properly require a physiotherapy service, which its budget had not provided for. Application of such objective criteria results in the reduction of some hospital budgets and the increase of others. In a word, the hospital's proper role in a regionalized scheme determines the prospective global budgetary payments it receives.

The Canadian hospital insurance progam has not only implemented the regionalization concept, it has slowed down the inevitable (and worldwide) rise in hospital costs. Although Canadians use hospitals more than Americans do (about 2,000 days per 1,000 persons per year, compared with about 1,300 days), their hospital expenditures have risen more slowly.[9] Canadian hospitals as a whole are very pleased with the entire system, and the high level of content in the population is reflected by the competition among the ten provinces to cover people for additional benefits each year—drugs, dental service, nursing home care, and so on.

FRANCE

France is one of several European nations in which group financing of health services began in hundreds of local voluntary mutual aid societies in the early nineteenth century and then matured into a nationwide social insurance program. The legislation mandating that all industrial workers and their dependents be insured was enacted in 1928; since then, coverage has been gradually extended to farmers, the self-employed, and other groups. Today, over 90 percent of the French people are protected by the mandatory national health insurance (social security) program, and most of the remainder buy insurance protection voluntarily. After World War II, the hundreds of local mutual aid societies were consolidated into a national framework, carrying out responsibilities for the social security system.

French hospitals are owned and operated mainly by units of local government; some 76 percent of the beds are under such sponsorship, and the balance are proprietary or voluntary, nonprofit. No hospital of any sponsorship, however, may be built or significantly modified without the approval of the Ministry of Health. This approval is based on the application of a ministerial plan that divides France into 21 regions, in each of which the hospitals are graded into three levels of function, as in the classical regionalization concept.[10]

The French hospital regions are composed of two to eight (averaging 4.5) *départements,* which are roughly equivalent to counties in the United States. The head of each department is a prefect, who is not locally elected but appointed by the central government. The prefect is aided by a departmental health officer, also centrally appointed. Among the health officer's functions is the annual review and approval of hospital budgets. In this review, he must apply central ministry standards appropriate to the functional category into which each hospital fits under the national regional plan. From this budget, a per diem cost is calculated for each hospital. This amount is then chargeable to the social security system for each patient-day of care provided to an insured person. For nonsurgical or nonmaternity cases, the patient must copay 20 percent, but if he is poor this fraction is paid by the municipality. Thus, as in Canada, but by a different process, the national health insurance system enforces the regionalization concept designed by the Ministry of Health.

Cooperative relationships among the three levels of hospitals in each region have been voluntary in France, but a 1970 law was intended to promote closer coordination. Grants are given to establish hospital syndicates, which will share certain specialized services, thereby avoiding costly duplication. Hospitals in a syndicate receive allotments for education of professional personnel, preventive services, and expansion of outpatient ambulatory services. Thus, through the financial leverage of both the social security funds and the Ministry of Health, France is attempting to organize its hospitals into functioning regional networks. Ownership of each institution remains local, under either public or private management.

NORWAY

Medical care financing in Norway, as in France, started with local mutual aid societies or "sickness funds"; mandatory enrollment of wage earners was enacted in 1910. After being gradually extended, social insurance coverage of the entire population was required by law in 1956. By 1972, the concept of medical care as a social right had become so firmly established in Norway that no political party would think of reducing it, and funding was shifted to general revenues.[11]

Hospitals in Norway, both general and special, are overwhelmingly public entities. Some 90 percent of the short-term general hospital beds are owned and controlled by local provincial governments. In all of these, the entire medical staff consists of carefully chosen specialists who work on salary, usually full-time. These hospital posts carry great prestige, and appointment to them is made by the local governments from a competitive list of applicants screened by the national Directorate of Health Services.

Since 1969, the Norwegian Ministry of Social Affairs, which includes both the Directorate of Health Services and the Institute of National Insurance, has been taking steps to coordinate the nation's hospitals into five integrated regions. With a national population of only 4 million, Norway's regions contain 500,000 to 1 million persons each and a total of 19 provinces. Under the national plan, hospitals are classified as regional, provincial, or local and have corresponding staffs and functions. All hospital construction planned in a region must be approved by the national government. Each hospital's budget, moreover, must be reviewed and approved by the Directorate of Health Services, and the criteria for approval depend on the hospital's function in its region.

Payment for hospital care (until recently) came 75 percent from the national insurance program and 25 percent from the provincial government; the patient paid nothing, unless he chose one of the few nonpublic hospitals, in which case he paid the 25 percent local share. (Since the nonpublic hospitals, which account for 10 percent of hospital beds, are much more modestly staffed and equipped, they tend to be used only for simple conditions such as normal childbirths and minor elective surgery.)

Based on the central government's budget review, a cost per patient-day is calculated for each hospital, and this determines the payments made by the health insurance system. As of 1978, however, Norway shifted to a global prospective payment system similar to Canada's. Actually, 90 percent of budgeted costs are to be paid this way (and are to be shared equally between national insurance and the provincial government), and the remaining 10 percent will vary with the specific number of patient-days of care provided. Because Norway has salaried hospital doctors, there is no financial incentive for unjustified or prolonged hospitalizations. In fact, all decisions on hospital admission are made by the hospital specialist. When the patient is discharged, a report is sent back to the referring community practitioner.

Thus one sees in Norway a country in which hospital regionalization is promoted by the national government and enforcement is accomplished through payments made by the health insurance system and the local governments.

ENGLAND

The regionalization concept has been carried further in England than in any of the countries just described.[12] When the national health service was launched in 1948, it had three main parts: (1) general practitioner care with other ambulatory services, (2) environmental and preventive health services, and (3) hospital and specialist services. Each sector grew from distinct historical antecedents. The hospital system was an outgrowth of the wartime scheme through which each hospital had an assigned role in emergency care of bomb victims. As recommended in the Beveridge Report in 1942, every resident of Britain is entitled to all necessary services free, except for small copayments on drugs and dental prostheses.

On the appointed day in July 1948, all but a few hospitals, along with their associated assets and liabilities, were taken over by the Minister of Health. For administration, the hospitals (both general and special) of England and Wales were placed under the control of 15 regional hospital boards. Within each region (averaging about 3 million people), groups of hospitals with a total of 1,000 to 2,000 beds were operated by hospital management committees. From the national budget to finance the NHS (about 80 percent from the general treasury) global allotments were made to each hospital region for both operating and capital expenses. The regional boards, in turn, allotted funds to cover the approved budgets of the hospital management committees. These funds had to cover all operating expenses, including the salaries of the medical staffs—full-time specialists as well as doctors in training.

When the NHS was reorganized in 1974, the three main sectors were united under the control of 90 area health authorities. In this way, much closer integration is achieved among the preventive, ambulatory, and hospital services. The financing of hospitals, however, remains on essentially the same global budgetary basis, with the regional hospital boards being replaced by regional health boards. In spite of all the fiscal constraints due to overall economic difficulties, British hospitals are in much more stable financial condition than previously, although most physical plants are rather old. The NHS as a whole has kept its expenditures to under 6 percent of the GNP, compared with more than 9 percent in the United States. British health indexes, on the other hand, are somewhat better than their U.S. counterparts.

CHILE

Most of the economically less developed countries of the world have also organized their hospitals in regionalized frameworks, and

Chile illustrates one in which the arrangements were especially comprehensive. Prior to 1952, when the Chilean national health service was formed, Chile was served by three major public subsystems of medical care plus a private sector. The oldest was the *beneficencia*, or welfare network of hospitals. Second was the Ministry of Health array of hospitals and health centers, the latter mainly for preventive services. Third was the social security system for employed (mostly urban) workers, which operated various polyclinics. With the establishment of the national health service, the resources of all three programs were acquired by the Ministry of Health and were integrated under the administration of 13 health zone authorities.[13]

Within each zone, health areas were set up around the major general hospitals. The health centers, polyclinics, and small health posts in these areas functioned as satellites, administratively and functionally, of the central facility. Both treatment and preventive services are rendered in all ambulatory care units, and the head of the hospital also serves as the general director of the health area. Financial support comes through global allotments made to each health zone authority, which in turn makes grants to the hospitals and other health facilities. Nationally, the funds are derived mostly from general revenues, with some coming from the social security fund, which still pays cash benefits (for old age, invalidism, and so on) to workers. Because the Chilean middle class constituted a market for private medical practice, only about 70 percent of the population of Chile was entitled to national health services without charge. Coverage was being extended gradually to 100 percent, until the military coup of 1973 reversed the trend. (This account, in fact, describes the Chilean national health service before its substantial "privatization" by the military government.)

POLAND

In any review of regionalized hospital systems, it is appropriate to include a Socialist country, and I have chosen Poland because in 1976 I had the opportunity of undertaking a five-week study there. Poland adopted a Socialist political system after World War II; while its agriculture and a few other activities remain largely private, the health services have become essentially nationalized, very much in accordance with the Soviet model (see chapter 18).[14]

Before World War II, a certain percentage of Polish workers had social insurance protection for medical care, there were several rural health cooperatives, and there were some municipal hospitals for the poor. Most people, however, had to purchase medical care privately. The human and physical resources for health care were then decimated by the war. With peace, the overwhelming need was to train thousands of doctors, nurses, and medical auxiliaries (*feldshers*) and to construct hospitals and health centers. The years since 1945 have been tumultuous and full of change.

Conversion of the system to its present form did not occur overnight. Local public hospitals were not transferred to the central Ministry of Health until 1948. The social insurance program for medical care was absorbed by Ministry of Health only in 1951, and in that year the local pharmacies were also nationalized. Extension of the benefits of the public medical system to the peasants, thereby achieving 100 percent coverage, did not occur until 1972.

Poland today is divided into 49 provinces for general civil administration, including administration of the health services. The nation is served by ten strategically placed medical academies or schools under the supervision of the Ministry of Health. Thus, each medical academy, and the large hospital with which it is linked, serves as the professional center of a region made up of about five provinces. The provinces, in turn, are divided into integrated health areas (ZOZs), which always contain a central district hospital, sometimes one or two smaller hospitals, and numerous health centers for primary care and polyclinics for ambulatory specialist care.

The medical or surgical specialist heading each department in the main hospital is responsible also for corresponding services in the ambulatory care facilities throughout the ZOZ. Thus the chief of pediatrics, for example, supervises all child health services, preventive and curative, in the primary health care centers. Provinces vary in size and may contain as few as three or as many as 33 ZOZs. In all of them, however, the supervisory hierarchy continues upward in each health discipline from the ZOZ to the main provincial hospital and from there to the major medical center associated with one of the ten medical academies or schools. Thus the educational centers in Poland, as in most other Socialist countries, stand at the apex of a pyramid of health services. The professors are expected to supervise and monitor the quality of health care throughout their region, in addition to their teaching duties. Research, on the other hand, is conducted mainly in separate specialized research institutes.

All Polish health personnel, including physicians and dentists, are required to work for salaries in the public system at least seven hours a day. Private practice has never been forbidden, and many doctors and dentists still provide care to the small portion of the population who are willing and able to pay privately rather than use the public system. Most of this private care, however, is given through medical cooperatives, in which fees are regulated and doctors may work no more than two hours a day. In the public system, which provides all the hospital service and 80 to 90 percent of the ambulatory care, there are no charges to patients except small ones for drugs. The costs are met by the central government, which makes global allotments to each provincial health authority; allotments are supplemented by limited contributions from industrial enterprises to support special occupational health services for workers.

CONCLUSION

From these relatively brief accounts of regionalized health care systems in six countries, it is evident that the concept outlined at the start is being applied, with varying degrees of thoroughness, throughout the world. With more or less similarity, one would find parallel policies being pursued in almost any country one might examine.

It appears that the principal way in which various regional health systems differ is the degree of autonomy exercised by hospitals. This, in turn, seems to depend on the method of financing. In countries like Canada or France, where the classical social insurance mechanism predominates, each hospital retains a good deal of autonomy. In others, like England or Poland, where general revenue financing predominates, hospitals are part of a public network and each facility plays the role designated for it by a public authority. The regional networks of institutions also include peripheral units for care of the ambulatory patient.

Even in the less structured systems and countries, the trend of regionalization is toward defining the role of each hospital more specifically, in accordance with the theoretical regional model. The national health insurance support systems are clearly being used as leverage to influence hospital functions.[15] The thrust of this worldwide movement in the health services is toward the attainment of national *systems* of health service, which are designed to meet human needs more rationally and economically than are traditional private markets for medical care.

NOTES

1. R. F. Bridgman and M. I. Roemer, *Hospital Legislation and Hospital Systems*, public health paper no. 50 (Geneva: World Health Organization, 1973).

2. L. S. Rosenfeld and H. B. Makover, *The Rochester Regional Hospital Council* (Cambridge, Mass.: Harvard University Press, 1956).
3. W. J. McNerney and D. C. Riedel, *Regionalization and Rural Health Care* (Ann Arbor: University of Michigan, 1962).
4. K. D. Yordy, "Regionalization of Health Services: Current Legislative Directions in the United States," in *The Regionalization of Personal Health Services*, E. W. Saward, ed. (New York: Prodist, 1976), 201–22.
5. M. I. Roemer and R. C. Morris, "Hospital Regionalization in Perspective," *Public Health Reports* 74 (October 1959):916–22.
6. M. S. Blumberg, *Shared Services for Hospitals* (Chicago: American Hospital Association, 1966).
7. L. S. Rosenfeld and I. Rosenfeld, "National Health Planning in the United States: Prospects and Portents," *International Journal of Health Services* 5 (1975):441–53.
8. R. Roemer and M. I. Roemer, *Health Manpower Policy under National Health Insurance—The Canadian Experience* (Washington, D.C.: Health Resources Administration, 1977).
9. S. Andreopoulos, ed., *National Health Insurance: Can We Learn from Canada?* (New York: Wiley & Sons, 1975).
10. Bridgman and Roemer, *Hospital Legislation.*
11. M. I. Roemer and R. Roemer, *Manpower in the Health Care System of Norway* (Washington, D.C.: Health Resources Administration, 1977).
12. R. Levitt, *The Reorganised National Health Service* (London: Croom Helm, 1976).
13. M. I. Roemer, *Medical Care in Latin America* (Washington, D.C.: Pan American Union, 1963).
14. M. I. Roemer and R. Roemer, *Health Manpower in the Socialist Health Care System of Poland* (Washington, D.C.: Health Resources Administration, 1978).
15. M. I. Roemer, *Comparative National Policies on Health Care* (New York: Marcel Dekker Co., 1977).

23

Coordinating Health Services and Manpower Policy

An important component of national health planning is estimating the numbers and types of health manpower required to meet population needs. Yet all too often, policies on the training of doctors, nurses, and other personnel are formulated with little consideration of health service requirements. In the late 1970s, the World Health Organization set out to promote closer coordination in countries between requirements for health services and manpower development programs. This chapter reviews the ways in which such coordination is being attempted in various countries.

The social tasks of (1) organizing the provision of health services to populations and (2) systematically preparing health personnel have evolved along quite separate paths. In recent years, however, as the need for a comprehensive and planned approach to a nation's health problems has become increasingly recognized, the two paths of social action have gradually been converging.

BACKGROUND

The organized provision of health services has been undertaken by a variety of social entities. Churches played a key role in the estab-

---

This chapter is an adapted and substantially revised version of "National Experience in Coordination of Health Services and Manpower Development," Annex 1 in Report on Consultation on Health Services and Manpower Development, World Health Organization, Geneva, September 6–8, 1976 (HMD/77.1), 18–32.

lishment of hospitals. Workers and other groups of citizens organized the first societies for collective economic support (through insurance) of the costs of sickness, these efforts later coming under governmental insurance laws. Various components of local or national government undertook actions for environmental sanitation, in order to control communicable disease. In the great majority of countries there eventually arose a central ministry of health, with continually expanding responsibilities involving both preventive and curative health services. Other governmental, as well as nongovernmental, agencies have arisen at national and local levels for the provision or financing of health services to selected populations.

The systematic education of manpower for providing health services has evolved along a separate path. Education of physicians was the first formal effort, originating in Salerno, Italy, in the ninth century. Universities arose in most of the main cities of Europe during the next several centuries, and many of them included faculties of medicine. Since the universities were an outgrowth of the Renaissance, their key role was seen as the accumulation and transmission of classical knowledge. To play this role, they adopted a position of independence from the Christian churches, the government, and other social entities. Even when universities came to be financed mainly or entirely from public funds (government at different levels), the tradition of autonomy persisted.

Thus, the education of physicians by universities was regarded as a responsibility solely of the professors in the faculties of medicine. The numbers of candidates prepared and the content of their education were matters solely for the decision of the faculty. The rise of capitalism and laissez-faire economics, meanwhile, created an environment in which physicians did their work as a "liberal profession"—free to practice their art and sell their services wherever and however they chose. After the fourteenth century, some countries enacted licensure laws specifying requirements for the practice of medicine, but it was several more centuries before governments put further constraints on the numbers of persons trained as physicians or the content of their education. The autonomy of the universities and the freedom of the medical market were the dominant realities.

The zealous guarding of university autonomy had substantial justification. The early struggles of great scientists such as Galileo and Copernicus against repression by the centers of power are well known. Only by freedom from external interference—whether from church, government, or other sources—could there be an uninhibited search for knowledge and an objective pursuit of truth. The actual approach to these objectives has not always been consistent with the ideal, but the idea of academic freedom for the community of scholars in a university has been a central principle in the development of institutions of higher education. Yet this same freedom has often isolated scholars from the real world.

It was only in the early twentieth century that social pressures led to estimates of the *needs* of a population for the services of physicians or other health personnel. Apothecaries or pharmacists had originated in the Middle Ages as specialists in drugs, which they sold directly to patients (as does the traditional herbalist in Asia to this day). Not until the nineteenth century was the pharmacist obligated to follow the prescriptions of doctors for most drugs. Formal education of nurses arose in nineteenth century England, not in universities, but in hospitals. A wide variety of other specialized health personnel (laboratory technicians, physical therapists, record clerks, and so on) soon followed, schooled in diverse types of educational institutions. For physicians and these many other types of health personnel, there slowly emerged a recognition that certain minimal numbers were needed to operate hospitals or to render various sorts of health services to the population.

The most dramatic departure from the free market concept of production and use of health manpower came with the Russian Revolution of 1917. Here for the first time a national government decided that its population needed a certain number (or ratio) of physicians, nurses, pharmacists, *feldshers,* and others. In virtually every category, the quantity estimated as necessary exceeded the available supply, so the government formulated health manpower plans and established schools for training large additional numbers of health personnel. A five-year plan for all aspects of the economy, including health services and health manpower, was launched in 1928.

When in 1929 the world was struck with a massive depression—a severe crisis of the prevailing economic system—many other nations undertook cautious efforts at planning. In the 1930's, much national legislation was enacted to extend the scope of governmental health programs, both preventive and curative. Ministries of health became more important, and insurance systems were extended. Popular demands for health protection became major political issues, to which national governments had to respond. World War II postponed social progress, but after the war national planning of all sectors of the economy, including health service, became a widely accepted principle. In the many new, developing nations, liberated from colonial status, national planning became a very high priority.

The emergence of a nationwide perspective on social needs had special impact in the field of health. It led national governments to consider what specific steps would be necessary to assure the provision of a wide variety of health services to whole populations. The degree to which those steps were actually taken, of course, varied greatly with a nation's political commitment, the stage of its economic development, its cultural features, and other factors. In virtually all formulations of the national need for health services, however, there was included a component for the training and rational use of health manpower.

Since health manpower planning and production evolved separately from the provision of health services, the existing organized entities in these two fields were usually separate. This meant that coordination of plans and actions was necessary if health manpower were to be produced and used in a manner and to an extent appropriate to the needed health services. Here again, the extent of this coordination has varied greatly among nations, depending on power relationships at different times and places. In almost all countries, nevertheless, some degree of coordination in certain facets of health services and health manpower has been achieved.

The relationships between health services and manpower development (HSMD) are in active ferment throughout the world. The degree of HSMD coordination varies from the very limited in some countries to the very great in others. The picture changes every day, but it may be helpful in understanding the HSMD concept to consider various expressions of it actually found in different countries.

NATIONAL EXPERIENCES IN COORDINATION

A wide range of HSMD activities may be coordinated to advantage. Manpower development has been considered by WHO to involve (1) planning, (2) production, and (3) management, or use, of health personnel. Coordination with the health service system of a country may occur within each of these sectors. Somewhat more specifically, coordinating actions in these three components of manpower development may be undertaken as follows:

— Health manpower planning
  1. Ministry of health planning analyses
  2. Health policy coordinating councils

— Health manpower production
  3. Education financed by health authorities
  4. Health ministry regulation of manpower
  5. Educational programs under health authorities

— Health manpower management
  6. University participation in health services
  7. Control of manpower development by health authority

In some countries, only the first one or two of these seven forms of coordination are implemented. In others, perhaps the first four, five, or even six forms are implemented to some degree. In a relatively few countries, the seventh form of coordination may be implemented. The following are concrete illustrations of national policies and practices in each of these seven types of action.

Ministry of Health Planning Analyses

As a part of general health planning efforts, estimates of national needs for health manpower in all categories are made in many countries. This includes most of the highly developed countries and most of the developing countries.

In *India*, for example, the five-year plan for 1970–75 prepared by the Ministry of Health and Family Planning called for allocation of 115,553 million rupees, of which 9,822 million went for education and research.[1] Underlying these figures are estimates of additional health manpower needed, the training of which would be conducted by many schools and universities under various public and private auspices.

Australia has a hospitals and health services commission within its Ministry of Health, and among its many functions has been health manpower planning.[2] After determining the current supply of each type of personnel, estimates have been made of additional numbers needed to reach desirable ratios (which, in turn, have been designated by various advisors). Health manpower planning is a prominent function of the *Canadian* Ministry of National Health and Welfare. A health manpower directorate in this ministry has used data from the federal-provincial health insurance program to determine the rates of health care utilization by the population.[3] Committees of medical specialists then propose an optimal time allotment for each type of case and a reasonable number of working hours in the doctor's week; from this they calculate the numbers of each type of specialist needed.

One of the most extensive studies, mainly for the purpose of health manpower planning, was done in *Colombia*, during 1964–67. This "Study on Health Manpower and Medical Education in Colombia" was a combined effort of the Ministry of Public Health and the Association of Medical Schools in that country. It included compilation of data on most types of health manpower, as well as a national survey of morbidity and utilization of health services by the population. The information produced by this research contributed to Colombia's health manpower planning over the subsequent years.

Dissemination of the conclusions drawn from these health manpower planning analyses, and the transmission of them to educational authorities, is intended to influence the educational programs of universities and other institutions for training health personnel. Health ministry estimates of the need for additional dentists, for example, provide powerful arguments to a university dental faculty for acquiring greater resources (from a ministry of education or from general university funds) for dental education. Estimates of health manpower needs, of course, also shape the decisions of general national planning commissions. The impact of planning proposals on the programs of academic institutions may be mediated in a variety of ways.

One may cite other illustrations of the relationship between manpower planning by a health ministry and actions in manpower production by an education ministry. In *Sweden*, the Ministry of Health and Social Affairs has a permanent committee for national health planning, which has projected the need for physicians to the year 1990. This requires that the number of medical school graduates be increased to 1,000 per year; the Ministry of Education has accepted the recommendations and intends to augment the financing of the universities accordingly.[4] Similar projections of manpower supply and need to the year 1990 have been made by the Ministry of Health and Welfare in *Japan*.[5]

In *Algeria*, the planning of educational programs for health personnel has been deliberately assigned to the Institute of Public Health, under which there is a committee representing not only the health services, but also the schools for primary, secondary, and higher education, the schools for training allied health personnel, and the consumers of health services.[6] Thus the manpower planning decisions made by the institute may be expected to incorporate the viewpoints of the schools that will have to do the training.

Health Policy Coordinating Councils

Coordination of the many sectors of the health field has long been facilitated by the establishment of national or local councils, on which are representatives of the several ministries and other organizations concerned. These councils typically include representatives of educational authorities and, among other things, consider matters involving the relationship of health services to manpower development. Sometimes the councils are advisory to the ministry of health or other ministries, and sometimes they may have clear policymaking powers.

In *Iran*, for example, in 1976 there was established a High Council of Health representing the Ministry of Higher Education and Science, the Social Welfare Ministry, and other organizations, as well as the Ministry of Health. Among the council's functions was the coordination of activities in manpower development with those in the health services. The decisions of this council were evidently more than advisory, since they affected the programs of the several ministries.[7] A similar National Health Council has been appointed in *Thailand*, specifically oriented toward the coordination of health services and health manpower production. In *Venezuela*, a National Council of Health has been appointed by the president, with delegates from the Association of Medical Schools, as well as the Institute of Social Security, the Ministry of Public Health, and other agencies providing health care. This council is expected not only to set policies relevant to health, but also to supervise their implementation.

In *Sri Lanka*, a national committee that was established in 1964 to focus principally on general manpower development includes representatives of the health services.[8] This Planning Committee on Manpower and Education has, among other things, set targets for the output of health personnel. For 1970, its goal for training would yield a ratio of one doctor per 3,000 persons and one nurse for each 4.5 hospital beds.

There are, of course, countless national advisory bodies, representing various interest groups, on selected components of health services. In the *United States*, for example, a National Advisory Council on Mental Health gives advice to the Department of Health and Human Services on both services and personnel training in the field of mental health. The scope of the health policy councils noted here, however, is much broader. Such bodies are being established in an increasing number of countries in recognition of the complex relationships among the many sectors influencing health and health services. Comprehensive health advisory councils may also be established at local levels, especially in federated nations. In *Canada*, such bodies have been established in all ten provinces.

Education Financed by Health Authorities

With respect to the production of health manpower, ministries of health or other health authorities may play a direct or indirect role.

Financial support for the education of health personnel may be provided extensively by health authorities, even when the educational programs are conducted by universities or schools that are independent or supervised generally by an education authority. This strategy for influencing health manpower production has been extensively applied in the *United States*, both at national and state levels. During World War II, in order to increase the supply of nurses, a program of grants to nursing schools—for both expansion of faculties and fellowships for students—was launched by the national health authorities. In about 1960, with the widespread recognition that more physicians and dentists were needed, grants were given to medical and dental schools (both private and public) to increase their capacities for training personnel. This indirect approach to influencing health manpower production has been necessary in the United States because of the strong traditions of the universities as independent bodies. The medical faculties, moreover, are often closely associated with the private medical profession, which has long been apprehensive of what it sees as governmental interference in medical affairs. In the 1970's, grants were given to all schools of medicine, dentistry, optometry, and certain other fields on a flat per-student basis, thereby providing a strong incentive for the schools to increase their enrollments.

Canada does not have a national ministry or department in the field of education, a policy resulting from the cultural division between French-speaking and English-speaking Canadians. Departments of education function at the provincial level, however, and they provide the main financial support for the medical schools. To enlarge the capacities of the medical schools, the Ministry of National Health and Welfare has established a fund for capital grants to construct or expand medical school facilities in all the provinces.

Selective financial grants by health agencies have also been used to influence the content of curriculums in medical schools. In *Belgium*, the National Institute of Sickness and Invalidity Insurance (part of the social security system) has given subsidies to the medical faculties specifically for strengthening teaching in the field of family medicine. In *Australia*, the Hospitals and Health Services Commission (within the Ministry of Health) has allotted grants to the medical schools for programs of continuing education focused on the needs of general practitioners.

A widespread impact of health ministries on health manpower education is, of course, through their financial support of teaching hospitals affiliated with medical schools. In most *Latin American* countries, the principal settings in which medical students are taught clinical disciplines are large urban hospitals financed mainly by ministries of health.[9] Sometimes these hospitals are owned by charitable societies, but their financial support is still mainly governmental. The availability of patients for teaching purposes is naturally a constraint on the number of medical students who can be properly trained, so the health ministry has obvious influence on the output of physicians. In *Great Britain*, the teaching hospitals have an especially large role in the training of medical students. They are key facilities in the health regions of the national health service, in spite of the control of medical schools by the universities.[10] This sort of dynamic is found to some extent in nearly all countries.

Health Ministry Regulation of Manpower

Through their authority for regulating health manpower, ministries of health may influence the content of professional education. A striking illustration of this is seen in *Norway*, where the curriculum in the nursing schools must meet national standards set by the Ministry of Church and Education.[11] In designing those standards, however, the latter ministry consults thoroughly with the health services directorate in the Ministry of Social Affairs. Also, when the nursing schools submit their curriculums to the Ministry of Education for approval, they are routinely transmitted to the health authorities for comment.

The widespread authority of ministries of health to register or license all or many types of health personnel exerts an indirect influence on their preparation. Such registration is usually the requirement in developing countries, such as for physicians in *Malaysia*.[12] It is the policy in *Colombia, Sweden*, and *Japan*; the first two of these countries also recognize specialty qualifications of physicians through their health ministries.[13] In *France*, the Ministry of Health licenses nurses, and the proficiency of assistant nurses is certified by the health authorities at the departmental level.

The full potential of this registration or licensing power in health ministries has not been exploited. It might be used, for example, to improve geographic distribution of physicians and other personnel by restricting registration to those practitioners who would settle, for certain periods of time, in designated areas. This has, in fact, been done quite recently in certain provinces of *Canada* with respect to immigrant physicians, who are required to practice in isolated rural areas until citizenship is attained (a five-year period).

As a condition for licensure, all new graduates of medical schools in *Mexico* have long been obligated to work for six to 12 months in a rural area, under the direction of the local public health officer. *Colombia, Venezuela, Iran, Thailand, Malaysia*, and other developing countries have similar requirements. In *Norway*, all medical school graduates, in order to be licensed, must do an internship of 18 months, six of which must be spent working with a district doctor in a rural location. Improved geographic distribution of physicians on a more permanent basis has been encouraged through policies of the Ministry of Health in *Tunisia*, where for some years new medical graduates were authorized to practice only if they located outside the national capital, Tunis.[14] Somewhat similar objectives are achieved in the national health service of *Great Britain* through its policy of barring new GPs from NHS participation if they settle in overdoctored areas. Thus, the doctor who wishes to be paid for general practice work under the NHS must settle in an underdoctored area.

Despite these illustrations, registration of new physicians or other personnel within a ministry of health, or sometimes separate medical councils, is usually a pro forma matter, requiring only that the candidate be a graduate of an educational program approved by the education authorities. With regard to graduates of foreign schools, a health ministry generally applies more discrimination in the registration process.

Educational Programs under Health Authorities

Another linkage of health manpower production to health services occurs where a ministry of health is engaged directly in the training of personnel. Many forms of such training are found throughout the world.

A striking form of such action is seen when a health ministry sets out to train a new type of health worker not previously "produced" by the regular educational institutions. This has been done, for example, by the South Australian State Public Health Department in *Australia* to produce school dental therapists.[15] These allied health workers, trained for two years following secondary school, are modeled after the dental nurse of *New Zealand*. It is noteworthy that in the pioneer program of New Zealand, started in 1920, the initiative was taken by the established dental school at the University of Dunedin. In Australia, however, the concept of briefly trained dental workers to treat children was not embraced by the university dental faculty; therefore, the health authority simply established a training institution of its own and registers the graduates for work exclusively in the school dental program.

Another such innovative manpower training program has been operated since the 1940's in the Province of Saskatchewan, *Canada*, under the Department of Public Health. In this thinly settled prairie region, there are many small hospitals (under 50 beds) in which the need for laboratory and X-ray diagnostic services is not great enough to justify employment of technicians in each of these two fields. The established educational programs were preparing only fully qualified laboratory technicians and fully qualified X-ray technicians. The Department of Public Health, therefore, designed and operated its own course for training combined technicians who could carry out relatively simple diagnostic procedures in both fields.

More generalized auxiliary personnel for primary health care in rural areas have been trained by ministries of health in many developing countries. The Public Health College and Training Center in Gondar, *Ethiopia*, is a good example. This center was established by the Health Ministry, with the aid of WHO, UNICEF, and USAID, to prepare community health officers (with three years of study following secondary school), community nurses (with two years of study after primary school), and community sanitarians (with one year of study after six years of primary school). The Gondar College has no connection with the Ministry of Education or other educational institutions, but its graduates meet an obvious need for the staffing of rural health centers. In *Malaysia*, the Rural Health Training Centre at Jitra, in the state of Kedah, was started in 1953 by the Ministry of Health to provide assistant nurses, assistant midwives, and sanitary overseers for staffing a national network of rural health centers and subcenters.[16] Indeed, throughout *Africa, Latin America,* and *Asia* there are scores of such training programs for village health workers conducted by ministries of health or local units of the national health authority.

Another contribution of health service systems to manpower development is so commonplace that it might be overlooked. This is the regular maintenance of facilities, mainly hospitals, that provide the practical or clinical aspects of training for the educational institutions producing physicians, nurses, laboratory technicians, physical therapists, and other types of personnel. Nurses are, of course, often educated entirely in hospitals and under the hospital administration; but even when the nursing school is independent, as it is in *Norway*, the bedside aspects of training are still provided in hospitals. Sometimes rural health centers of a health ministry participate in the training of medical students, as in the pioneer program of the University of Zagreb, *Yugoslavia*. Through their experience, medical, nursing, and other types of students become better acquainted not only with the practical aspects of clinical service, but to some extent with the organizational structure of the health care system as well.

Schools of public health offer a relatively new type of manpower training, typically at the postgraduate level, and these programs are often sponsored directly by a ministry of health rather than a university. Of the ten such schools in *Latin America*, five are under ministerial sponsorship and five are part of a university. In *Australia*, the

School of Public Health on the University of Sydney campus illustrates an interesting form of coordination; while located in this academic setting, the school is fully financed and controlled by the public health authorities.

Sometimes one category of training program in a country may relate to the ministry of health in several different ways. In *Peru*, for example, there were ten schools of nursing in 1963. Seven of these were controlled by hospitals, and three were separate institutions operated directly by the Ministry of Health. Meanwhile, additional advanced nursing schools were planned in provincial universities, to be affiliated with regional hospitals administered by the Ministry of Health.[17]

Finally, health ministries play an extensive role in the continuing education of medical and allied manpower. Not only is this often financed by health authorities, through special subsidies, but it is also often conducted directly by ministries themselves or bodies subordinate to them. Thus, in the *United States*, state or large municipal public health agencies often offer short courses for physicians on prevention-oriented subjects, such as multiphasic screening for chronic disease; dentists are offered instruction on fluorides in relation to dental health; nurses are offered instruction on emergency services. In the developing countries, such initiative for continuing education is often taken by health agencies in small towns serving rural regions, where academic institutions are lacking. Postbasic education of nurses in *Sri Lanka* is conducted by the Ministry of Health, although basic nurse training comes under the Ministry of Education. Continuing or postgraduate education is, of course, intended to produce more skilled personnel.

University Participation in Health Services

In the management, or use, of health manpower, primary responsibility rests with health agencies. In numerous ways, however, and in many special projects, educational institutions (mainly universities) are deeply involved in the delivery of health care.

University-controlled hospitals, while intended mainly to serve teaching purposes, still render a great deal of sophisticated medical service. One may be critical of the inordinately high investments often made in the construction and operation of such facilities, but it remains true that university hospitals provide a great deal of service, often of a life-or-death nature, to selected patients. Moreover, they typically serve as the peak of a pyramidal hierarchy of health facilities in a regional scheme, functioning not only as an ultimate referral center for different cases, but also as a source of technical leadership for the entire region or nation. The extent to which the university medical center attempts to spread knowledge throughout its region, as opposed to being simply an isolated center of excellence, varies. In *Sweden*, for example, the principal university hospitals serve as consultants to physicians in the smaller county or district hospitals in their regions.[18] This has also been the intention in many African countries, such as *Ghana*, although the heavy workloads of university hospital specialists often does not allow them much time to visit peripheral institutions.[19]

Besides this general health service role of university hospitals, there are several special projects in the world where very broad health care responsibilities are assumed by universities. A fine example is in the Negev Desert area of *Israel*, involving the Ben-Gurion University at Beersheva. To provide a full range of curative and preventive health services to the many thousands of people in this newly settled region, as well as higher education in medicine, the university, the health insurance system of the Israeli Labour Federation, and the Ministry of Health have formed a consortium. The dean of the medical faculty functions simultaneously as the regional director of health services.[20] This Beersheva project is serving, in a sense, as a pilot effort; if it is successful, it may eventually be applied throughout Israel.

In the northern part of *Nigeria*, at Zaria, the Ahmadu Bello University has established a health manpower training program of wide scope. To carry this program out effectively, the university has assumed administrative control of a number of surrounding hospitals, health centers, and dispensaries serving a population of about 1 million.[21] In *Ghana*, also, there is a special project near Accra (the national capital and site of the university) radiating from a health center in the village of Danfa; the management of health services in this region has been assigned to the medical faculty. Thus, the education of medical students and the provision of health services are integrated.

In *Latin America*, coordinated teaching-service areas (*areas docente-asistenciales*) have been under development for several years, with financial aid from the Kellogg Foundation of the United States. The objective is clearly educational, but the means to this end is involvement of universities in the actual delivery of services. As described by a Kellogg Foundation official:

> The program began in 1972 and has among its objectives the involvement of medical schools with the health care delivery system in adjoining areas; participation of clinical teachers in education and services at all levels of the system; curricular modifications to allow for clinical learning at various levels of the system to be equal in rank, in terms of academic credits, to experience in the university hospital; and development of a regionalized, multilevel health care system in the chosen area, in agreement with health authorities.[22]

The most highly developed of the seven HSMD coordinated projects is at the Universidad del Valle, in Cali, *Colombia*. The degree of actual university responsibility varies among the other six projects, in *Guatemala, Panama, Brazil, Bolivia, Venezuela,* and *Jamaica*. It would appear that the university tends to become more deeply involved in the direct management of services. Ultimate responsibility remains, by legal necessity, with the several ministries of health, but delegation of authority to the universities for day-to-day management has still been feasible.

In the *United States*, there have also been certain projects in which universities have taken responsibility for delivering health services to designated populations. One of the earliest (since the 1930's) was in Baltimore, Maryland, where the responsibility for public health administration in the eastern health district of that city was assigned to the Johns Hopkins University School of Hygiene and Public Health. With a faculty member appointed as director of this district of the city's public health service, many opportunities are available for practical field training of graduate students of public health. The financing of these services and the definition of the general scope of work, however, remain the responsibility of Baltimore's health department.

As part of the teaching of community medicine to medical students, some U.S. medical schools have taken responsibility for managing health centers providing comprehensive ambulatory services to low-income persons. This has been done by Tufts University in a slum area of Boston, Massachusetts, and by the University of Southern California in a section of Los Angeles with a population of about 20,000. These neighborhood health centers are financed by national health authorities and their administrative control has been shifting to organizations of local residents, but, in their initial years, leadership was taken by the medical schools. In the medical school at Kuopio, *Finland*, the department of community medicine is closely connected with the health service system of the surrounding area.

Another interesting type of responsibility assumed by universities for general health service to a population is illustrated in certain health maintenance organizations (HMOs) in the *United States*. These are health insurance entities providing comprehensive ambulatory and hospital services to their enrolled members, who pay monthly rates. In Boston, Massachusetts, the Harvard University medical school has sponsored such an HMO, using its faculty members as physicians for about 100,000 persons; the program serves also as a vehicle for teaching students—not only clinical medicine, but also social medicine. A similar HMO is sponsored by the Johns Hopkins School of Medicine at a planned community—Columbia, Maryland.

Control of Manpower Development
by Health Authority

At the farthest end of the spectrum of forms of HSMD coordination is the full integration of manpower planning, production, and management within a system of health services. Such integration has been in effect in the *Soviet Union* since about 1937.

It is noteworthy that after the Russian Revolution of 1917 all health services, both preventive and curative, were brought under the control of a Ministry of Health, except for the education of health personnel. The latter remained the responsibility of the universities and the Ministry of Education. Then, after 20 years of experience with this dichotomy, the government decided that the numbers and types of physicians and allied personnel being produced were not entirely consistent with the health needs of the population. Therefore, around 1937, the medical schools were withdrawn from the universities and reorganized as medical institutes under the direct control of the Ministry of Health; corresponding responsibility was assumed by this ministry for training pharmacists and all types of middle medical personnel.[23]

This organizational model has been emulated by other countries that have established a Socialist political structure in recent years. Modifications have been made, however, to adapt the model to individual circumstances.

In *Cuba*, after its 1959 revolution, nearly all aspects of health service were integrated under the Ministry of Public Health (MINSAP).[24] The training of all health personnel other than physicians and dentists was included in this consolidation of authority. The University of Havana, a prestigious institution (under general supervision by the Ministry of Education), retained its schools of medicine and dentistry. Two additional medical schools were incorporated into other universities, at Santiago de Cuba and Santa Clara.

To administer its wide range of health programs, MINSAP was organized initially into five directorates, each under a vice minister: (1) personal health care, (2) medical supplies, (3) medical training, (4) hygiene and epidemiology, and (5) economics. These were eventually consolidated into two directorates: hygiene and epidemiology, and personal health care and training. Experience had shown that the training of allied health personnel was most effective when it was closely linked to the hospitals, polyclinics, and other institutions providing personal health care. Medicine and dentistry remained university-based disciplines, however, partly because of a strong tradition and partly because of the need for other disciplines (in the natural sciences, social sciences, and languages) in the teaching programs. Clinical studies by medical and dental students are, of course, done in the MINSAP facilities. (After 1975, moreover, medical and dental education was indeed transferred to MINSAP control.)

The independence of the medical faculties in universities, while all other health manpower production comes under a health ministry, is also found in the People's Democratic Republic of *Czechoslovakia*.[25] In *Poland*, however, the fully integrated model is applied. The traditional university-based disciplines—medicine, stomatology, and pharmacy—have been regrouped under medical academies, which are controlled by the Ministry of Health. Nurses and all other middle medical personnel are trained in special schools, which are also under Ministry of Health supervision.[26] Poland's ten medical academies are supervised by one central department of the Ministry of Health, rather than by various provincial public health authorities, as in the Soviet Union.[27]

The very comprehensive integration of health manpower training with health services in *Poland* is considered by Polish leaders to be beneficial for both sectors. That is, the training programs are designed to meet the needs of the population, while the existence of educational responsibilities in almost all hospitals and other health facilities is stimulating to the daily performance of the health personnel.[28] There is an especially impressive program of postgraduate education, both for specialization and for continuing studies, directed by a national center in Warsaw (under the Ministry of Health) and implemented in all provinces throughout the country.[29]

Regarding the People's Republic of *China*, it may be noted that, in spite of many differences from the concepts of the Soviet Union, the integrated model of health manpower production and health service delivery is also applied.[30] The 110 schools of modern medicine, along with numerous schools of traditional Chinese medicine, are under the control of the Ministry of Health. Nearly all hospitals and health centers are engaged in training various types of health personnel. Even the more than 1.5 million barefoot doctors, who have captured the imagination of people everywhere, get part of their brief training at health centers and part from city physicians who come to the villages. The training of health manpower is very decentralized throughout the health service system.

These demonstrations of the full integration of health manpower production into the system of health services in the Socialist countries obviously warrant careful study by health policymakers from all nations. While the exact administrative arrangements for HSMD coordination must, of course, be adapted to the realities of each country, the

Socialist experience may have useful lessons. In the Polish pattern, for example, an outside observer might suspect that withdrawal of the medical schools from the universities, with their rich tradition in cities like Krakow and Warsaw, would reduce their scientific or scholarly status. The faculty members of the medical academies, however, state that their status is now greater than ever. Previously, they explain, they constituted only a single faculty in a large university with many competing faculties. Now, they have more academic independence and considerably more financial support through the Ministry of Health. Furthermore, they feel a greater collegial relationship with other physicians serving mainly in the health service system.[31]

Enrollment in the medical schools of the Socialist countries tends to be very large, so the teaching responsibilities of the faculty are heavy. It may be noted, however, that teachers are not expected to do much research, which comes under separate institutes. Faculty members are kept alert by widespread involvement not with research, as in most other countries, but with health service.

STRATEGIES FOR COORDINATION

This review of actual experience with several forms of HSMD coordination has been far from complete. Yet it may be enough to demonstrate that the HSMD concept is not simply theory; it has already been implemented in a great variety of ways throughout the world.

It is obvious that the approaches taken in various countries depend on the overall political and social conditions. In most countries, the development of higher education and of the health service system remain predominantly separate. Coordination of their activities usually requires special initiative and effort on the part of the educational institution, the health service agency, or both. This has usually meant articulation or coordination of the two systems only at selected points.

Seven types of actual coordination have been reviewed, and it is evident that there is no single, comprehensive formula that can be applied in all countries. Only in the Socialist countries, with their planned economies, has coordination of health services with manpower development been effectuated on a very large scale, although even in these societies there are significant variations because of local circumstances and history. In most countries, it would seem that progress in HSMD coordination requires initiative at different times and places, when an opportunity is presented. The views of the Organization for

European Cooperation and Development are probably representative of the attitude that would be found in most countries:

> We reject the notion of an educational enterprise slavishly subservient to current health care practices. Equally, we reject the notion of an educational enterprise pursuing its own aims independently of the needs of society and of health care systems. Instead we [wish] to identify means whereby education and health care can unite in a partnership aimed at a series of mutual changes, as improved health care systems of the future evolve . . . [There is a] need to establish mechanisms and processes in the organizations concerned (that is, health and education agencies) in such a way as to enhance their capability to respond more rapidly and effectively to the changing needs of the future.[32]

It should be clear that none of the seven forms of HSMD coordination reviewed above is mutually exclusive. Actions of two, three, or more types could be carried out simultaneously in a country, and this is, in fact, the case in many countries. One may speculate that simultaneous activities of several forms probably have a reinforcing effect such that, if numerous coordinating actions are taken, the whole range of functions in both the service and manpower systems is likely to become better coordinated.

NOTES

1. World Health Organization, *Fifth Report of the World Health Situation 1969–72* (Geneva, 1975), 143.
2. Committee on Health Careers (Personnel and Training), Report to the Hospitals and Health Services Commission, *Australian Health Manpower* (Canberra: Australian Government Publishing Service, 1975).
3. M. I. Roemer and R. Roemer, *Health Manpower under National Health Insurance: The Canadian Experience* (Washington, D.C.: Department of Health, Education, and Welfare, 1976).
4. S. A. Lindgren, "Sweden," in *Health Service Prospects: An International Survey*, I. Douglas-Wilson and G. McLachlan, eds. (London: The Lancet and the Nuffield Provincial Hospitals Trust, 1973), 116.
5. *Ibid.*, 223.
6. Organization for European Cooperation and Development (OECD), *Study of Education of the Health Professions in the Context of Health Care Systems* (Paris, 1975).
7. World Health Organization (WHO), "Report on Consultation on Health Services and Manpower Development, 6–8 September 1976" (Geneva, 1976).

8. L. A. Simeonov, *Better Health for Sri Lanka* (New Delhi: WHO Regional Office for South-East Asia, 1975).

9. M. I. Roemer, *Medical Care in Latin America*, studies and monographs 3 (Washington, D.C.: Pan American Union, 1963).

10. K. Barnard and K. Lee, eds., *NHS Reorganization: Issues and Prospects* (Leeds, England: University of Leeds, Nuffield Centre for Health Services Studies, 1974).

11. K. Evang, *Health Services of Norway* (Oslo: Universitetsforlaget, 1976).

12. M. I. Roemer, "The Development and Current Spectrum of Organized Health Services in a New Asian Country: Malaysia," in *Health Care Systems in World Perspective* (Ann Arbor, Mich.: Health Administration Press, 1976), 45.

13. R. Roemer, "Legal Systems Regulating Health Personnel," *Milbank Memorial Fund Quarterly* 46 (October 1968):431–71.

14. M. I. Roemer, *The Organization of Medical Care under Social Security: A Study Based on the Experience of Eight Countries* (Geneva: International Labour Office, 1969).

15. R. Roemer and M. I. Roemer, *Health Manpower in the Changing Australian Health Services Scene* (Washington, D.C.: Department of Health, Education, and Welfare, 1976), 41–42.

16. L. W. Jayesuria, *A Review of the Rural Health Services in West Malaysia* (Kuala Lumpur: Ministry of Health, 1967).

17. T. L. Hall, *Health Manpower in Peru: A Case Study in Planning* (Baltimore: Johns Hopkins Press, 1969).

18. A. Engle, *Perspectives in Health Planning* (London: Athlone Press, 1968).

19. F. T. Sai, "Ghana," in *Health Service Prospects*, 125–55.

20. WHO, *Report on Consultation.*

21. *Ibid.*

22. M. M. Chaves, *Strategies for Improving Health in Latin America* (Battle Creek, Mich.: W. K. Kellogg Foundation, 1976), 15–16.

23. H. E. Sigerist, *Medicine and Health in the Soviet Union* (New York: Citadel Press, 1947).

24. M. I. Roemer, *Cuban Health Services and Resources* (Washington, D.C.: Pan American Health Organization, 1976).

25. E. R. Weinerman, *Social Medicine in Eastern Europe* (Cambridge, Mass.: Harvard University Press, 1969).

26. J. Leowski, ed., *Health Service in Poland* (Warsaw: Polish Medical Publishers, 1974).

27. J. R. Missett, et al., "Undergraduate Medical Education in Poland: Variation on the Soviet Theme," *Journal of Medical Education* 49(October 1974):979–84.

28. J. Indulski and J. Kaminski, "The Role of the State in the Development of the Citizens' Health Protection," *Santé Publique* (Bucharest, Rumania) 18(1975):389–402.

29. E. Ruzyllo, "A Uniform Nationwide System of Continuing Medical Education, with Special Reference to Postgraduate Studies," *Materia Medica Polona* 4 (July–September 1972):140–51.

30. V. W. Sidel and R. Sidel, *Serve the People—Observations on Medicine in the People's Republic of China* (New York: Josiah Macy, Jr. Foundation, 1973).
31. M. I. Roemer, personal observation, Poland, October 1976.
32. OECD, *Study of Education.*

24

Health Care Insurance—
Its Worldwide Diversity

References to social insurance or social security support of medical care costs have been made throughout this book. Usually referred to as "health insurance," this economic mechanism has been a crucial feature of the health care system in many countries. The health insurance experience of one country often influences policy in other countries, but the methods of implementation differ greatly among nations. This chapter offers an overview of health insurance as a highly adaptable, worldwide strategy in health care systems.

The pattern of health insurance with which most Americans are familiar is the use of insurance to pay doctor, hospital, or related bills for services rendered along conventional lines. The doctor or hospital gives services to a patient, and the "third party," which carries the patient's insurance, simply pays a fee to the provider or may indemnify the patient for all or part of the fee he has personally paid. There may be numerous variations on this theme, but in nearly all of them the customary pattern of delivering the health service is unaffected: health insurance is regarded simply as a way of paying medical bills.

A wider view of the development of health insurance—or, as Europeans most often call it, sickness insurance—around the world indicates that this familiar U.S. conception is by no means universal. In

Based on a paper presented at George Washington University, Washington, D.C., May 1980.

fact, there is great diversity among the patterns of health services delivery under the insurance mechanism, whether statutory or voluntary. These patterns of delivery, as well as the exact procedures by which funds are raised, have evolved along several paths at different times and places.

BACKGROUND

After many decades in which working people enlisted in private insurance societies, Germany in 1883 enacted the first law mandating that certain types of low-income workers be insured to meet the costs of sickness. These costs were twofold: (1) compensation for the wages lost because of disabling illness and (2) the costs of medical care. This first social insurance law, which was enacted by the conservative government of Chancellor Otto Von Bismarck, required that employers share the costs of periodic premiums with the workers; the government also contributed on the ground that the program would relieve public agencies of welfare burdens they might otherwise have to bear.

For several decades a Socialist movement had been growing in Central Europe (the *Communist Manifesto* was issued in 1848), and by this legislation Bismarck hoped to attract the support of workers away from the expanding Social Democratic party. Recognizing this strategy, Socialists in the Bundestag (parliament) actually opposed the idea as paternalism and pauper's insurance. Coverage was, indeed, mandatory only for low-paid workers, on the assumption that workers with higher incomes, along with middle-class families, could pay for their medical services privately. This policy also satisfied the doctors, who would retain their private market of more affluent patients, while getting paid for services to poorer workers and their dependents who would otherwise seek free care in public outpatient facilities.

The idea of social insurance soon spread to other European countries—first to Austria-Hungary and eventually to every other country on the continent. As the popularity of the programs with the workers became apparent, the left-wing political parties changed their views and supported the concept, calling, in fact, for extension of both the persons covered and the benefits provided. While insurance for general medical care and short-term disability came first, it was soon followed by protection against wage loss and medical expenses of work injuries, financed solely by employers. Pensions for old age or permanent invalidity followed, along with survivors' benefits (life insurance) when the breadwinner died. As the social insurance funds enlarged, family allowances were added—that is, supplements to regular wages to help bear the costs of raising children. In the twentieth century, unemployment compensation—to replace part of the earnings lost during layoffs—became still another social insurance benefit.

In the health insurance sector, the range of benefits was extended along several lines. Initially, protection tended to be limited to out-of-hospital services of physicians and prescribed drugs; hospital care in this period, used infrequently anyway, was provided free in public hospitals for low-income persons. As the quality and importance of hospitalization increased with advances in medical science, insured families wanted greater amenities than those found in the large public wards, and benefits were added for furnishing hospital care in semiprivate rooms. Later, dental services became insured in some countries, as well as sometimes eyeglasses; there were typically various limitations on these services under insurance, requiring the patient to pay part of the costs.

The general health insurance idea was first extended outside Europe in 1921—to Japan. (Insurance for work-related injuries had been established in the United States in 1910, but this workmen's compensation was not broadened to general medical care until 1965, when Medicare for the aged was enacted.) Chile was the first developing country to adopt social insurance for general medical care of workers, in 1924. Both Japan and Chile were much influenced by Germany, although they did not emulate the German model of health care delivery. With the worldwide economic depression of the 1930's, several more countries adopted general health insurance for selected population groups; another leap in the number of countries with insurance coverage occurred after World War II. By 1979, there were 75 countries—some on every continent—with some form of social insurance for general medical care to part or all of their populations. This meant that nearly half of the world's 160 sovereign nations and all of those that were predominantly industrialized had statutory health insurance of one sort or another.

The diversity of patterns through which the idea of medical care insurance is implemented can be best appreciated by reviewing the main developments in different regions of the globe.

EUROPEAN MODELS

The pattern of medical care delivery associated with the pioneer German health insurance law was simply an extension of the private practice model, which had become firmly established by the 1880's. Since higher income persons got their medical care from individual doctors rather than at crowded and impersonal public outpatient clinics, it was natural for workers, contributing to the costs of their own insurance, to expect similar arrangements. Likewise, medications would be obtained from private pharmacies. The *Krankenkassen*, or sickness funds, that preceded the statutory program paid the full physician costs—that is, with no copayments or cost sharing by the patient—so the statutory program continued that policy. Indeed, the hundreds of *Krankenkassen* had become such vested interests by the 1880's that they could hardly be ignored in the formulation of the law. Although Bismarck had personally favored a unified national health insurance system, the funds had sufficient political strength to win a key role in the administration of the program. In effect, the law simply required that certain workers must be insured and that employers contribute to the costs of the insurance, but these requirements were ordinarily met by enrollment in existing *Krankenkassen*.

The *Krankenkassen* gradually came under increasing regulation by the central government. In Germany, and in the many countries emulating it, regulating authority was placed in the Ministry of Labor, since the economic protection of working people was the main purpose. The *Krankenkassen*, in turn, negotiated with doctors about the fees to be paid for their services. Various funds with similar political, religious, or occupational characteristics would often join together in federations, to achieve certain administrative economies and to increase their bargaining power with the doctors regarding fees.

In response, the physicians in Germany formed associations for the purpose of negotiating with the federations. Eventually there evolved a pattern in which a sickness fund paid to a medical association a flat amount periodically (usually every three months) for each enrolled member. The medical association then paid fees to the individual doctors, but since the monies were limited it had to exercise some surveillance over expenditures. This led to various systems for identifying abuse, by doctors and patients. If there was not sufficient money to pay all fees in a given quarter-year, doctors would have to accept less than full payment for services rendered in that period. (Eventually the mechanism was modified to assure full payment of medical fees.)

The great complexities of the German health insurance program led to the imposition of various constraints in the laws enacted by other countries later. The Belgian law of 1894 did not mandate coverage of any type of worker, but simply regulated the operations of the local sickness funds. It subsidized the funds in order to increase their stability and to help them enroll low-paid workers; not until a half-century later (1944) was enrollment made compulsory. Even though the funds were voluntary, however, they constrained utilization of medical care by requiring that patients pay a share, usually 25 percent, of all medical bills and prescriptions.

Legislation in the Scandinavian countries enacted between 1910 and 1915 imposed copayment requirements on the patient from the outset.

Eventually copayment was limited to the first two encounters in an episode of illness, on the ground that subsequent services were dependent on the decision of the doctor rather than the patient. Copayments were waived for indigent persons and pensioners and were not payable by anyone for hospitalization. In fact, Swedish hospitals were financed mainly by local provincial revenues for every resident, not just for the poor, both before and after social insurance. This included the services of hospital doctors—specialists almost entirely on full-time salaries from the hospital. Coverage in the Scandinavian countries was initially through enrollment of people in local societies, as in Germany. Eventually, however (in Norway, it was in 1930), the separate societies lost their autonomy and became branch offices of the national insurance institution. Coverage was made universal in 1956 in Norway and a little later in the other Scandinavian countries.

The national health insurance law in Great Britain was enacted in 1911, under Liberal Prime Minister Lloyd George. It mandated coverage only of low-income manual workers, not their dependents. Benefits were limited to general practitioners' services and prescribed drugs. Hospital and specialists' services had long been available to working-class people without charge at public general hospitals and some voluntary hospitals. Dependents of workers and others could voluntarily join the same friendly societies, as local insurance organizations were called, that covered the primary worker. Other organizations also sold private insurance for hospitalization, which would entitle the subscriber to a private or semiprivate room and the physician of his choice.

The response of the British program to the problem of cost control under insurance linked to private medical practice was to abandon fee-for-service remuneration. Instead, all covered workers were required to choose a GP from among those participating—virtually all doctors in any working-class area. Then the friendly society would pay a flat monthly amount for every worker on a doctor's list or panel, regardless of the specific services rendered to patients that month. A GP would naturally try to attract as large a panel of potential patients as possible, because his income depended on the length of the list. He had no financial incentive to render excessive services, while at the same time he had to keep patients satisfied or they would leave his panel for another doctor's. Aside from this built-in cost-control mechanism, the capitation pattern of general practice, which was retained after enactment of the national health service in 1948, had the great virtue of assuring every insured worker a primary care provider as the point of entry to the whole medical care system.

It was not until 1928 that France enacted social insurance for medical care of industrial workers, though there were hundreds of local mutual benefit societies operating before that time. The French medical profession was so strong and so individualistic, however, that it succeeded in having the insurance operate on an indemnity basis— that is, reimbursing the worker only after he had paid the doctor personally. Thus, the doctor was free to charge the patient whatever he wished, and the patient could then seek reimbursement from his mutual society at a rate of 80 percent of the official schedule. The doctor was not obligated to follow this fee schedule in his charges, however, so the patient might end up with less than 80 percent indemnification of actual charges. In later years, especially as economic conditions worsened, French doctors agreed to follow the official schedule of fees, but there have been recurrent controversies about this issue. Developments have been somewhat similar in Belgium, where the local health insurance funds also retain a great deal of autonomy.

Social insurance coverage for most medical care costs gradually spread throughout every country of Europe, although in the more agricultural countries of East Europe it was confined usually to industrial workers, who were a minority of the population. In Germany and France today, about 90 but not 100 percent of the population is mandatorily insured; most of the remaining people have voluntary health insurance, leaving only a handful without any insurance protection. Pensioners and other recipients of public assistance are typically enrolled in the regular statutory insurance system through governmental revenue subsidies.

INITIAL DEVELOPMENTS OUTSIDE EUROPE

The idea of mandatory health insurance for industrial workers spread to Japan and Chile in the 1920s, but the patterns of organization were different. In Japan, there were no workers' mutual aid funds, but the industrial establishments became the principal framework of the statutory insurance. Managerial paternalism was part of the Japanese tradition, and a fund was established in each major company to pay the medical expenses of its workers. For insurance of workers in smaller companies, separate funds were organized by groups of employers. Typically there was free choice of doctor and fee-for-service remuneration, as in Europe. For dependents, on the other hand, the benefits were usually only 50 or 60 percent of the official fees, related doubtless to the inferior status of women in Japan. Extension of mandatory health insurance to self-employed persons, to farmers, and to others occurred in Japan only after World War II. A separate national fund was established to cover these people.

Developments in Chile differed even more from those in Europe. Here, the mass of the population was really poor, and the market for private patients was small. Doctors could hardly demand fees for serving manual workers and were glad to be offered steady salaries. Hence, the health insurance program, which was one large national institution under the Ministry of Labor rather than a network of local sickness funds, employed doctors to work in health centers. These health centers were constructed by the institution and provided ambulatory care. Typically the doctors worked in the insurance program two or three hours per day and received monthly salaries. Hospitalization was provided in the existing governmental or charitable hospitals, with attendance also by salaried doctors. Since the workers were paying at least part of the costs, hospital amenities were somewhat better for them than for the indigent. Dependents were not covered at all in the original Chilean program, so a sick wife might be served in a large open ward of the hospital while her insured husband occupied a semiprivate room.

Not only were dependents excluded in the initial Chilean legislation, agricultural workers were excluded, despite their being more numerous than industrial workers. White-collar workers, on the other hand, organized small voluntary health insurance societies for themselves. Later these were consolidated in the governmental National Medical Service for Employees, which is still separate from the program for manual workers.

Brazil started a national health insurance institute for industrial workers in 1931. Soon after, six other national institutes were established for transport workers, commercial employees, governmental civil servants, railroad and utility workers, maritime workers, and bank employees. Each of these organizations had its own medical personnel and facilities. Not until the 1970s, under a military government that was bent on efficiency and economy, were the seven separate health insurance institutes integrated into one national social insurance program.

Peru passed a law to cover industrial workers with health insurance in 1936. At first, like Chile and Brazil, the program provided ambulatory care in special health centers and used existing hospitals for inpatient care. Then, in 1939, the Peruvian social security program built in Lima the first general hospital exclusively for insured workers. The governmental and charitable hospitals in Peru were deemed inadequate to provide high quality care for insured persons. Soon afterward, a separate health insurance program for white-collar employees was launched; it also had its own special hospitals, which were more spacious and better equipped than the workers' hospitals. The Peruvian pattern of separate "social security hospitals," as they are called, then spread rapidly throughout Latin America. It was adopted in Brazil and eventually in 18 of the 20 Latin American countries that had launched social insurance programs for medical care by 1970. In nearly all these countries until about the last decade, however, the health insurance system covered only a small percentage of the national population—typically between 5 and 15 percent.

White-collar employees not only had a separate insurance system with different facilities and personnel, they often had a "dual choice" pattern of medical care delivery. To adjust to employees' tastes, and to satisfy national medical associations with their increasing political strength, these middle-class employees could use the insurance body's health centers and hospitals, if they wished, without charge. If they preferred, however, they could consult a private physician and pay part of the medical and hospital charges themselves—usually 33 to 50 percent of the total.

The Latin American pattern of providing medical care to insured persons in health centers and hospitals built and controlled by the insurance organization, with doctors and other health personnel employed by the organization, may be described as the direct pattern of medical care delivery under health insurance. It may be contrasted with the indirect pattern used in Europe, under which the insurance system paid for medical services rendered by independent personnel or facilities, or sometimes only indemnified the insured person for expenses that he personally incurred. Broadly speaking, since about 1940 the direct pattern has been used in the lower income, developing countries, while the indirect pattern has been implemented in the wealthier, industrialized countries. This generalization, however, requires special qualifications with respect to certain types of services, particularly hospitalization.

DEVELOPMENTS AFTER WORLD WAR II

The second World War was a watershed for medical care organization, along with most other social issues. The health insurance concept spread to all other continents and changed its character in Europe, as well.

In 1945, Turkey started a statutory health insurance program for employed workers in the main cities, Istanbul and Ankara. The direct pattern of medical care delivery was used. Soon other Middle Eastern countries did the same: Iran in 1949, Iraq in 1956, Tunisia in 1960, and Lebanon in 1963. In Tunisia, the strategy of organization had one important difference. A former French colony on North Africa's Mediterranean coast, Tunisia was a very poor country. The social insurance body, instead of building its own facilities and engaging its own personnel, contracted with the Ministry of Health to provide medical services for insured workers through the ministry's health facilities and personnel; with the additional money from social insurance, these resources could be expanded. Thus the doctors and other medical personnel serving insured people were part of the same corps that served the general population. They were not paid higher salaries and furnished more favorable working conditions, serious points of contention between health ministries and the separate social security systems in Latin America.

A similar policy was implemented in India's public insurance program for certain industrial workers, which had been started in 1948. Reflecting the weak industrial development of that country, the program was limited to (1) employees of private firms (2) with 20 or more workers (3) using electrical power and (4) covering only workers earning under 500 rupees per month (about $100 U.S. at the time). The Employees State Insurance Corporation (ESIC), which administered the program, covered about 15 million workers at 356 industrial locations, some 3 percent of the Indian population at that time.

As was the case in Tunisia, but not in most other developing countries, ESIC attempted to have an integrated approach with the Indian Ministry of Health. In the main, it used its funds to contract with the ministry for service to insured workers by regular ministry personnel and facilities. In some places that had heavy concentrations of covered workers, ESIC funds were used to enable the Ministry of Health to construct new facilities. In other places, workers could select a participating GP, who was paid on a capitation basis (as in Great Britain); this usually occurred in large cities. Cooperation between the social insurance program and the Ministry of Health in India has clearly been beneficial for both.

The nationwide health insurance program that took shape in Israel when it became an independent nation in 1948 was unique. The Federation of Jewish Workers had been organized in Palestine around 1900; bringing ideas from Europe, these workers organized a sickness insurance fund, the *Kupat Holim,* in 1912. Under the British mandate over Palestine after World War I, the *Kupat Holim* grew rapidly. By the time of Israel's statehood, despite its voluntary character, the program covered at least half the population; by 1960, this proportion reached 85 percent. At the same time, governmental social insurance in Israel was limited to maternity cash grants for working women or the wives of working men. Unlike voluntary health insurance in Europe or North America, however, the *Kupat Holim* delivered medical care by the direct pattern. All doctors and other health personnel were and are salaried employees of the organization, and they provide service in health centers and hospitals owned by it. Because of the Federation's great political strength, the *Kupat Holim* has been able to maintain its independence. Only in the 1970s were serious steps taken in Israel to develop a governmentally controlled health insurance program; in the scheme being planned, the administrative structure and resources of the *Kupat Holim* will continue to play a role.

Canada also took governmental action to establish social insurance for medical care after World War II. Saskatchewan had suffered greatly during the 1930s, and in 1944 it elected a semi-Socialist government, the Cooperative Commonwealth Federation. By 1946, legislation had been passed to extend to the population of the entire province insurance for virtually unlimited care in general hospitals. In Canada, as in the United States, there was a growing voluntary insurance movement for hospital care at the time, but the Saskatchewan Hospital Services Plan was the first such statutory program covering an entire population. Soon the province of British Columbia followed suit. The experience proved so favorable that by 1957 the national government enacted legislation to share approximately half the cost of any provincial program of hospitalization insurance meeting federal standards. Within a few years, social insurance for general hospitalization and for outpatient diagnostic services was nationwide in Canada.

In 1962, Saskatchewan again did the pioneering, with a social insurance program for ambulatory and inpatient physician care. In spite of a strike by physicians that obstructed the start of the program for 23 days, it soon proved so successful that by 1966 the national government again took legislative action to share in the costs of any such provincial program; all provinces had joined in the scheme by 1971. The indirect pattern of medical care delivery is used in Canada, with physicians paid on the basis of a fee schedule negotiated in each province. Hospitals, however, are paid by the provinces on the basis of a flat prospective budget (rather than by either per diem or individual item billing), which greatly simplifies administration and promotes economical management.

Australia also had voluntary insurance for medical care for some years, but in 1950 it enacted its first social insurance law in the health field. Initially, the sole benefit was payment for costly and lifesaving drugs prescribed for anyone—the only national health insurance program to start that way. Strictly speaking, this was not insurance, since it was financed by general revenues for the entire population. Gradually the pharmaceutical benefits were extended to virtually all prescribed drugs. In 1953 legislation was enacted to encourage greater enrollment in voluntary insurance plans by governmental sharing in the costs of hospitalization of insured persons. In 1970 the amount of this subsidy was made greater for low-income families, to enable voluntary insurance plans to enroll such families at lower premiums.

In 1972, after 20 years of relatively conservative government, the Labour party was elected to power in Australia, and in 1974 universal national health insurance with quite comprehensive benefits was enacted. A fiscal crisis developed in 1976, however, leading to the defeat of the Labour party. The more conservative Liberal-Farmers coalition government then took action to dismantle the new national health insurance program. By 1979 the Australian health insurance system had been returned essentially to its previous voluntary form. This is the only instance that I know of where an established national health insurance program has been undone for a period. The Labour party was returned to power, however, in 1983 and took steps to reinstate nationwide health insurance.

SOCIALISM AND SOCIALIZED HEALTH CARE

Until World War II, all the countries considered so far had health insurance with somewhat less than 100 percent population coverage. The first country to achieve universal coverage for both curative and preventive health services was the Soviet Union after the Russian Revolution of 1917. Socialized medicine was not accomplished all at once, however. In the cities, certain industrial workers, comprising about 12 percent of the population, had had health insurance protection previously; this coverage was gradually extended to the entire urban population through insurance contributions made by all enterprises. The rural population of the USSR was initially served by a separate public medical system developed from the district *zemstvo* medicine program started under the Czars. This program made great use of *feldshers*, who were supervised by relatively few physicians and financed by central revenues.

Not until 1937 were the urban and rural programs unified into one national health service financed from general public revenues and offering equal benefits to all. Doctors and all other health personnel were on full-time salary, working in governmental health centers, polyclinics, and hospitals. Responsibilities were delegated through a regionalized network of facilities in each province, and the delivery of therapeutic and preventive services was integrated by teams of personnel. Private medical practice was never abolished in the Soviet Union, and a little of it still exists. As the public system became stronger, however, the market for private patients naturally diminished. The Soviet strategy had been to train vast numbers of medical personnel—proportionately more than in Western Europe or the United States—but to pay them relatively modest salaries.

With World War II, the Soviet health services, along with the entire national economy, suffered massive setbacks. The period from 1945 to 1960 was one of reconstruction. By 1970 enough doctors had been trained to eliminate the need for new *feldshers*. (Ironically, this was just when the United States was starting to train physicians' assistants (from Vietnam war veterans) and later nurse-practitioners, mainly to provide primary care to the poor in rural areas and urban slums.)

The several countries of Eastern Europe that adopted a Socialist form of government after World War II emulated, in large part, the Soviet pattern of health care. Typically, they started by extending the previous social insurance programs, eventually developing a unified national system financed by general public revenues. A hallmark of all these systems was centralized planning, which led to massive increases of personnel and facilities. Another key feature was unification of virtually all health-related activities (including manpower training, research, and drug production) and all preventive and treatment services under a single national ministry of health. Special efforts were made in all the Eastern European Socialist countries to equalize the distribution of personnel between urban and rural areas.

The Liberation of China and the country's development into a socialized economy began in 1949. In the first decade of the People's Republic, much guidance was offered by and accepted from the Soviet Union. In the cities, health insurance was extended for the industrial workers, with partial copayments required for dependents, as in Japan. A separate system was developed for the huge rural population, based largely on the structure of the agricultural communes. The latter are essentially local units of government built around cooperative ownership and control of land, each containing between 10,000 and 50,000 people. Each commune supports at least one health center, which is staffed by both modern and traditional Chinese doctors along with other personnel. Several communes make up a county, of which there are 2,200, each having a hospital.

With the Great Proletarian Cultural Revolution of 1965–70, there was a dramatic shift of emphasis from the urban to the rural population's health care. The barefoot doctor was created to serve the people at the level of the production brigade (of about 1,500 members), into which communes are divided. The barefoot doctor is a peasant, chosen and trusted by the people, who receives brief training (three to six months) in preventive services, family planning, environmental sanitation, health education, and initial treatment of common ailments. Most barefoot doctors are young men or women who are paid the same way as other peasants, on the basis of the work they do. The barefoot doctor and his or her store of drugs and supplies are often supported by a cooperative fund of the production brigade, but patients may also have to pay small fees into this fund for specific treatments. The cooperative fund may also pay charges for services rendered at the health centers or hospitals, although these facilities are under the network controlled by the Ministry of Health. China is still a very poor country and has not yet attained the economic strength to offer everyone health services without charge.

Since the death of Chairman Mao Tse-tung in 1976 and the formation of a new government, China has been stressing longer training of the barefoot doctors and fuller use generally of modern scientific technology. Nevertheless, even up to 1976 China had made remarkable achievements in its people's health, largely through greatly improved nutrition, effective communicable disease control and environmental sanitation, successful family planning, and wide extension of primary health care.

Another Socialist health care pattern is illustrated in Cuba, which had its Revolution in 1959. Unlike most Latin American countries, Cuba had not developed a general statutory health insurance program for industrial workers, but had only maternity service benefits for workers' wives and for working women. About 7 percent of the population, predominantly middle-income people in the main cities, belonged to voluntary prepaid medical care plans or *mutualistas*. These were organized mainly by groups of doctors, who usually also owned a hospital and other facilities. These medical care societies continued to operate as one division of the Ministry of Public Health until around 1970, when they became fully integrated into the national system.

Based on advice principally from Czechoslovakia, Cuba developed a health care system based largely on the Soviet model. It trained only a few *feldsher*-type medical assistants, however, but it greatly increased the output of doctors. (The need for doctors was especially urgent because about half the country's doctors fled after the revolution.) Several hundred polyclinics, staffed by teams of doctors and allied personnel, constitute the basic framework of the Cuban system. Each unit provides complete ambulatory care to about 25,000 people. Priority in development of resources has gone to the rural areas. As in the Soviet system, all health services are financed from general revenues except out-of-hospital drugs, for which small charges are payable at governmental pharmacies. All health-related activities, including personnel training, are supervised by the Ministry of Public Health. After 20 years of the socialized system, the Cuban health record (life expectancy, infant mortality, and so on) has become the best of any Latin American country.

EVOLUTION OF NATIONAL HEALTH SERVICES

The four Socialist countries just described established their health care systems, which cover their entire populations and are financed from general revenues, after a social revolution. Even after such a sudden and comprehensive change in the power structure, a socialized system, with its integrated organization and control of all personnel and facilities, cannot take shape overnight. It takes years to create the needed resources and to organize them into a unified, comprehensive framework. The People's Republic of China is still in a relatively early stage of this developmental process.

Free enterprise, or capitalist, countries may develop many of the features of socialized systems, but a longer period of evolution is required. By "many of the features," I refer to universal population coverage or integration of preventive and curative services or general revenue financing or salaried employment of doctors and others in teams or centralized planning to meet population needs—but not necessarily all of these features. The evolutionary path seems to pass invariably through a stage of national health *insurance*, which serves to establish the value and feasibility of collective financing, even though it is based on a relatively conservative form of taxation. Then some political change within the setting of parliamentary democracies is usually necessary to move from the stage of insurance to a national health service.

National health services differ from country to country, but the best known one is doubtless Great Britain's. National health insurance covering GPs' services and drugs for manual workers (not their dependents) had been enacted, it will be recalled, in 1911. Over the subsequent decades, public and voluntary hospitals had developed, local public health services had expanded, and voluntary health insurance had grown. During World War II, England organized its hospitals into regional networks to make more efficient the emergency care of war casualties. The British people, civilian as well as military, suffered greatly during the war, and to raise morale Prime Minister Winston Churchill and President Franklin Roosevelt formulated goals for the war as early as August 1941. In the Atlantic Charter they declared that the war was intended not only to defeat fascism, but also to assure all people "freedom from want." This included access to comprehensive health care for everyone, the specific requirements of which were outlined in 1942 in the Beveridge Report.

Immediately after the war, in spite of the great leadership of Churchill and the Conservative party during the war, the Labour party was elected to power. In 1946, some 35 years after statutory health insurance had begun, the national health service was enacted, with a starting date of July 1948. Essentially, the NHS offered comprehensive health services to everyone, with financial support coming mainly (though not entirely) from general revenues. Three parallel administrative structures were established, based largely on existing arenas of power, to provide care: (1) ambulatory care, including GP services, prescribed drugs, and dental and optical care, was provided through a network of local executive councils; (2) hospital and specialist services were provided through regional hospital boards, each controlling the facilities and their personnel and serving about 3 million people; and (3) public health, visiting nurse, ambulance, and certain other services were provided through several hundred existing local government authorities. Medical specialists, along with all other personnel in hospitals, were salaried and employed full-time or nearly full-time by the regional boards, a pattern similar to that found in Socialist countries and in Britain, to a lesser extent, before the NHS. The GPs, dentists, and pharmacists, however, remained in private practice while being paid by the government. Thus, the indirect pattern of medical care delivery was retained in Britain for ambulatory care, even though GPs were paid by capitation rather than fee-for-service.

It took another 26 years before the three components of the British NHS were integrated under a network of area health authorities and regional health boards in 1974. In each area health authority there is a community medicine specialist who is expected to supervise and integrate all health services of the three previous components. A community health council of local citizens is also chosen for advisory purposes. This integrated administration is expected to place greater emphasis on preventive services by incorporating them in the services of hospitals and ambulatory care providers, as well as in the traditional local public health authorities. Private practice has never been forbidden in Great Britain, and in recent years, with severe economic constraints on the financing of the NHS, it has expanded for a small class of affluent people. Voluntary health insurance, in fact, has increased to support private medical fees.

Action by New Zealand to cover all of its population with entitlement to general medical care was actually taken earlier than in Britain. In 1939, this small country in the South Pacific (with a population of about 2 million) enacted a health program with many features of a national health service, even though it was described as national health insurance. Unlike the European health insurance systems, New Zealand's system placed responsibility for heath care not in local sickness funds under a Ministry of Labor, but in the Ministry of Health, which also supervised the preventive services and hospitals. Almost all hospitals were publicly controlled under regional authorities, and specialists in these were predominantly full-time salaried employees. General practitioners remained in private practice, but they were paid on a fee-for-service basis, and cost sharing was required of the patient. Financial support for ambulatory services and drugs in New Zealand is drawn from an earmarked social security fund, but the hospital and specialist services, which involve an increasing majority of all costs, are supported from general revenues. There is also a growing movement to establish health centers throughout New Zealand for delivery of ambulatory care by teams of health personnel.

The Scandinavian countries, particularly Sweden and Norway, are further examples of the evolution of national health insurance programs toward 100 percent population coverage and financial support predominantly from general revenues. In Norway, the first health insurance legislation, in 1909, simply provided that certain standards be met by local sickness funds, which were to be supervised by a national social insurance authority. In 1930, the local funds were converted into branch offices of the National Insurance Institution, a component of the Ministry of Social Affairs. By the 1940s, a majority of the population was covered by health insurance, but it was still not compulsory for everyone. Extension to universal coverage occurred finally in 1956. After World War II, hospitals and their staffs of salaried specialists were expanded; their services were financed partially by general revenues of local provincial governments and partially by the National Insurance Institution. An increasing share of total health expenditures in recent years has come from general revenues rather than social insurance. This applies also to ambulatory medical care, which is provided by a national network of salaried district doctors, and to dental care of children furnished by publicly employed dentists.

In the less economically developed world, Chile illustrates well the evolution of a health care system from the national insurance model to one with many characteristics of a national health service. Mandatory health insurance, it will be recalled, started in Latin America with the Chilean legislation of 1924. Coverage was limited, however, to industrial workers, not including their dependents or the much larger population of agricultural workers or peasants. Then in 1952, borrowing the term from Great Britain, Chile launched its *Servicio Nacional de Salud*. The nation's three main subsystems of health care were unified under this service: (1) the social security program and its polyclinics for industrial workers, with coverage extended to their dependents; (2) the network of charitable or "beneficencia" hospitals for the poor; and (3) all hospitals, health centers, and personnel of the Ministry of Health. It was estimated that some 70 percent of the Chilean population was covered by the service. Financial support continued from the social security fund, but most of the costs were met from general revenues.

The principal exclusions were white-collar employees, who were often in voluntary health insurance plans. In 1968, however, coverage was extended to these middle-class people on a dual-choice basis—that is, permitting the use of private doctors and hospitals with substantial cost sharing, as explained earlier. With the election of the Popular Unity government of Salvador Allende (himself a physician and former Minister of Health) in 1970, coverage was extended to virtually the entire population. In 1973, the Allende government was overthrown by a military coup, and financial support of the national health service was greatly reduced. In line with the conservative economic policies of the military government, the service's public sector program was weakened and private medical care was strengthened. The legal structure of the national health service, however, remains.

Other countries have taken similar action to unify their separate medical care insurance programs with the programs of their ministries of health and other agencies. In the 1970s, this was accomplished in Costa Rica, and major steps toward this end were taken in Venezuela. In the Middle East, the social security health care program of Iraq (started in 1956) was brought under the Ministry of Health in the late 1970s, and similar consolidation has recently been brought about in Libya. Greece enacted legislation for a unified health system in 1983. These strategies of integration are essentially moves toward the concept of a national health service.

Perhaps the most internationally important demonstration of this evolutionary process occurred recently in Italy. As in other European countries, voluntary mutual aid societies for medical care had grown up in Italy since the nineteenth century. After World War II, with the fall of fascism, coverage was made mandatory for most industrial workers, and the numerous mutual societies were converted into local branches of a national health insurance system. By the 1970s, coverage reached over 90 percent of the population, although the range of benefits differed among local societies. Then, in 1977 Italy's several left-wing political parties gained substantial strength in the parliament. In 1978, a national health service was legislated, under which 100 percent of the population would be covered and financial support would be shifted gradually to general revenues. Physicians would be free to remain in private practice or to be employed in hospitals and health centers on salary. The whole system will be administered by a greatly strengthened Ministry of Health, which will manage all health resources and programs through Italy's 20 political regions (see chapter 25).

HEALTH INSURANCE IN THE UNITED STATES

This worldwide overview of national health insurance developments has so far deliberately omitted the United States. Before suggesting any lessons to be drawn from international experience, it may be helpful to review the development of U.S. health insurance in outline form:

1. 1798—mandatory health insurance of merchant seamen to support a network of marine hospitals at major ports
2. Nineteenth century—voluntary health insurance through deductions from the wages of workers in isolated industries to support physician and hospital care
3. Late nineteenth and early twentieth centuries—voluntary insurance for physician care to members of fraternal orders in large cities, mainly European immigrants
4. 1910—workmen's compensation under state laws to meet costs of medical care and wage losses in injured industrial worker's, with all states covered by 1950
5. 1915–20—efforts to enact social insurance for low-paid workers in many state legislatures, none of which was successful

6. 1929—origin of voluntary insurance for hospital care, later called Blue Cross and sponsored by hospitals

7. 1939—equivalent rise of voluntary insurance for physician care during hospitalization, sponsored by state medical societies

8. 1939—introduction in July of the first national health bill by Senator Robert Wagner, sponsor of the Social Security Act of 1935 (the bill was dropped at the onset of World War II in September)

9. 1943–52—introduction of and debate on national health insurance and public health bills in successive drafts, with bitter nationwide controversy

10. 1943—origin of large, comprehensive health insurance programs based on prepaid group medical practice, for example the Health Insurance Plan of Greater New York and the Kaiser-Permanente Health Plan in California

11. 1945 and onward—commercial insurance companies stimulated to massive sales of group insurance for hospital and medical expenses of inpatient care (done previously on a small scale, but greatly accelerated) with the threat of national health insurance

12. 1955—origin of insurance for major medical expenses, to protect against catastrophic costs of a wide range of medical services, but with substantial deductibles and copayments

13. 1957–64—recognition of inadequate voluntary health insurance protection for the aged, rising problem of chronic illness and its costs among the aged, and introduction of various proposals for national health insurance protection of the elderly

14. 1965—enactment of Medicare (for national insurance of the medical and hospital costs of the aged) and Medicaid (for greater public support, from both federal and state revenues, of medical care for the poor)

15. 1970–75—introduction of 23 wide-ranging national health insurance bills in Congress, associated with a critical escalation of all health care costs

16. 1973—legislation to promote health maintenance organizations as a strategy for constraining costs by modifying incentives in the medical care system

17. 1976–80—a new era of debate about national health insurance, emphasizing benefits for catastrophic illnesses and incorporation of private health insurance carriers in any national program

18. 1981—emphasis on competition among private health insurance plans

This is hardly a comprehensive account of U.S. health insurance developments over the last 183 years, but it may be enough to provide a framework for suggesting some major lessons from foreign experience.

LESSONS OF THE INTERNATIONAL EXPERIENCE

Perhaps the overriding lesson of the international health insurance experience is that policies are intimately linked with overall economic and political developments. The rise of the insurance mechanism to cover health care costs was basically an outgrowth of the Industrial Revolution, the emergence of a large working class dependent on wages for survival, and recognition of the value of cooperation to cope with risks, such as the costs of sickness.

Beyond this, there have been several social trends which can be identified in the forms that health insurance organization have taken in numerous countries. I would suggest that these give us certain insights about necessary, or at least probable, directions to be taken by health insurance in the United States' future:

1. The growth of voluntary health insurance leads inevitably to statutory insurance, because of both the strength and weakness of voluntary programs: on the one hand, voluntary health insurance demonstrates the feasibility and value of the idea of health insurance; on the other hand, its operation leaves various inadequacies and inequities that can be corrected only by governmental action.

2. In affluent, industrialized countries, health insurance starts typically as a mechanism for paying charges under the medical care delivery patterns that previously existed; in time, the rise in expenditures (due to both advanced technology and rising rates of utilization) leads to increased measures of regulation or control.

3. In less developed countries, where the market for private medical care is small, health insurance usually starts with a

direct pattern of medical care delivery, under which physicians and others work as employees in an organized framework.

4. The rapid development of completely socialized systems of health service, in which all people are entitled to care as a civic right and all health personnel and facilities are governmental, depends on major social revolutions.

5. In the absence of social revolutions, national health services, with everyone entitled to comprehensive care supported mainly by general revenues, are achieved only after many years of experience with more limited forms of national health insurance, and after political developments conducive to change.

6. Even without development of full-scale national health services, the general trend of national insurance systems is toward wider population coverage and broader scope of medical services; this is true both under the indirect pattern of medical care delivery in industralized countries and the direct pattern in the developing countries.

7. Mounting pressures for economy in all countries have been leading to greater emphasis on preventive and ambulatory services and less relative use of costly hospital services.

8. Considerations of both efficiency and effectiveness have led everywhere to increased rationalization of health care delivery under insurance, involving greater use of auxiliary personnel working with doctors in teams.

9. Under insurance, the increasing visibility of expenditures has led to demands for assurance that the money is wisely spent; this, in turn, has led to increasing control and monitoring of the quality of phsyician performance, hospital management, drug production and distribution, and, ultimately, the health outcomes of the medical care system.

10. As a greater share of a nation's health care expenditures comes under insurance mechanisms, there are rising political pressures for overall planning of health care systems, including planning of the supply of health resources (personnel and facilities) to be produced, their geographic distribution, and the patterns under which they function.

11. In the interests of social equity, as well as economy, the deployment of resources under national health insurance systems is increasingly based on principles of regionalization,

with patients being transported to the facilities and personnel most appropriate for their care.

12. General medical care is being regarded in most countries as a basic social right that should depend on need rather than affluence; the extension of health insurance both heightens sensitivity to this concept and provides practical methods for implementing it.

13. Implementation of egalitarian concepts leads to increased use of general revenues for national health insurance.

14. With health insurance monies coming visibly from the entire population, most countries have found it increasingly necessary to give the average citizen a voice in the determination of national and local health policies.

This roster of 14 major lessons from health insurance developments around the world is admittedly rather general. Only brief reference has been made to specific health insurance techniques, such as capitation remuneration of doctors, copayment as a constraint on utilization of services, prior authorization of elective surgery as a constraint, prospective budgeting of hospital costs, statistical or medical chart audits of professional performance, the use of drug formularies, or the many other administrative techniques that evolve for the efficient operation of health insurance programs. All these administrative devices vary in their applicability at different times and places.

These 14 trends, however, may serve to demonstrate that health insurance in all countries is more than simply a method for paying medical bills. The spreading of medical care costs over populations and over time has doubtless been the initial objective of health insurance, voluntary or governmental, everywhere. It is just as clear, however, that in time health insurance dynamics operate to modify the structure and function of health care systems in the direction of improved efficiency, effectiveness, and equity.

25

Methodologies for National Health Planning

Free market operations in health care have led to so many difficulties and inequities that countries of widely divergent ideologies have undertaken deliberate planning of health resources and services. Much of this has not been identified as planning, although it has the basic attribute of purposeful intervention in the health care market. This chapter examines various approaches to national health planning taken by different types of countries.

National health planning—or, more accurately, the planning of a nation's health resources and services in order to reach certain goals—is now a worldwide practice. If one may speak of planning eras or periods, the world is now some 40 years into the health planning era that started in the midst of World War II.

ERAS OF HEALTH PLANNING

Soon after the onset of World War II, in 1939, work began in Great Britain on the study that produced the epochal Beveridge Report, which led to the establishment after the war of the British national health service.[1] In this period also, the Bhore Commission of India

This chapter is an adapted and substantially revised version of "Health Services Planning: Methodologies of Different Nations," in HOPE Conference Report—Urban and Rural Health Care in the Americas, October, 1979, 9–17.

(which was not yet independent) was designing a comprehensive health care system for that huge and impoverished country.[2] Political discussions were starting in Chile, which led in 1952 to the amalgamation of several separate health programs into the *Servicio Nacional de Salud*.[3] In the United States, the studies that resulted in the 1946 Hill-Burton Act were begun.[4]

World War II was clearly a cataclysm in the global network of nations, with capitalism and imperialism having reached a breaking point. This was expressed in the rise of fascism, a strategy for coping with the distributional problems of private enterprise by converting industrial control into brutal state power, and destroying all free actions of workers, farmers and other people.[5] In response, Britain, France, pre-Communist China, the United States, and Soviet Russia joined to defeat the Fascist Axis powers. If this great struggle was to have more than a negative purpose, however, it had to envisage greater social benefits for the mass of the population. This required planning for the years after the war, planning that would modify the workings of the market through deliberate allocation of resources on the basis not of personal wealth, but of human needs.[6] Thus, in the midst of World War II, there began the current era of health services planning.

The world had its first great upheaval 25 years earlier during World War I.[7] Out of the ashes of that conflict emerged the world's first Socialist nation, the USSR. When the Soviet Union became stabilized, it launched in 1928 its first five-year plan, encompassing all aspects of the economy, including health care.[8] Although this promptly identified planning with communism in the minds of most leaders of Western Europe and the United States, only a year later a massive collapse of the world capitalist economy ushered in the Great Depression of the 1930s. In response, the United States enacted the Social Security Act of 1935, thereby joining Europe in repelling the onslaughts of the business cycle with a vast program of compulsory social insurance.[9] Thus, the period from about 1920 to 1940 constituted a planning era that was marked particularly by the rise of socialism and the extension of social insurance in the United States and elsewhere.

A rough outline of the long-term development of health care planning is shown in table 25.1. The main achievements (and there were many besides the ones mentioned) in each of these eras have not typically been identified as outcomes of planning. Yet each embodied the crucial feature of the process we now describe as planning: that is, the deliberate intervention in the socioeconomic market by collective actions to reduce the human tragedies resulting from unfettered market operations.

Table 25.1   Development of Health Care Planning

Period	Health Planning Feature
1500–1800	Origin of hospitals (Christian) Rise of the universities (medicine)
1800–1880	Organized public health services for community prevention
1880–1920	Rise and growth of social insurance for disability and medical care Flowering of medical science and expansion of hospitals
1920–1940	Socialism and five-year plans Extension of social insurance Medical specialization and technology
1940–1980	Worldwide extension of comprehensive national health planning

The first public health acts legislated in Great Britain and Europe in the early nineteenth century imposed social measures to prevent the spread of contagious disease through dirty water and unregulated disposal of human waste.[10] In 1883, Germany enacted the first health insurance, perhaps motivated by political opposition to a rising Socialist movement.[11] Nevertheless, this set in motion a worldwide movement for systematic group financing of medical care for sickness. Such actions constituted planning as surely as the decision of a U.S. health planning agency in 1980 to build (or not to build) a 100-bed hospital in a rural county.

With some further oversimplification, one can identify in the modern world five general approaches to health planning, linked to five types of countries:

1. Socialist
2. Welfare state
3. Transitional developing
4. Entrepreneurial developing
5. Advanced free enterprise

These approaches, as well as the WHO approach to health planning, will be discussed below.

SOCIALIST HEALTH PLANNING

Since governmental intervention in market operations is most complete in Socialist countries, it is appropriate to discuss their approach to health planning first. Centralized planning of all sectors of the economy and of social life is, of course, the hallmark of socialism. In the health services more than in other fields, the private sector has dwindled to very small proportions, so central planning has an especially comprehensive scope.

The basic health planning model was formulated by the Soviet Union soon after its establishment in 1917. The crucial principle was that health service would be a government function provided without charge to all persons.[12] To implement this principle, virtually all health personnel would become salaried civil servants, health facilities would be taken over and operated by the government, drugs and supplies would be produced by public enterprises, and all health services—as well as medical research and professional education—would be directed by a central ministry of health. Preventive and therapeutic services would be integrated, with emphasis on prevention. Deliberate measures would be taken to achieve equitable distribution of resources, in order to overcome the traditional handicaps of rural people. In the process of development, priority would be accorded to children and industrial workers.

After 60 years, the Soviets have not yet fully achieved their objectives, but progress since Czarist Russia has been enormous.[13] The Socialist planning methodology has been relatively simple. As applied in modern Poland, it may be summarized as a sequence of technical, economic, and political decisions. Technical judgments, based largely on empirical studies, are made about the health needs of the population— that is, the need for health personnel, hospital beds, primary care facilities, drugs, and so on. Economic assessments are then made to determine the nation's ability to produce the needed resources within a certain time. Political decisions finalize the standards to be established for short-term and long-term targets, in light of the competing needs of the society.

While this summary is oversimplified, the planning process itself is simple and straightforward compared with the complexities of planning in countries with mixed private and public economies. None of the Socialist countries (including China and Cuba) has ever prohibited private medical practice, and it exists to some extent in all of them. The publicly planned services, however, have been so extensively developed that the market for privately purchased care has dwindled to very small proportions. The planning process, moreover, is not conducted solely in Moscow, Havana, or Peking. While basic policies and goals are established centrally, their implementation depends largely on actions and adaptations carried out at the provincial and local levels. This is particularly true in the huge and heterogeneous People's Republic of China.[14]

WELFARE STATE HEALTH PLANNING

Nations classifiable as welfare states are numerous and varied, so only selected examples of them can be considered. Perhaps the most important common denominator in their health planning strategies is that, whereas health care receives public economic support, the delivery of care is only partially put under public control. Within this broad definition, of course, there are countless variations.

The initial planning of the British national health service, for example, was designed to preserve the sovereignty of four major power groups: the general medical practitioners (about half the doctors), the hospitals and specialists, the local public health authorities, and the medical schools with their teaching hospitals.[15] The GPs would remain, as they do to the present day, in private practice. The specialists had long served in salaried appointments in hospitals, and this concept was simply extended; part of their time could be devoted to private, paying patients. As during the critical days of World War II, the hospitals were placed under the control of regional boards. Local public health authorities and medical training centers retained much independence. It was only in 1974 that these four separate channels of governance were integrated into some 90 area health authorities.[16] The most sweepingly planned feature of the NHS has remained its overwhelming support (about 85 percent) from national general revenues and the availability of services, almost entirely without charge, to every resident (see chapter 12).

In Canada, with its highly autonomous provinces, planning has been much more decentralized. A system of universal hospital insurance, followed by universal insurance for physician care, was pioneered by one cooperatively oriented province, Saskatchewan.[17] Eventually, national legislation was enacted along the same lines, and then a great deal of both national and provincial planning was stimulated to yield appropriate numbers and distribution of health manpower and hospital beds.[18] Only recently has the formula for federal matching of provincial expenditures been modified to induce greater cost containment.[19] Likewise, only after the personal problems of medical care costs and accessibility were solved has Canadian leadership called for greater emphasis on health promotion and prevention (see chapter 13).[20]

One might offer many other examples of the health planning process in other industrialized welfare states, but I will discuss only a third, the plans recently legislated in Italy.[21] After a century or more of multiple semi-autonomous health insurance funds, with wide differences in benefits, depending on the earnings of their members, Italy launched in 1978 a national health service. It is modeled largely after the British NHS, with support from general revenues replacing variable insurance contributions by workers and employers. Most specialists, based in hospitals, will be on salary, but GPs will receive capitation payments according to the number of persons registered on their lists. The whole system will be administered by a single, unified Ministry of Health. Administrative functions will be delegated to Italy's 20 regions, which in turn are subdivided into local health units of 50,000 to 200,000 people. Local health units will supervise organized preventive services and administer hospitals and ambulatory care facilities.

All this is to be brought about gradually, as local health insurance funds are dismantled and the physicians, both specialists and generalists, become employed in the local health units. Such employment will not be compulsory, but working conditions and financial rewards are expected to make it attractive. Those physicians preferring to remain in private practice may do so, with the specialists being paid by the ministry on a fee-for-service basis and GPs being paid by capitation. Drugs will be provided at only about 8 percent of their cost if they are on the official drug list, which contains some 800 products. The target date for achieving national uniformity in benefits, both therapeutic and preventive, was sometime in 1982, but the shift in financing from health insurance contributions to general revenues may take longer than this.

Italy illustrates particularly well a central feature of planning—namely, its political foundations. After the fall of fascism and the establishment of the 1948 Italian Republican Constitution, the previously voluntary mutual aid societies were converted into agencies for managing mandatory governmental insurance.[22] Their coverage by the 1970s, in spite of the unevenness noted earlier, grew to over 90 percent of the population. Discussion of further development into a unified national health service, with various commissions recommending such a change, was widespread by 1960,[23] but the diverse political parties in the Italian Parliament could not reach agreement.

It was only in 1977, when the Italian Communist party (PCI) had become a substantial opposition to the ruling Christian Democrats, that a majority vote was cast for a national health service. The PCI engaged the services of British medical consultants to design the plan.[24] The planning was not based on any sophisticated analysis of morbidity, manpower resources, or such, but simply on commonsense emulation of the health care experience and trends of other European countries. The crucial decisions were made, in other words, not on the basis of careful operations research or systems analysis, but on the basis of political judgment with the votes to back it up. The course of health events in Italy remains to be seen, but it will obviously depend mainly on the relative strengths of competing political parties.

HEALTH PLANNING IN TRANSITIONAL, DEVELOPING COUNTRIES

By "transitional, developing countries," I refer to those primarily agricultural countries which have, for various reasons, launched major socially financed health care programs for significant sections of their population. Although an upper class still receives a disproportionately large share of the available services privately, important equalization measures have been taken. The majority of medical manpower is publicly employed full-time or part-time, most health services are provided in organized settings, most hospital beds are in governmental facilities, and substantial health expenditures are derived from the public sector. Illustrative of such countries are all but a few of the Latin American republics, some of the Middle East countries (such as Iran and Egypt), Malaysia and Singapore in Asia, and perhaps India. With rapid changes occurring in all countries, both developing and industrialized, one cannot be too rigid about applying a scheme of classification such as this.

Colombia is a country of this type. Its per capita gross domestic product in 1976 was about $600 (U.S.).[25] Since 1946, it has had a social security system for industrial, commercial, and some agricultural workers. Services are provided to covered persons and their dependents through hospitals and health centers, which have salaried medical and allied personnel and are under the direct control of the Colombian Social Security Institute.[26] While only a small fraction of the population is covered, coverage has been expanding. Between 1967 and 1970, for example, coverage rose from 10 to 16 percent of the economically active people.[27] The majority of the Colombian population, however, is rural and is served by the health posts, health centers, and hospitals of the Ministry of Health. Of the nation's 45,300 hospital beds (about two per 1,000 people), 80 percent are in public facilities.

Health planning in Colombia is part of a general social and economic development plan. The major health priority is to provide better primary care to the rural population; this is done through trained auxiliary personnel working at health posts, which are linked to health centers. In the mid-1960s, an extensive national household survey was made in Colombia, yielding information on morbidity and the types of health services received. One of the important findings was that, contrary to previous belief, only 17 percent of ambulatory care encounters in rural areas were with a traditional healer, and only 3.4 percent in cities.[28] The great majority of sickness episodes reported were not treated at all.

To implement the planning objective of better delivery of primary care to the rural population, several schools have been established for training young women and men from the villages, often persons with no more than four or six years of elementary education. They are taught the rudiments of environmental hygiene, communicable disease prevention with immunizations, family planning services, treatment of common diseases, and the importance of referring difficult cases to a medically staffed health center or hospital. Colombia, like other Latin American countries, had been skeptical about the training of health auxiliaries in "second-class medicine" until the spectacular impact of China's barefoot doctors was broadcast after 1971.

The Colombian Social Security Institute is using its more abundant funds to extend coverage to larger numbers of workers with stable employment, along with their dependents. While socially insured people in this type of country have a clear advantage over the noninsured and the low-income rural population, the evidence suggests that social security programs in Latin America do *not* inhibit the growth of ministry of health services. On the contrary, extension of ministerial health services and social security health services go hand in hand. The latter programs, moreover, channel into reasonably organized health care systems money that might otherwise be spent much less prudently in the private sector.[29]

A second example of health planning in a transitional, developing country is Malaysia, a former British colony that gained independence in 1957. Even before independence, planning was started on a rural health services scheme. In 1953, a model rural health center was established, largely as a training unit, in a northern province that had experienced much antigovernment guerrilla warfare.[30] Fifteen years later, I had the opportunity to evaluate the accomplishments of this program for the World Health Organization.[31]

The planning strategy in Malaysia was relatively simple. A Ministry of National and Rural Development was responsible for mapping out resources in the 70 administrative districts of the country. For each area with a rural population of 50,000, there was intended to be a main health center staffed by a physician, a professional nurse, and others. Peripheral to each main center would be four subcenters staffed entirely by auxiliaries and serving 10,000 people each. As satellites to each subcenter, there would be five midwife clinics serving 2,000 people each. To cover the entire rural population with this model would require 100 main health centers, 400 subcenters, and 2,000 midwife clinics. After 15 years, about 40 percent of the goal has been achieved.

Subsequent planning called not only for additional construction of facilities, but also for training of auxiliary personnel as well as physicians. A medical school had been established in 1959; as its first graduates were turned out, a law was passed to require two years of rural service. This permitted physician staffing of the subcenters as well as the main centers. The training of auxiliary personnel at the midwife clinics was broadened to include infant health care. The scope of health administration at the district level was extended to include responsibility for curative services in the district hospitals as well as ambulatory and preventive services in the rural health units. Step by step, more of the rural population is being covered by publicly financed health care—85 percent being reached by 1982. In the cities, specialist services are provided by salaried hospital doctors at relatively well developed public facilities for both inpatients and outpatients. Private medical care is limited mainly to the services of urban GPs (see chapter 9).

As a third example of this transitional type of developing country, there is the Caribbean island of Barbados.[32] The health manpower resources of this small island are relatively plentiful, and the Barbados Labour party elected to power in 1976 proposed launching a national health service. The planning task was to determine precisely the number and types of personnel needed, how much the scheme would cost, and how could the necessary funds be raised. The government decided that the program should be developed not all at once, but in stages.

The first stage would be primary health care for everyone as a social right.[33] Based on prior utilization data assembled from several sources, and assuming a certain future increase, one could estimate that primary care would be accessible to everyone through about 70 primary care teams. Each team would consist of a general physician, a medical practice nurse, a community nurse, and a clerk. The teams would be located partly in polyclinic buildings, partly in private group practices, and partly as separate private units. The doctors would remain in private practice but would be paid by capitation; the other team members would be on government salaries. Hospital and specialist services were already available, without charge, at one large public general hospital (see chapter 6).

Financing this primary care service, it was estimated, would cost about B$9 million ($4.5 million U.S.). Fortunately, there already existed a national insurance program that provided work injury compensation, old-age pensions, and certain other benefits; counting dependents, a survey showed that coverage would be 82 percent of the population. Accordingly, it was not difficult to calculate that 82 percent of the estimated costs could be raised by increasing the national insurance tax on both workers and employers by 0.8 percent. The remaining 18 percent of costs would come from the general budget of the Ministry of Health.

As might have been expected, opposition to the new plan was promptly forthcoming from the private Barbados Association of Medical Practitioners. The association behaved little differently from the British Medical Association when the NHS was first outlined or from the American Medical Association until the very day in July 1965 that Medicare was signed into law. The ultimate implementation of Barbados health planning will depend on the political courage and determination of future governments.

HEALTH PLANNING IN ENTREPRENEURIAL, IMPOVERISHED COUNTRIES

By "entrepreneurial, impoverished countries," I refer to those nations which, while rural and with a very low average standard of living, have done relatively little to mobilize financial resources for organized health services needed by the mass of the population. Most of the countries of Africa would belong in this category, as well as several of the countries of Asia. These countries tend to be characterized not only by the very low percentage of GNP spent on health, but also by a relatively small share of health expenditures coming from public, as opposed to private, sources (see chapter 10).

In Senegal, a small African country with about 5 million persons, the total per capita health expenditure is not known, but the trend of health outlays as a percentage of the *government's* budget is significant. In 1970–71, the Ministry of Health was allotted 9.1 percent of the total government budget; by 1976–77, this had declined to 6.0 percent.[34] In the Republic of Korea, a national survey of household expen-

Table 25.2 Source of Funds for Health Care, Thailand 1978

Source	Percent
Ministry of Public Health	22.9
Other government agencies	10.0
Foreign aid and voluntary groups	1.6
Private households	65.5
Total	100.0

Table 25.3 Distribution of Private Households' Expenditures on Health Care, Thailand 1970

Purpose	Percent
Private doctors	44.9
Government hospital fees	24.8
Drug sellers	20.8
Traditional healers	7.0
Health center fees	2.3
Other	0.2
Total	100.0

ditures was carried out in 1975; of the nation's total expenditures for health purposes, 86.6 percent was derived from private sources and 13.4 percent from public sources.[35] Under such circumstances, it is obvious that there must be enormous inequities in the distribution of health care resources. Governmental health planning, moreover, is typically very much handicapped by being restricted to a small fraction of the total resources.

In 1978, I studied for WHO the health care system of another Asian country of this type, Thailand.[36] On the basis of household interview data on private health expenditures and official reports from numerous government agencies, it was possible to conclude that health funds were derived as shown in table 25.2.

The unfortunate reality was that virtually all systematic health planning activities, and these were considerable, were confined to the Ministry of Public Health program, which involved less than one-fourth of the total expenditures. Among private households (based on a survey done in 1970), expenditures were distributed as shown in table 25.3. One may be surprised at the private expenditures for government hospitals and health centers, but official policy in Thailand requires payments from all but the most destitute patients for drugs and diagnostic tests done in public facilities (see chapter 7).

Planning in Thailand calls for providing all 570 districts of the country (in 71 provinces) with district hospitals of ten to 30 beds, all 5,500 subdistricts (or clusters of villages) with health centers for ambulatory care, and all 49,000 villages with midwifery stations. These goals, as of late 1978, had been achieved 56 percent, 73 percent, and 4 percent, respectively. More important, however, was the fact that the rates of utilization of health centers and district hospitals by the people were very low; most people, even though they are very poor, tend to bypass these public facilities and seek care from private doctors, untrained drug sellers, or traditional healers.[37]

The problems of health planning in countries of this type were candidly described by the former director of medical services of Ghana in 1973.

> In 1963 a Planning Commission including two doctors was set up, and a comprehensive national development plan was written. This plan, which was not implemented, was very ambitious. It aimed to provide for very rapid development of hospital services and at the same time for promotive, protective, and preventive services—an almost impossible task. . . . After the coup of 1966 this plan was shelved . . . [A new committee] reporting two years later stated that the emphasis should be on the promotive and protective services . . . and training of health personnel. Nothing was done to implement this committee's report. In 1971 another committee was set up [for] devising a health-sector plan. . . . This committee reported towards the end of 1971 . . . when the Government which ordered it was overthrown by another military coup. . . . Thus the latest attempt to produce a health plan can be regarded as stillborn.[38]

Since 1973, Ghana has gone through several more military coups, so one cannot be too surprised about continued frustration with national health planning efforts.

HEALTH PLANNING IN
ADVANCED FREE ENTERPRISE COUNTRIES

Finally we come to the type of country that is best illustrated by the United States. One might also place Australia and the Union of South Africa in this category. All three are countries with substantial health care resources, reflecting their overall affluence. Governmental support for health care, however, has been limited largely to high-cost hospital services and to the care of the poor and other selected populations or disease categories. Ambulatory medical service for the majority of the population is still mainly a private matter, although buffered somewhat by voluntary insurance.

As of 1980, the health planning policy of the United States assigned most responsibilities to some 200 local health systems agencies, which had very limited authority.[39] The agencies were expected to be influenced by national guidelines, but these were permissive rather than directive. In practice, the agencies had very little impact outside the approval or denial of hospital bed construction. This situation has been socially accepted because of the spiraling costs of hospital care and the recognition that hospital bed supply is a major determinant of hospital utilization under medical care patterns in the United States.[40] It is true that, since the Social Security Act of 1935, federal grants to the states for services such as preventive maternal and child health services and venereal disease control constituted a form of support for planning, not labeled as such. With respect to health manpower distribution, improved medical care for the poor, extended preventive service, coordination of ambulatory services, and the many other aspects of comprehensive health planning, health systems agencies have been unable to do very much. Furthermore, under the Reagan Administration, the local HSAs are being gradually dismantled, leaving health planning functions only at the state level.

Perhaps the more important instrumentality for general health care planning in the United States is the legislation supporting extension of health maintenance organizations or HMOs.[41] Built on the principle of local initiative, nongovernmental sponsorship, and free competition, the HMO establishes a subsystem of comprehensive health services in which the incentives of the key decision makers, physicians, are modified. Incentives are geared toward maximizing prevention-oriented services and the most prudent possible use of hospitalization and costly procedures, rather than maximizing the latter, as under fee-for-service patterns. Although HMOs entail possible abuses, they can be construed as a way of promoting built-in planning and self-regulation in a pluralistic, free enterprise economy.[42] Health systems agencies, however, have had little interest in promoting HMOs.

The relative weakness and great decentralization of health planning in the United States may be attributed not only to a traditional aversion to strong central authority, derived from the days of the American Revolution, but also to a continued failure to achieve political consensus on a system of comprehensive national health insurance. This issue has been debated since 1939, but final action has been taken only on limited voluntary health insurance for employed persons and on social insurance for persons with work-related injuries (workmen's compensation) and for the aged (Medicare).[43] It has only been through the leverage provided by national systems of health care financing that other industrialized nations (the welfare states) have been able to plan health resources to meet social needs.[44] Perhaps the most optimistic view of current U.S. efforts in local health planning is that they are providing useful experience for thousands of consumers on planning boards and are providing a framework for requirements to be expected after some form of national health insurance legislation is enacted.[45]

Recent events in Australia dramatize the relationship between national health insurance and health planning in an affluent, free enterprise setting. In 1972, the Labour party was elected to power. In 1974, a law was passed to replace the local voluntary health insurance programs (which were very much like those in the United States) with a national health insurance system that provided the entire population with comprehensive services. As the nation was tooling up for this new program, a great deal of planning was done on health services regionalization, measures to meet health manpower requirements, encouragement of community health centers, improved organization of hospitals, and so on.[46] Then, for many economic and social reasons, the Labour party lost its political control in 1976. Action was promptly taken to modify the national health insurance law step by step. To underscore a purely fiscal interpretation of the law, it was given a new label, Medibank. By 1979, the law was virtually dismantled.[47] With this, most national planning, which would have gradually modified the Australian health care system, has steadily declined. When the Australian Labour Party regained power in 1983, active health planning was resumed.

THE WORLD HEALTH ORGANIZATION APPROACH TO PLANNING

The World Health Organization encourages an approach to national health planning that has evolved significantly—especially in its application to the developing countries.

The WHO convened its first expert committee on national health planning in 1967.[48] (Perhaps it is not accidental that this was just one year after the United States enacted its first comprehensive health planning legislation, thereby purging the subject of its Socialist connotations and endowing it with respectability.) The committee's report was very generalized and relativistic: that is, it suggested that each country must develop its own methods, which would be appropriate to its particular social and political setting. As summarized a few years later in another WHO document, a health plan was defined simply as:

... a predetermined course of action that is firmly based on the nature and extent of health problems, from which are derived priority goals. The heart of the planning process is the analysis of alternative means of achieving the preselected goals in the face of a variety of constraints.[49]

The planning process, in other words, required accurate information on health problems (diseases, mortality, and so on) and the formulation of various possible solutions. The planner's duty was to provide these background data and an array of alternative solutions, leaving to policymakers the decisions on which actions to take.

This methodology was refined and taught to national health planners at several training centers around the world. It was perhaps most thoroughly implemented in a training program of the Pan American Health Organization (PAHO), formulated at the Center for Development Studies (CENDES) in Venezuela, and later disseminated in courses given by the Latin American Insitute for Economic and Social Planning in Santiago, Chile. This PAHO-CENDES method was taught to over 2,500 Latin American health planners.

The PAHO-CENDES method required that disease problems be measured on the basis of mortality rates and quantified according to (1) magnitude, (2) importance, and (3) their vulnerability.[50] The costs of various choices of corrective action were then to be estimated and cost-benefit ratios calculated. The rationality of this—and of other, similar health planning techniques—can hardly be challenged, but unfortunately the PAHO-CENDES method was never successfully applied, in Latin America or elsewhere. Not only were the necessary statistical data seldom available, but even when the final cost-benefit ratios of various health action plans could be estimated, political decisions on health programs were made on wholly different grounds.

After several years of disappointing and frustrating experiences of this sort, the WHO finally abolished its unit on national health planning, along with several other organizational units devoted to strictly scientific quantification of health problems for the purpose of furnishing guidance on policy decisions. In their place, WHO established in the office of the director-general a unit to develop and promote a strategy defined as "country health programming."[51]

The essential strategy of country health programming is the formation in each country of a national group or council made up of the top decision makers on health policies and programs. While all possible information on health problems and resources should be fed to this council, stress should be placed on active discussion and *decisions* on immediate, practical steps to be taken toward the goal of comprehensive health services for entire populations. To promote the concept of national commitment to such a goal, WHO, along with UNICEF, started by sponsoring an International Conference on Primary Health Care in September 1978, at Alma Ata in the Soviet Union.[52] The purpose of the conference was both political and inspirational. Excessive attention to precise data collection, analysis, and formulation of alternative policy options would be replaced by promotion of action, as rapidly as possible, to extend at least minimal general health services, preventive and curative, to the billions of impoverished people in developing countries now without such care.

Thus, the Declaration of Alma Ata returns to the forthright tone of the 1948 WHO Constitution with words such as these:

> Governments have a responsibility for the health of their people which can be fulfilled only by the provision of adequate health and social measures. A main social target of governments, international organizations and the whole world community in the coming decades should be the attainment by all peoples of the world by the year 2000 of a level of health that will permit them to lead a socially and economically productive life. Primary health care is the key to attaining this target as part of development in the spirit of social justice.[53]

Abandoning previous caution on political matters, the Alma Ata Declaration of nearly all the world's nations goes on to state:

> All governments should formulate national policies, strategies and plans of action to launch and sustain primary health care as part of a comprehensive national health system and in coordination with other sectors. To this end it will be necessary to exercise political will, to mobilize the country's resources and to use available external resources rationally.[54]

To someone who started work with WHO in 1950, when the organization was barely two years old and when its approach to achieving health improvement was almost wholly technical (trying to spread ideas through demonstration projects in selected localities), the change in posture is especially dramatic.[55] Lest there be any doubt about the WHO director-general's judgment of current international health requirements, in a message sent in late 1978 to all regional offices he calls on the six global regional directors to "assume a stronger political role" in their work.[56] Recent WHO strategies refer to the value of a "managerial process for national health development," but there is no less emphasis on the need for political commitment and political will.[57]

Thus, the approach to health planning proposed by the World Health Organization today has evolved from a highly technical toward a frankly political one. Planning is intended to correct the failures of the free market to achieve equity. While certainly not rejecting the value of information and analysis, the objective of health planning should be to stimulate political decisions that will move nations as rapidly as possible toward the goal of health for all. The nature of the goal and the responsibilities of governments, according to WHO and UNICEF, need no longer be argued. The task of planning is to achieve the political consensus necessary for the distribution of health services everywhere in a spirit of social justice.

NOTES

1. W. Beveridge, *Social Insurance and Allied Services* (New York: Macmillan Co., 1942).
2. Government of India, Health Survey and Development Committee, *Report*, 4 vols. (New Delhi, 1946).
3. H. Duran, *Sintesis de la Historia de las Acciones de Salubridad en Chile* (Santiago: Escuela de Salubridad, 1954).
4. Commission on Hospital Care, *Hospital Care in the United States* (Chicago, 1946).
5. A. J. P. Taylor, *The Origins of the Second World War* (New York: Wiley, 1972).
6. G. Myrdal, *Beyond the Welfare State: Economic Planning and Its International Implications* (New Haven: Yale University Press, 1960).
7. C. L. Becker, *Modern History: The Rise of a Democratic, Scientific, and Industrialized Civilization* (New York: Silver, Burdett & Co., 1935), 680–723.
8. H. E. Sigerist, *Socialized Medicine in the Soviet Union* (New York: Norton & Co., 1937).
9. E. M. Burns, *Social Security and Public Policy* (New York: McGraw-Hill, 1956).
10. G. Rosen, *A History of Public Health* (New York: MD Publications, 1958), 206–33.
11. H. E. Sigerist, "From Bismarck to Beveridge: Developments and Trends in Social Security Legislation," *Bulletin of the History of Medicine* 8 (April 1943): 365–88.
12. G. A. Popov, *Principles of Health Planning in the U.S.S.R.*, public health paper no. 43 (Geneva: World Health Organization, 1971).
13. I. P. Lidor et al., *Soviet Public Health and the Organization of Primary Health Care for the Population of the U.S.S.R.* (Moscow: Mir Publishers, 1978).
14. V. W. Sidel and R. Sidel, *Serve the People—Observations on Medicine in the People's Republic of China* (New York: Josiah Macy, Jr. Foundation, 1973).
15. A. Lindsey, *Socialized Medicine in England and Wales: The National Health Service 1948–1961* (Chapel Hill: University of North Carolina Press, 1962).
16. R. Levitt, *The Reorganised National Health Service* (London: Croom Helm, 1976).
17. M. G. Taylor, *Health Insurance and Canadian Public Policy: The Seven Decisions that Created the Canadian Health Insurance System* (Montreal: McGill-Queen's University Press, 1978).

18. R. Roemer and M. I. Roemer, *Health Manpower Policy under National Health Insurance—The Canadian Experience*, DHEW Publication (HRA) 77–37 (Washington, D.C.: Health Resources Administration, 1977).

19. M. Lalonde, *A New Perspective on the Health of Canadians: A Working Document* (Ottawa: Health and Welfare Canada, 1974).

20. R. J. Van Loon, "From Shared Cost to Block Funding: The Politics of Health Insurance in Canada," *Journal of Health Politics, Policy, and Law* 2 (Winter 1978):454–78.

21. F. B. McArdle, "Italy's National Health Service Plan," *Social Security Bulletin* 42, no. 4 (April 1979): 38–42.

22. S. Z. Koff, "Emergency Medical Services in Crisis: An Italian Case Study," *Milbank Memorial Fund Quarterly—Health and Society 53* (Summer 1975):377–401.

23. M. I. Roemer, personal observation, Italy, August 1960.

24. H. Faulkner, British general practitioner, personal communication, October 1976.

25. Pan American Health Organization, "Colombia," in *Proposed Program and Budget Estimates, 1980–81* (Washington, D.C., 1979), 157–61.

26. Social Security Administration, "Colombia," in *Social Security Programs Throughout the World 1977* (Washington, D.C., 1978), 50–51.

27. M. I. Roemer, "Development of Medical Services under Social Security in Latin America," *International Labour Review* 108 (July 1973):1–23.

28. Ministry of Public Health of Colombia and Colombian Association of Medical Schools, *Study on Health Manpower and Medical Education in Colombia. Vol. II: Preliminary Findings* (Washington, D.C.: Pan American Health Organization, 1967).

29. M. I. Roemer and N. Maeda, "Does Social Security Support for Medical Care Weaken Public Health Programs?" *International Journal of Health Services* 6, no. 1 (1976):69–78.

30. L. W. Jayesuria, *A Review of the Rural Health Services in West Malaysia* (Kuala Lumpur: Ministry of Health, 1967).

31. M. I. Roemer, "The Development and Current Spectrum of Organized Health Services in a New Asian Country: Malaysia," in *Health Care Systems in World Perspective* (Ann Arbor, Mich.: Health Administration Press, 1976), 39–59.

32. _____, *A National Health Service in Barbados: Developing the Primary Care Phase* (Bridgetown: Ministry of Health and National Insurance, 1979).

33. Barbados Ministry of Health and National Insurance, *Development Plan 1977–82* (Bridgetown, 1977).

34. World Health Organization, *Financing of Health Services*, technical report series 625 (Geneva, 1978), 95.

35. C. K. Park, *Financing Health Services in Korea* (Seoul: Korea Development Institute, 1977).

36. M. I. Roemer, *The Health Care System of Thailand* (New Delhi: World Health Organization, South-East Asia Regional Office, 1981).

37. F. A. Day and B. Leoprapai, *Patterns of Health Utilization in Upcountry Thailand* (Bangkok: Mahidol University, Institute for Population and Social Research, 1977).

38. F. T. Sai, "Ghana," in *Health Service Prospects: An International Survey*, I. Douglas-Wilson and G. McLachlan, eds. (London: The Lancet and The Nuffield Provincial Hospitals Trust, 1973), 148.

39. L. S. Rosenfeld and I. Rosenfeld, "National Health Planning in the United States: Prospects and Portents," *International Journal of Health Services* 5, no. 3 (1975):441–53.

40. M. I. Roemer and M. Shain, *Hospital Utilization under Insurance* (Chicago: American Hospital Association, 1959).

41. J. L. Dorsey, "The Health Maintenance Organization Act of 1973 (P.L. 93-222) and Prepaid Group Practice Plans," *Medical Care* 13 (January 1975):1–9.

42. M. I. Roemer and W. Shonick, "HMO Performance: The Recent Evidence," *Milbank Memorial Fund Quarterly* 51 (Summer 1973):271–317.

43. E. Feingold, *Medicare: Policy and Politics* (San Francisco: Chandler Publishing Co., 1966).

44. M. I. Roemer, "Social Insurance as Leverage for Changing Health Care Systems," *Bulletin of the New York Academy of Medicine* 48 (January 1972):93–107.

45. W. Shonick, *Elements of Planning for Areawide Personal Health Services* (St. Louis, Mo.: Mosby Co., 1976).

46. R. Roemer and M. I. Roemer, *Health Manpower in the Changing Australian Health Service Scene*, DHEW Publication (HRA) 76–58 (Washington, D.C.: Health Resources Administration, 1976).

47. R. M. Southby and E. Chesterman, *Australia: Health Facts 1979* (Sydney: University of Sydney, School of Public Health and Tropical Medicine, 1979).

48. World Health Organization, *National Health Planning in Developing Countries*, technical report series no. 350 (Geneva, 1967).

49. H. E. Hilleboe, A. Barkhuus, and W. C. Thomas, Jr., *Approaches to National Health Planning*, public health papers no. 46 (Geneva: World Health Organization, 1972), 9.

50. J. Ahumada et al., *Health Planning: Problems of Concept and Method*, scientific publication no. 111 (Washington, D.C.: Pan American Health Organization, 1965).

51. World Health Organization, *Sixth General Programme of Work Covering a Specific Period (1978–1983)* (Geneva, 1976), 71–72.

52. _____, *Primary Health Care: A Joint Report by the Director-General of the World Health Organization and the Executive Director of the United Nations Children's Fund* (Geneva and New York, 1978).

53. World Health Organization and United Nations Children's Fund, *Alma Ata 1978: Primary Health Care* (Geneva, 1978), 3.

54. *Ibid.*, 5.

55. M. I. Roemer, *A Health Demonstration Area in El Salvador* (Washington, D.C.: Pan American Health Organization, 1951).
56. World Health Organization, *Study of WHO's Structure in the Light of Its Functions*, background paper prepared by the Director-General (New Delhi: Regional Office for South-East Asia, 1978), 14.
57. _____, Managerial Process for National Health Development, Geneva, 1981.

Bibliography of Comparative Studies of National Health Care Systems

Abel-Smith, B., *An International Study of Health Expenditures*, public health paper no. 32 (Geneva: World Health Organization, 1967).

_____, *Poverty, Development, and Health Policy*, public health paper no. 69 (Geneva: World Health Organization, 1978).

Abel-Smith, B. and A. Maynard, *The Organisation, Financing and Cost of Health Care in the European Community* (Brussels: European Economic Community, 1978).

American Public Health Association, *Primary Health Care: Bibliography and Resource Directory* (Washington, D.C.: American Public Health Association, 1982).

Anderson, O. W., *Health Care: Can There Be Equity?—United States, Sweden, and England* (New York: John Wiley & Sons, 1972).

Banta, D., and K. B. Kemp, eds., *The Management of Health Care Technology in Nine Countries* (New York: Springer Publishing, 1982).

Basch, P. F., *International Health* (New York: Oxford University Press, 1978).

Behrman, S. J., L. Corsa Jr., and R. Freeman, eds., *Fertility and Family Planning: A World View* (Ann Arbor, Mich.: University of Michigan Press, 1969).

Blanpain, J., *National Health Insurance and Health Resources* (Cambridge, Mass.: Harvard University Press, 1978).

Bowers, J. Z., and E. F. Purcell, eds., *The Impact of Health Services on Medical Education: A Global View* (New York: Josiah Macy Jr. Foundation, 1978).

Bridgman, R. F., and M. I. Roemer, *Hospital Legislation and Hospital Systems*, public health paper no. 50 (Geneva: World Health Organization, 1973).

Brocklehurst, J. C., ed., *Geriatric Care in Advanced Societies* (Lancaster: Medical and Technical Publishing, 1975).

Bryant, J., *Health and the Developing World* (Ithaca, N.Y.: Cornell University Press, 1969).

Bullough, B., and V. Bullough, *The Emergence of Modern Nursing* (New York: Macmillan, 1969).

David, H. P., ed., *International Trends in Mental Health* (New York: McGraw-Hill, 1966).

Douglas-Wilson, I., and G. McLachlan, eds., *Health Service Prospects: An International Survey* (London: The Lancet and The Nuffield Provincial Hospitals Trusts, 1973).

Elling, R. H., *Cross-National Study of Health Systems: Concepts, Methods, and Data Sources—A Guide to Information Sources* (Detroit, Mich.: Gale Research, 1980).

_____, *Cross-National Studies of Health Systems: Countries, World Regions, and Special Problems—A Guide to Information Sources* (Detroit, Mich.: Gale Research, 1980).

_____, *Cross-National Study of Health Systems* (New Brunswick, N.J.: Transaction Books, 1980).

Evang, K., *Health Services, Society, and Medicine* (London: Oxford University Press, 1960).

Fry, J., *Medicine in Three Societies: A Comparison of Medical Care in The USSR, USA, and UK* (New York: American Elsiever, 1970).

Fry, J., and W. A. J. Farndale, eds., *International Medical Care: A Comparison and Evaluation of Medical Care Services Throughout the World* (Oxford: Medical and Technical Publishing, 1972).

Fulcher, D., *Medical Care Systems: Public and Private Health Coverage in Selected Industrialized Countries* (Geneva: International Labour Office, 1974).

Glaser, W. A., *Health Insurance Bargaining: Foreign Lessons for America* (New York: Gardner Press, 1978).

_____, *Paying the Doctor: Systems of Remuneration and Their Effects* (Baltimore, Md.: Johns Hopkins Press, 1970).

_____, *Social Settings and Medical Organization: A Cross-National Study of the Hospital* (New York: Atherton Press, 1970).

Holmes, A. C., *Health Education in Developing Countries* (London: Thomas Nelson & Sons, 1964).

Ingle, J., and P. Blair, *International Dental Care Delivery Systems* (Cambridge, Mass.: Ballinger Publishing, 1978).

Ingman, S. R., and A. E. Thomas, eds., *Topias and Utopias in Health: Policy Studies* (The Hague: Mouton Publishers, 1974).

International Development Research Centre, *Low-Cost Rural Health Care and Health Manpower Training: An Annotated Bibliography with Special Emphasis on Developing Countries* (7 volumes) (Ottawa, Canada, 1975-80).

Kent, P. W., ed., *International Aspects of the Provision of Medical Care* (London: Oriel Press, 1976).

King, M., ed., *Medical Care in Developing Countries* (Nairobi, Kenya: Oxford University Press, 1966).

Kleczkowski, B. M., M. I. Roemer, and A. van der Werff, *National Health Systems and Their Reorientation Towards Health for All,* public health paper no. 77 (Geneva: World Health Organization, 1984).

Kleinman, A. et al., eds., *Culture and Healing in Asian Societies: Anthropological, Psychiatric and Public Health Studies* (Cambridge, Mass.: Schenkman Publishing, 1978).

Kohn, R., and K. L. White, *Health Care: An International Study* (London: Oxford University Press, 1976).

Lee, K., and A. Mills, eds., *The Economics of Health in Developing Countries* (New York: Oxford University Press, 1983).

Leichter, H. M., *Comparative Approach to Policy Analysis: Health Care Policy in Four Nations* (New York: Cambridge University Press, 1979).

Maxwell, R. J., *Health and Wealth: An International Study of Health-Care Spending* (Lexington, Mass.: Lexington Books, 1981).

_____, *Health Care: The Growing Dilemma* (New York: McKinsey & Co., 1975).

Maynard, A., *Health Care in the European Community* (London: Croom Helm, 1975).

McLachlan, G., ed., *Public/Private Mix for Health: The Relevance and Effects of Change* (London: Nuffield Provincial Hospitals Trust, 1982).

Muller, M., *The Health of Nations: A North-South Investigation* (London: Faber & Faber, 1982).

Newell, K. W., *Health by the People* (Geneva: World Health Organization, 1975).

Pannenborg, C. O., A. van der Werff, G. B. Hirsch, and K. Barnard, eds., *Reorienting Health Services: Application of a Systems Approach* (New York and London: Plenum Press, 1984).

Paul, B., *Health, Culture and Community* (New York: Russell Sage Foundation, 1955).

Raffel, M. W., ed., *Comparative Health Systems: Descriptive Analyses of Fourteen National Health Systems* (University Park, Penn.: Pennsylvania State University Press, 1984).

Roemer, M. I., *Comparative National Policies on Health Care* (New York: Marcel Dekker, 1977).

_____, *Health Care Systems in World Perspective* (Ann Arbor, Mich.: Health Administration Press, 1976).

_____, ed., H. E. Sigerist,*On the Sociology of Medicine* (New York: MD Publications, 1960).

_____, *The Organization of Medical Care under Social Security: A Study Based on the Experience of Eight Countries* (Geneva: International Labour Office, 1969).

Roemer, M. I., and R. Roemer, *Health Care Systems and Comparative Manpower Policies* (New York: Marcel Dekker, 1981).

Rosen, G., *A History of Public Health* (New York: MD Publications, 1958).

Sand, R., *The Advance to Social Medicine* (London: Staples Press, 1952).

Sidel, V. W., and R. Sidel, *A Healthy State: An International Perspective on the Crisis in United States Medical Care* (New York: Pantheon Books, 1977).

Sigerist, H. E., *Civilization and Disease* (Ithaca, N.Y.: Cornell University Press, 1943).

Silver, G. A., *Child Health: America's Future* (Germantown, Md.: Aspen Systems, 1978).

Simanis, J., *National Health Systems in Eight Countries* (Washington, D.C.: U.S. Social Security Administration, 1975).

U.S. Social Security Administration, *Social Security Programs Throughout the World* (Washington, D.C.: U.S. Social Security Administration, 1980).

Virgo, J. M., *Health Care: An International Perspective* (Edwardsville, Ill.: International Health Economics and Management Institute, 1984).

Weinerman, E. R., *Social Medicine in Eastern Europe: Organization of Health Services and the Education of Medical Personnel in Czechoslovakia, Hungary, and Poland* (Cambridge, Mass.: Harvard University Press, 1969).

World Health Organization, *Sixth Report on the World Health Situation 1973-1977*, Vol. 1 and 2 (Geneva: World Health Organization, 1980).

Index

Acupuncture, 311

Aged, care of, 7–8, 18, 33, 242; Great Britain, 179; Kenya, 111; Norway, 160; Thailand, 95; U.S., 240, 242, 387

Alma Alta Conference and Declaration, 10, 406

Ambulatory care, 319–34; Barbados, 76, 78; Canada, 198–203, 204; China, emphasis on, 312; Cuba, 295–96, 382; developing countries, 144, 147, 149–50, 151, 328–31; dispensaries, 319–22; facilities, 19, 32; financing, 17, 20, 37; Great Britain, 174–76, 188, 383; Guatemala, 55, 57, 59, 61–64, 67, 68; industrialized countries, 251–53, 331–33; Kenya, 113, 114; New Zealand, 384; Norway, 166–67; Poland, 286, 346; Soviet Union, 275–77, 279, 281–82, 326–27; Thailand, 91, 100; under-developed countries, 329–30. *See also* Health centers; Health posts; Health stations; Primary care

Apothecaries, 14, 29, 320, 351

Australia: aged, care of, 8; continuing education, 356; dental care, 168, 230, 358; financing in, 245, 331; flying doctor service, 229; GPs, 247; health centers, 166, 226, 229, 234, 326; health expenditures, 146; hospital care pattern, 167, 226; insurance, 21, 245, 331, 379; life expectancy, 263–64; nurses, 231, 232, 233; planning, 353; public health schools, 359–60

Barbados, planning health care in, 75–86, 399–400; administrative requirements, 80–81; cost estimates, 82–83; existing structure, 76; funds, source of, 83–84; health manpower resources, 79–80; primary care in, 76–79

Barefoot doctors (China), 10, 21, 236, 310, 311, 314, 315, 328, 364, 381

Belgium: cost sharing in, 242, 373; health centers and polyclinics, 235, 331, 332; health expenditures, 146; health personnel, 231, 232, 233, 234, 235, 332; health status indicators, 263, 266; hospital care pattern, 167; insurance in, 243, 372–73, 374; medical education, 356

Bevan, Aneurin, 173

Beveridge, Sir William, 173

Beveridge Report (Great Britain), 173, 344, 383, 391

Biggs, Herman, 324

Birth control. *See* Family planning

Birthrates: China, 315; developed countries, 259; Malaysia, 140

Blue Cross, 387

Brazil: coordination of services and manpower, 362; health indicators related to income, 43, 294; insurance, 375; medical education, 147, 362

Buddhism: and care in Thailand, 89, 100, 102

Canada, 193–220; ambulatory care,

—Barbados plan, 82–84
—cooperative systems, 37
—rising: Canada, 215; Great Britain, 189; U.S., 241, 257
Cost sharing, 371; Belgium, 373; Chile, 385; China, 309, 381; Cuba, 300, 382; France, 374; New Zealand, 384; U.S., 387. *See also* Copayment obligations
Cuba, 293–303, 381–82; aid to other countries, 298, 302; ambulatory services, 295–96, 328; health expenditures, 298–300; health indicators and income, 43, 45, 47, 294; health personnel, 296; medical training, 363–64; private practice, 394; recent changes, 296–99; Soviet aid to, 301
Czechoslovakia: aid to Cuba, 293, 381; medical education, 327, 364

Dawson Report (Great Britain), 174, 323–24, 333
Deathrates: China, 307; Cuba, 300; developed countries, 259
Delivery of services, 31, 35, 38, 149–50. *See also* Ambulatory care; Hospitals
Dental care: Australia, 230; Barbados, 85; Canada, 202, 230; Great Britain, 171, 172, 175, 181–82, 383; Guatemala, 60, 72; insurance for, 371; Norway, 157, 158–59, 160, 162, 168, 230, 385; Thailand, 90; United States, 236
Dental nurses: Barbados plan, 85; Canada, 202, 205, 230; New Zealand, 168, 233, 358
Dentists: Australia, 233; Barbados, 85; Belgium, 233; Canada, 205, 233; Cuba, 297–98; Great Britain, 175, 182; Guatemala, 60; Kenya, 110, 115, 124; Norway, 159, 233; Thailand, 104; U.S., 233, 356
Depression of 1930s: effect on health

center movement, 325; effect on health planning, 351, 371, 392
Developing countries, 4, 6, 36; brain drain from, 298; health centers, 326, 328–31; health expenditures, 49–50, 145–46, 299; health indicators, and income distribution, 41–51; insurance in, 9, 18, 22, 388–89; licensing, 357; planning, 397–400; rural care, 10, 252, 359; sources of health care support, 18–19, 21, 34, 143–52, 330
Disabled, care for, 14, 17, 95, 111, 158, 202
Distribution of health personnel. *See* Geographic distribution of health personnel
Doctors. *See* Physicians
Drugs, 32, 149; Australia, 379; Barbados, 85; Canada, 202, 206, 218, 230; China, 311; Cuba, 298, 300, 382; developing countries, 147–48; Great Britain, 175, 181, 382, 383; Guatemala, 60–61, 66–68; in history of medicine, 13, 14, 15, 20, 321, 351; Italy, 396; Kenya, 110, 114, 115, 117, 118, 126, 127; Malaysia, 132, 134; Norway, 159, 161, 162, 165, 167, 230; Poland, 230, 285; private financing of, 18, 20; regulation of, 254; rural supply, 230; Soviet Union, 276, 327; Thailand, 91, 93–94, 103, 104. *See also* Drug sellers; Pharmacies
Drug sellers, 150; Kenya, 127; Thailand, 103–4, 402

Emergency care: Kenya, 111; Soviet Union, 279; Thailand, 91, 94, 99
England: health indicators, 263, 266; regionalization concept, 344. *See also* Great Britain
Environmental sanitation, 8, 16, 17, 260; ancient Rome, 14, 144; Barbados, 81, 84; China, 311, 314, 381;

About the Author

MILTON I. ROEMER has been a professor in the School of Public Health at the University of California, Los Angeles, since 1962. He taught previously at Cornell and Yale Universities. He earned the M.D. degree in 1940 and holds master's degrees in sociology and public health. Dr. Roemer has served at all levels of health administration—county, state, national, and international (with the World Health Organization). In 1948, he published *Rural Health and Medical Care* with Dr. F. D. Mott; it was the first comprehensive American study of this subject. Since then he has published 28 books and more than 300 articles on the social aspects of health service. In 1974, he was elected to the Institute of Medicine of the National Academy of Sciences. As an international consultant, Dr. Roemer has studied health care organization in 55 countries—principally for the World Health Organization, USAID, and other agencies. In 1977, he received the International Award for Excellence in Promoting and Protecting the Health of People from the American Public Health Association. In 1983, APHA awarded Dr. Roemer its highest honor, the Sedgwick Memorial Medal for Distinguished Service in Public Health.